Bayer

Pharmaceutical Division

Jo Ellen Schweinle, MD
Strategic Projects Director &
Clinical Assistant Professor
Yale University School of Medicine

Dear Doctor:

Bayer Corporation, Pharmaceutical Division, maker of Cipro® I.V. (ciprofloxacin) and Cipro® (ciprofloxacin HCl) Tablets, is pleased to present you with Sabiston's *Review of Surgery*.

Thoroughly revised and updated, this new edition challenges the reader on all aspects of surgery. The hundreds of questions and answers are page-referenced to the parent-text, the new 15th edition of Sabiston's *Textbook of Surgery*, one of the most respected surgical references available.

Residents and medical students will find *Review of Surgery* an ideal resource when taking qualifying exams, while practicing surgeons will find it helpful in studying for recertification. We trust that you will find this book to be a valuable addition to your medical library, as well.

Cordially,

J Schweinle, M.D.

Jo Ellen Schweinle, MD
Strategic Projects Director &
Clinical Assistant Professor
Yale University School of Medicine

Bayer Corporation
400 Morgan Lane
West Haven, CT 06516-4175
Phone 203 812-6592
Fax 203 812-6547

REVIEW OF
SURGERY

DAVID C. SABISTON, Jr., M.D.
James B. Duke Professor of Surgery
Director of International Programs
Duke University Medical Center
Durham, North Carolina

W.B. SAUNDERS COMPANY
A Division of Harcourt Brace & Company
Philadelphia London Toronto Montreal Sydney Tokyo

W.B. SAUNDERS COMPANY
A Division of Harcourt Brace & Company

The Curtis Center
Independence Square West
Philadelphia, Pennsylvania 19106

REVIEW OF SURGERY, Second Edition

ISBN 0–7216–8671–0

Printed in the United States of America.

Last digit is the print number: 9 8 7 6 5 4 3 2

CONTRIBUTORS

JOHN G. ADAMS, Jr., M.D.
University of Missouri–Columbia School of Medicine

N. SCOTT ADZICK, M.D.
University of Pennsylvania School of Medicine

ROBERT W. ANDERSON, M.D.
Duke University Medical Center

PAUL S. AUERBACH, M.D., M.S.
Sterling Healthcare Group

ERLE H. AUSTIN III, M.D.
University of Louisville Medical School

WILLIAM H. BAKER, M.D.
Loyola University Chicago Stritch School of Medicine

CLYDE F. BARKER, M.D.
University of Pennsylvania School of Medicine

ROBERT H. BARTLETT, M.D.
University of Michigan School of Medicine

JAMES M. BECKER, M.D.
Boston University School of Medicine

FOLKERT O. BELZER, M.D. (deceased)
University of Wisconsin Medical School

MICHAEL E. BEREND, M.D.
Duke University Medical Center

JOHN J. BERGAN, M.D.
Loma Linda University Medical School and Uniformed Services University of the Health Sciences

AMITAVA BISWAS, M.D.
Harvard Medical School

R. RANDAL BOLLINGER, M.D., Ph.D.
Duke University Medical Center

R. MORTON BOLMAN III, M.D.
University of Minnesota

WILLIAM Z. BORER, M.D.
Thomas Jefferson University

JOHN BOSTWICK III, M.D.
Emory University School of Medicine

GENE D. BRANUM, M.D.
Emory University School of Medicine

KENNETH L. BRAYMAN, M.D., Ph.D.
University of Pennsylvania School of Medicine

ALYSON J. BREISCH, R.N., M.S.
Duke University School of Nursing

MURRAY F. BRENNAN, M.D.
Cornell University Medical College

GERT H. BRIEGER, M.D., Ph.D.
The Johns Hopkins University School of Medicine

JOHN H. CALHOON, M.D.
University of Texas Health Science Center at San Antonio

JOHN L. CAMERON, M.D.
The Johns Hopkins University School of Medicine

DAVID N. CAMPBELL, M.D.
University of Colorado Health Sciences Center

GRANT W. CARLSON, M.D.
Emory University School of Medicine

C. JAMES CARRICO, M.D.
University of Texas Southwestern Medical Center

JAMES CERILLI, M.D.
University of Rochester Medical Center

RAVI S. CHARI, M.D.
University of Toronto

WILLIAM G. CHEADLE, M.D.
University of Louisville School of Medicine

LAURENCE Y. CHEUNG, M.D.
University of Kansas School of Medicine

W. RANDOLPH CHITWOOD, Jr., M.D.
East Carolina University School of Medicine

BRYAN M. CLARY, M.D.
Duke University Medical Center

PIERRE A. CLAVIEN, M.D., Ph.D.
Duke University Medical Center

JOEL D. COOPER, M.D.
Washington University School of Medicine

JAMES L. COX, M.D.
Washington University School of Medicine

FRED A. CRAWFORD, Jr., M.D.
Medical University of South Carolina

ROBERT D. CROOM III, M.D.
University of North Carolina School of Medicine and University of North Carolina Hospitals

THOMAS A. D'AMICO, M.D.
Duke University Medical Center

MARK G. DAVIES, M.D., Ph.D.
Duke University Medical Center

R. DUANE DAVIS, Jr., M.D.
Duke University Medical Center

RICHARD H. DEAN, M.D.
Bowman Gray School of Medicine

HAILE T. DEBAS, M.D.
School of Medicine, University of California, San Francisco

JEROME J. DECOSSE, M.D., PH.D.
Cornell University Medical College

E. PATCHEN DELLINGER, M.D.
University of Washington School of Medicine

MARK E. DENTZ, M.D.
Duke University Medical Center

ARNOLD G. DIETHELM, M.D.
University of Alabama School of Medicine

GERARD M. DOHERTY, M.D.
Washington University

ROGER R. DOZOIS, M.D.
Mayo Medical School

ANDRÉ DURANCEAU, M.D.
University of Montreal

DAVID W. EASTER, M.D.
University of California, San Diego

JAMES M. EDWARDS, M.D.
Oregon Health Sciences University

JOSEPH R. ELBEERY, M.D.
East Carolina University School of Medicine

STEVE EUBANKS, M.D.
Duke University Medical Center

SAMIR M. FAKHRY, M.D.
University of North Carolina School of Medicine

JOHN A. FEAGIN, M.D.
Duke University Medical Center

AARON S. FINK, M.D.
Emory University School of Medicine

JOSEF E. FISCHER, M.D.
University of Cincinnati College of Medicine

ROBERT D. FITCH, M.D.
Duke University Medical Center

WILLIAM R. FLINN, M.D.
University of Maryland Medical School and Hospital

M. WAYNE FLYE, M.D., PH.D.
Washington University School of Medicine

THOMAS J. FOGARTY, M.D.
Stanford University School of Medicine

DOUGLAS L. FRAKER, M.D.
University of Pennsylvania School of Medicine

ALLAN H. FRIEDMAN, M.D.
Duke University Medical Center

DAVID FROMM, M.D.
Wayne State University

HERBERT E. FUCHS, M.D., PH.D.
Duke University Medical Center

DAVID A. FULLERTON, M.D.
Northwestern University

STANLEY A. GALL, JR., M.D.
St. John's Hospital

WILLIAM E. GARRETT, JR., M.D., PH.D.
Duke University Medical Center

WILLIAM A. GAY, JR., M.D.
Washington University School of Medicine

J. WILLIAM GAYNOR, M.D.
Children's Hospital of Philadelphia

COHAVA GELBER, PH.D.
Duke University Medical Center

ANNETINE C. GELIJNS, PH.D.
Columbia University School of Public Health, College of Physicians and Surgeons

GREGORY S. GEORGIADE, M.D.
Duke University Medical Center

FARID GHARAGOZLOO, M.D.
Georgetown University School of Medicine

DONALD D. GLOWER, M.D.
Duke University Medical Center

J. LEONARD GOLDNER, M.D.
Duke University Medical Center

RICHARD D. GOLDNER, M.D.
Duke University Medical Center

CLEON W. GOODWIN, JR., M.D.
U.S. Army Institute of Surgical Research

JOHN GORECKI, M.D.
Duke University Medical Center

LAWRENCE J. GOTTLIEB, M.D.
University of Chicago School of Medicine

JOHN P. GRANT, M.D.
Duke University Medical Center

PAUL D. GREIG, M.D.
University of Toronto

KATHERINE P. GRICHNIK, M.D.
Duke University Medical Center

HERMES C. GRILLO, M.D.
Harvard Medical School

JAY L. GROSFELD, M.D.
Indiana University School of Medicine

FREDERICK L. GROVER, M.D.
University of Colorado Health Sciences Center

J. CAULIE GUNNELLS, JR., M.D.
Duke University Medical Center

JEFFREY A. HAGEN, M.D.
University of Southern California, Los Angeles

PER-OTTO HAGEN, M.D.
Duke University Medical Center

CARL E. HAISCH, M.D.
East Carolina University

JOHN D. HAMILTON, M.D.
Duke University Medical Center

CHARLES B. HAMMOND, M.D.
Duke University Medical Center

WILLIAM T. HARDAKER, JR., M.D.
Duke University Medical Center

ALDEN H. HARKEN, M.D.
University of Colorado

DAVID H. HARPOLE, JR., M.D.
Duke University Medical Center

JOHN M. HARRELSON, M.D.
Duke University Medical Center

MARQUIS E. HART, M.D.
University of California, San Diego

JEFFREY S. HEINLE, M.D.
Boston Children's Hospital and Brigham and Women's Hospital

JULIO HOCHBERG, M.D.
West Virginia University Health Sciences Center

WILLIAM L. HOLMAN, M.D.
University of Alabama at Birmingham

RICHARD A. HOPKINS, M.D.
Brown University School of Medicine

J. DIRK IGLEHART, M.D.
Duke University Medical Center

SUZANNE T. ILDSTAD, M.D.
University of Pittsburgh School of Medicine

ANTHONY L. IMBEMBO, M.D.
University of Maryland School of Medicine

GLYN G. JAMIESON, M.D.
University of Adelaide

MICHAEL E. JESSEN, M.D.
University of Texas Southwestern Medical Center at Dallas

OLGA JONASSON, M.D.
Northwestern University

R. SCOTT JONES, M.D.
University of Virginia School of Medicine

ROBERT H. JONES, M.D.
Duke University Medical Center

GREGORY J. JURKOVICH, M.D.
University of Washington

LARRY R. KAISER, M.D.
University of Pennsylvania School of Medicine

STEVEN S. KANG, M.D.
Loyola University Chicago Stritch School of Medicine

KEITH A. KELLY, M.D.
Mayo Medical School

ALLAN D. KIRK, M.D., PH.D.
University of Wisconsin Health Center

JAMES K. KIRKLIN, M.D.
University of Alabama at Birmingham School of Medicine

STUART J. KNECHTLE, M.D.
University of Wisconsin School of Medicine

THEODORE C. KOUTLAS, M.D.
East Carolina University School of Medicine

THOMAS J. KRIZEK, M.D.
University of South Florida

TERRY C. LAIRMORE, M.D.
Washington University School of Medicine

GREGORY J. LANDRY, M.D.
Oregon Health Sciences University

BERNARD LANGER, M.D.
University of Toronto

JEFFREY H. LAWSON, M.D., PH.D.
Duke University Medical Center

ALAN T. LEFOR, M.D.
University of Maryland School of Medicine

GEORGE S. LEIGHT, JR., M.D.
Duke University Medical Center

L. SCOTT LEVIN, M.D.
Duke University Medical Center

JONATHAN J. LEWIS, M.D., PH.D.
Cornell University Medical College

R. ERIC LILLY, M.D.
Duke University Medical Center

JAMES E. LOWE, M.D.
Duke University Medical Center

H. KIM LYERLY, M.D.
Duke University Medical Center

GREG J. MACKAY, M.D.
The Nalle Clinic

RAYMOND G. MAKHOUL, M.D.
Medical College of Virginia

JOHN A. MANNICK, M.D.
Harvard Medical School

JAMES F. MARKMANN, M.D., PH.D.
University of Pennsylvania School of Medicine

G. ROBERT MASON, M.D., PH.D.
Loyola University Chicago Stritch School of Medicine

DOUGLAS J. MATHISEN, M.D.
Harvard Medical School

JAMES R. MAULT, M.D.
Duke University Medical Center

RICHARD L. McCANN, M.D.
Duke University Medical Center

DONALD E. McCOLLUM, M.D.
Duke University Medical Center

JOHN C. McDONALD, M.D.
Louisiana State University School of Medicine

DAVID C. McGIFFIN, M.D.
University of Alabama at Birmingham

ANTHONY A. MEYER, M.D., PH.D.
University of North Carolina School of Medicine

WILLIAM C. MEYERS, M.D.
University of Massachusetts Medical Center

GREGORY L. MONETA, M.D.
Oregon Health Sciences University

FRANK G. MOODY, M.D.
The University of Texas Medical School, Houston

A. R. MOOSSA, M.D.
University of California, San Diego

JON F. MORAN, M.D.
East Carolina University School of Medicine

ALAN J. MOSKOWITZ, M.D.
Columbia University, College of Physicians and Surgeons, School of Public Health

JOSEPH A. MOYLAN, M.D.
University of Miami School of Medicine

GORDON F. MURRAY, M.D.
West Virginia University Health Sciences Center

DAVID L. NAHRWOLD, M.D.
Northwestern University Medical School

ALI NAJI, M.D., PH.D.
University of Pennsylvania School of Medicine

ELAINE E. NELSON, M.D.
Stanford Medical Center/Kaiser Permanente

JEFFREY A. NORTON, M.D.
Washington University School of Medicine

JAMES A. NUNLEY, M.D.
Duke University Medical Center

JOHN A. OLSON, JR., M.D., PH.D.
Washington University School of Medicine

SUSAN L. ORLOFF, M.D.
University of California, San Francisco

MARK B. ORRINGER, M.D.
University of Michigan Medical School

ALBERT D. PACIFICO, M.D.
University of Alabama at Birmingham School of Medicine

THEODORE N. PAPPAS, M.D.
Duke University Medical Center

DAVID F. PAULSON, M.D.
Duke University Medical Center

JOSE A. PEREZ, M.D.
Duke University Medical Center

WILLIAM S. PIERCE, M.D.
College of Medicine, The Pennsylvania State University

JEFFREY L. PLATT, M.D.
Duke University Medical Center

HIRAM C. POLK, JR., M.D.
University of Louisville School of Medicine

WALTER J. PORIES, M.D.
East Carolina University School of Medicine

JOHN M. PORTER, M.D.
Oregon Health Sciences University

BASIL A. PRUITT, JR., M.D.
University of Texas Health Science Center at San Antonio

SCOTT K. PRUITT, M.D., PH.D.
Duke University Medical Center

CEMIL M. PURUT, M.D.
Duke University Medical Center

MICHAEL F. REED, M.D.
Harvard Medical School

KEITH REEMTSMA, M.D., MED. SC.D.
Columbia University College of Physicians and Surgeons

J. G. REVES, M.D.
Duke University Medical Center

NORMAN M. RICH, M.D.
Uniformed Services University of the Health Sciences

WILLIAM J. RICHARDSON, M.D.
Duke University Medical Center

LAYTON F. RIKKERS, M.D.
University of Wisconsin Clinical Science Center

MICHELLE L. ROBBIN, M.D.
University of Alabama at Birmingham School of Medicine

CARY N. ROBERTSON, M.D.
Duke University Medical Center

MICHAEL S. ROHR, M.D., PH.D.
Bowman Gray School of Medicine

ROLANDO ROLANDELLI, M.D.
Medical College of Pennsylvania and Hahnemann University

FRANCIS E. ROSATO, M.D.
Jefferson Medical College of Thomas Jefferson University

ERIC A. ROSE, M.D.
Columbia University, College of Physicians and Surgeons

JOEL J. ROSLYN, M.D.
Medical College of Pennsylvania and Hahnemann University

PABLO RUBINSTEIN, M.D.
Fred H. Allen Laboratory of Immunogenetics, New York Blood Center

DAVID C. SABISTON, JR., M.D.
Duke University Medical Center

JAMES D. ST. LOUIS, M.D.
Duke University Medical Center

PHILIP R. SCHAUER, M.D.
University of Pittsburgh School of Medicine and Medical Center

BRUCE D. SCHIRMER, M.D.
University of Virginia School of Medicine and Health Sciences Center

STEVE J. SCHWAB, M.D.
Duke University Medical Center

STEWART M. SCOTT, M.D. (deceased)
Duke University Medical Center

SEAN P. SCULLY, M.D., PH.D.
Duke University Medical Center

MARK W. SEBASTIAN, M.D.
Duke University Medical Center

H. F. SEIGLER, M.D.
Duke University Medical Center

GEORGE F. SHELDON, M.D.
University of North Carolina School of Medicine

G. TOM SHIRES, M.D.
Texas Tech University School of Medicine

G. TOM SHIRES III, M.D.
University of Texas Southwestern Medical Center at Dallas

JOSEPH B. SHRAGER, M.D.
Massachusetts General Hospital

KAREN S. SIBERT, M.D.
Duke University Medical Center

DONALD SILVER, M.D.
University of Missouri–Columbia School of Medicine

NORMAN A. SILVERMAN, M.D.
Case Western Reserve School of Medicine

RICHARD L. SIMMONS, M.D.
University of Pittsburgh School of Medicine

KEVIN M. SITTIG, M.D.
Louisiana State University School of Medicine

CRAIG L. SLINGLUFF, Jr., M.D.
University of Virginia School of Medicine

MILTON M. SLOCUM, M.D.
University of Missouri–Columbia School of Medicine

JAMES B. SNOW, Jr., M.D.
National Institutes of Health

HANS W. SOLLINGER, M.D., Ph.D.
University of Wisconsin School of Medicine

JAMES H. SOUTHARD, Ph.D.
University of Wisconsin Medical School

KEVIN P. SPEER, M.D.
Duke University Medical Center

THOMAS L. SPRAY, M.D.
University of Pennsylvania School of Medicine

ROBERT J. STANLEY, M.D.
University of Alabama School of Medicine

DELFORD L. STICKEL, M.D.
Duke University Medical Center

DAVID J. SUGARBAKER, M.D.
Harvard Medical School

BRUCE A. SULLENGER, Ph.D.
Duke University Medical Center

R. SUDHIR SUNDARESAN, M.D.
Washington University School of Medicine

SCOTT J. SWANSON, M.D.
Harvard Medical School

TIMOTHY TAKARO, M.D.
Duke University Medical Center

JAMES L. TALBERT, M.D.
University of Florida College of Medicine

MARK TEDDER, M.D.
Duke University Medical Center

ANGUS W. THOMSON, Ph.D., D.Sc.
University of Pittsburgh School of Medicine

ROBERT D. TIEN, M.D., M.P.H.
Duke University Medical Center

DENNIS A. TURNER, M.D., M.A.
Duke University Medical Center

DOUGLAS TYLER, M.D.
Duke University Medical Center

ROSS M. UNGERLEIDER, M.D.
Duke University Medical Center

JAMES R. URBANIAK, M.D.
Duke University Medical Center

THOMAS PARKER VAIL, M.D.
Duke University Medical Center

PETER VAN TRIGT III, M.D.
Cardiovascular and Thoracic Surgeons of Greensboro

STEVEN N. VASLEF, M.D., Ph.D.
Duke University Medical Center

ROBERT B. WALLACE, M.D.
Georgetown University Medical Center

HENRY L. WALTERS III, M.D.
Wayne State University School of Medicine

JOHN L. WEINERTH, M.D.
Duke University Medical Center

SAMUEL A. WELLS, Jr., M.D.
Washington University School of Medicine

H. BROWNELL WHEELER, M.D.
University of Massachusetts Medical School

ANTHONY D. WHITTEMORE, M.D.
Harvard Medical School

ROBERT H. WILKINS, M.D.
Duke University Medical Center

DOUGLAS W. WILMORE, M.D.
Harvard Medical School

WALTER G. WOLFE, M.D.
Duke University Medical Center

BRUCE G. WOLFF, M.D.
Mayo Medical School

ROBERT J. WOOD, M.D.
Emory University School of Medicine

CHARLES J. YEO, M.D.
The Johns Hopkins University School of Medicine

KARL A. ZUCKER, M.D.
University of New Mexico School of Medicine

PREFACE

The purpose of this *Review of Surgery* is to provide medical students, residents, and practicing surgeons an opportunity to review the field of surgery in preparation for many types of examinations. The questions have been written by authorities in the field, and they have also provided the appropriate answers. In addition, the page numbers for additional information concerning each question are cited where they appear in *Textbook of Surgery: The Biological Basis of Modern Surgical Practice,* fifteenth edition, the reference source for the *Review.*

Medical students will find this text useful in preparing for written and oral examinations in surgery while in medical school. For residents, it provides a reliable review of the literature for both *in-service* training examinations and for the basic and clinical science questions on formal certifying examinations. It will also be found useful by those in surgical practice in preparation for recertification examinations. The *Review* also includes questions and answers in the fields of neurosurgery, orthopedics, otolaryngology, pediatric surgery, plastic and maxillofacial surgery, and urology, and is useful for preparation for specialty board examinations as well, including those in pediatric surgery, vascular surgery, and colorectal surgery.

A prime strength of the *Review* is that the contributors are national and international authorities and are thoroughly familiar with their fields. They have provided the most important questions as well as the appropriate answers. It should be emphasized that *basic science* features are stressed, since this aspect is an advancing part of the entire field of surgery, and questions are increasingly asked concerning this area of surgical practice.

Finally, it is a privilege to express appreciation to all those who have contributed to these texts, as they are deserving of much praise.

David C. Sabiston, Jr., M.D.

CONTENTS

CHAPTER 1

THE DEVELOPMENT OF SURGERY

1. In the Hippocratic Oath it is stated, "I will not use the knife, not even on sufferers from stone, but will withdraw in favor of such men as are engaged in this work." Yet some of the outstanding books among the Hippocratic works are about surgery and the training and qualifications of the surgeon. This discrepancy can be explained by:

A. There was no surgery in ancient Greek times.
B. The precepts of the Hippocratic Oath were followed by only a small group of physicians.
C. The Oath is only one of many Hippocratic medical writings, some of which are specifically about surgeons and surgery.
D. The admonition about surgery is due to a mistranslation.

DISCUSSION: The Oath, perhaps the best known of the ancient Greek medical works ascribed to Hippocrates, is one of 70 surviving works. Some are book length and others, such as the Oath, much shorter. All the Hippocratic writings are in the same Ionian dialect, but there are so many inconsistencies in content and precepts that it is clear the books were written by an unknown number of medical writers and in the third century B.C. collected together under the name of one of the most famous medical teachers of a century earlier. One postulate is that the Oath was sworn only by the followers of Pythagoras, who were known to be opposed to abortion, suicide, and surgery, all of which are proscribed in the Oath but discussed quite openly in other Hippocratic writings.

Textbook: Page 1 ANSWER: B, C.

2. The significance to surgery of the publication in 1543 of the *Fabrica* of Vesalius was:

A. Its illustrations.
B. It was the first textbook of anatomy published.
C. The dissections carried out by Vesalius were on human, not animal, bodies.
D. It appeared as a printed volume.

DISCUSSION: Vesalius was one of the earliest of the Renaissance anatomists to stress careful human dissection, not merely dutiful following of earlier writers such as Galen, whose anatomy was based upon animal, and not human, dissection. The printing of books, especially those with illustrations, allowed faithful reproductions to be used by many students. Hand-drawn and hand-printed manuscripts could not be as widely disseminated for teaching as books would be in the sixteenth century.

Textbook: Page 3 ANSWER: A, C, D.

3. By 1800, much of the anatomy of the human body had been described. What obstacles remained to confine surgery to a relatively few operations, usually performed only in emergencies?

A. Knowledge of histology.
B. Control of postoperative infection and bleeding.
C. Control of pain.
D. Lack of skilled surgeons.

DISCUSSION: Although the structure of the body was quite well understood, surgeons as yet had little or no means to overcome four great obstacles to successful operations: pain, blood loss, shock, and infection.

Textbook: Pages 4–5 ANSWER: B, C.

4. What was the main significance for the surgeon of the introduction of anesthesia in the late 1840s?

A. Allowed the surgeon more time for an operation.
B. Led to conservative surgery.
C. Reduced the threat of shock.
D. Made patients more willing to submit to surgery.

DISCUSSION: Probably the single most important benefit of anesthesia for the surgeon was the great reduction in the need for speed in operations. Surgeons could now begin to devise better operative procedures, such as resection of a portion of bone for a tuberculous lesion, thereby saving the limb rather than amputating as was necessary in preanesthesia times. This became known as *conservative surgery* in the 1860s. Anesthesia also helped to prevent blood loss and excessive pain leading to shock, and it helped to reduce people's great fear of surgery.

Textbook: Pages 4–5 ANSWER: A, B, C, D.

5. Beginning in 1867, Joseph Lister published many papers describing and advocating his method of antiseptic surgery. His results were startlingly favorable. Why did it take two decades for antisepsis to win wide approval?

A. Those who opposed Lister did not understand or accept the germ theory of disease.
B. Lister was widely believed to be a quack.
C. Those who opposed Lister could not duplicate his results.
D. Those who opposed him were allergic to carbolic acid.

DISCUSSION: The slow acceptance of antiseptic surgery provides an excellent example of resistance to change and innovation. There were many reasons for the slow acceptance of Lister's techniques. In the hands of many surgeons, especially those who had little or no understanding of the new theory of germs, the method did not achieve the results Lister promised. Others thought the method too cumbersome, expensive, or time consuming or were irritated by the exposure to carbolic acid. Only with the natural evolution of antiseptic to aseptic surgery in the 1880s was the concept of surgical cleanliness fully understood and accepted.

Textbook: Page 5 ANSWER: A, C.

6. What role did the work of the French physiologist Claude Bernard have in the development of surgery?

A. Bernard was a follower of Lister's antiseptic technique.
B. Bernard was a disciple of Louis Pasteur.
C. Bernard's physiologic concepts and experiments led to our understanding of the body's internal regulating systems.

DISCUSSION: Bernard's concept of the *milieu interieur,* or the necessary internal equilibrium of the body, was a key to understanding the regulatory mechanisms so important in the care of surgical patients. His widely read *Introduction to Experimental Medicine* (1865) became a classic in the philosophy of medicine, and the development of medical science as laboratory research has been as pervasive an influence for surgical science as for medicine as a whole.

Textbook: Page 10 ANSWER: C.

7. Why can one ascribe a "school of surgery" to William S. Halsted?

A. Because Halsted founded his own medical school.
B. Because Halsted, along with his medical colleague William Osler, began a residency system that trained a generation of surgeons for academic positions all over the country.
C. Because the Halsted system of post-graduate training included clinical as well as laboratory experiences for the residents.

DISCUSSION: Halsted (1852–1922) was the first professor of surgery in the new Johns Hopkins Hospital and Medical School. He and his colleague William Osler established in 1889 a residency system for post-graduate training. From the experiences of the residents, which included clinical as well as experimental work, came a whole generation of surgical teachers who initiated similar programs elsewhere.

Textbook: Pages 7–8 ANSWER: B, C.

8. What were some of the important influences upon the professionalization of surgery in the last 100 years?

A. More medical school graduates wanted to become surgeons.
B. Surgeons earned more money.
C. Improved techniques and growing knowledge of physiology allowed for an ever-widening scope of surgery that in turn required increasingly specialized training.
D. Surgical journals, textbooks, and specialty societies that helped to train surgeons.

DISCUSSION: Surgical training programs, surgical journals (beginning with the *Annals of Surgery* in 1885), surgical textbooks, and surgical associations that are local, national, and international in membership all helped to provide surgeons the special knowledge and techniques to make theirs a specialty in name and in fact. The certification provided by the American Board of Surgery and the many surgical subspecialty boards that began in the 1930s provided a rationale and prescribed standards for the training of surgeons.

Textbook: Page 14 ANSWER: C, D.

9. Which design feature and analytic techniques can be employed in a randomized controlled clinical trial to avert selection, measurement, and confounding biases?

A. Concurrently treated comparative control groups.
B. Random assignment of treatment to patients.
C. Blinding of researchers and patients to treatment assignments.
D. Standard follow-up evaluations for the experimental treatment and control groups.
E. Analysis of primary hypothesis by intention-to-treat analysis.
F. All of the above.

DISCUSSION: Each of the design features listed may be included in a clinical trial to avoid bias. The experience of a comparative control group treated concurrently provides the expected rate of the study outcome under the null hypothesis of no effect of the investigational intervention. Without such a group, any improvement in the treatment group, regardless of whether or not it was treatment induced, could be interpreted as a treatment effect. Random assignment of treatment is used to ensure that the treatment and comparative control groups are equally constituted with respect to achieving the study outcome. To make sure that groups that are equally likely to achieve the study outcome are compared, analysis by the intention-to-treat principle is used. This principle dictates that outcomes are analyzed according to the treatment that patients are assigned to at randomization, regardless of whether or not they actually received it. The standard follow-up evaluations and blinding of patients and researchers help to avoid deferential care to a particular group, which could affect the measured outcome of the study.

Textbook: Pages 38–39 ANSWER: F.

10. Which of the following statements about the technique of meta-analysis are true?

A. It is a process for formally reviewing and statistically combining the results of research conducted previously.
B. It is applicable to the results of experimental and nonexperimental (epidemiologic) research.
C. It can increase statistical power for estimates of therapeutic effect by pooling results for different studies.
D. The results of studies are combined by calculating a weighted average of study-specific results.
E. The results of studies are combined by pooling the data from each and calculating average treatment outcomes.

DISCUSSION: Meta-analysis is a process for formally reviewing and statistically combining the results of previously conducted research and is applicable to experimental and epidemiologic data. One advantage to combining studies is that the estimates of treatment effect are derived from a larger patient experience and may achieve statistical significance, whereas the estimate of treatment effect from the individual study may not have. The only valid way to combine the results of different experiments is to keep the comparison of treatment groups within the original studies. Thus, the studies are combined by calculating a weighted average of study specific results, rather than simply pooling the data and calculating a treatment.

Textbook: Pages 43–44 ANSWER: A, B, C, D.

11. Which of the following lists of research designs is ordered in increasing susceptibility to bias?

A. Randomized controlled trial, case-control study, cohort study, case series, case reports.
B. Cohort study, case-control study, randomized controlled trial, case series, case reports.
C. Randomized controlled trial, cohort study, case-control study, case series, case reports.
D. Randomized controlled trial, cohort study, case-control study, case reports, case series.

DISCUSSION: The randomized controlled trial (RCT) is the strongest design for minimizing the biases that can enter into a clinical study. While the cohort study design cannot ensure that comparative cohorts are equally at risk for the study outcome, as an RCT can, it offers more control than the retrospective case-control design for guarding against measurement, selection, and confounding biases. The individual case reports or series of cases offer the weakest form of evidence. Neither has a defined population or comparison group, and neither guards against selection bias, measurement bias, or confounding. By contrast, the case series, which is a cross-sectional prevalence survey of a defined population, can minimize the effects of selection bias. However, these studies also lack a control group and therefore cannot put the findings into context.

Textbook: Pages 44–46 ANSWER: C.

12. Which of the following statements concerning quality of life are false?

A. Overall quality of life is an all-inclusive concept that incorporates the ability of the individual to function physically, emotionally, and socially.
B. Health-related quality of life (HRQOL) includes those factors of physical, emotional, and social functioning that immediately affect the health of the individual.
C. Instruments for measuring HRQOL fall into two broad categories, generic and disease specific.
D. Quality-adjusted life years (QALYs) is a complex outcome measure that captures features of both the survival and quality of life of the individuals being evaluated.
E. None of the above.

DISCUSSION: Overall quality of life is an all-inclusive concept that incorporates the ability of the individual to function physically, emotionally, and socially. In contrast, health-related quality of life is a more limited definition that includes only factors that immediately affect the health of the individual. Instruments that measure these concepts can be of the generic type or disease specific. The former assess the general aspects of HRQOL that are applicable to a variety of populations and, thus, allow broad comparisons of the relative impact of disparate health care interventions. The latter type is geared to a particular disease or population and focuses on the functional limitations or disabilities produced by the disease or population of interest. As stated, quality-adjusted life years combines survival and quality of life into a single measure, the QALY.

Textbook: Pages 46–47 ANSWER: E.

13. Which of the following statements about economic analysis of medical interventions are true?

A. One objective is to measure the resources consumed in relation to the health benefits provided.
B. The analysis can be undertaken from the perspective of society, the health care system, third-party payers, providers, and patients.
C. Cost-effectiveness and cost-benefit analyses differ in that only for cost-effectiveness analysis are all costs and health effects expressed in monetary terms, which allows the

calculation of a net monetary outcome of a health care intervention.
D. Two different types of costs can be examined within an economic evaluation: direct costs, which include resource categories directly related to the intervention being studied (e.g., personnel, medications, diagnostic testing, outpatient visits, cost of managing side effects), and indirect costs, which include earnings gained or lost by patients and society and the economic value of intangible costs such as pain and suffering.

DISCUSSION: All of the statements are correct except C. Statement C confuses the definitions of cost-effectiveness and cost-benefit analysis. It is cost-benefit analysis that expressed all of the health care resources consumed and health effects produced by a given health care intervention in monetary terms, which allows the calculation of a net monetary outcome of that intervention.

Textbook: Pages 50–51 ANSWER: A, B, D.

14. Which of the following statements about cohort and case-control study designs are true?

A. Case-control studies discern the association between a suspected risk factor and the development of disease by examining diseased and nondiseased patients and establishing prior exposures to the suspected risk factor.
B. The epidemiologic concept of cohort refers to a group of individuals who, at the time of their assembly, have characteristics in common.
C. In a cohort study design, groups of patients are followed over time to see whether the outcome event of interest develops.
D. Relative risk can be measured directly from a cohort study but only a proxy for relative risk, the odds ratio, can be measured in a case-control study.
E. All of the above.

DISCUSSION: Cohort studies evaluate patient groups or populations with different exposures to a suspected risk factor to determine the risk of developing a particular disease or outcome over time. The ratio of the incidence of disease in two such groups during a defined period of time is the relative risk of developing this disease related to the risk factor exposure. In case-control studies, patients who have a disease (cases) and a group of otherwise similar people who do not have the disease (controls) are selected and evaluated to determine the frequency of prior exposure to the suspected risk factor for the disease. The ratio of the odds of prior exposure to the suspected risk factor in cases and controls approximates the relative risk of developing disease related to exposure to the suspected risk factor. This approximation holds true only when the disease in question is rare.

Textbook: Pages 41–43 ANSWER: E.

15. Regulation of gene expression can take place at the level of:

A. Transcription.
B. Translation.
C. mRNA transport and splicing.
D. Posttranslational modifications.
E. All of the above.

DISCUSSION: Although a mammalian cell possesses the genetic instructions to make thousands of different proteins, only a subset of those proteins, perhaps 10% to 20%, are found in any single cell. This suggests that in each type of cell some genes are expressed whereas others are silent. Moreover, different sets of genes are expressed in different types of cells, and among those genes that are expressed the outputs of gene products can vary up to 1 millionfold. This means that in addition to the presence of the sequences that encode a protein, each gene must contain instructions that regulate production of the protein in correct amounts, at the correct times, for each cell type. Gene expression can be regulated at several points including transcription, mRNA transport and splicing, translation, and at the posttranslational level.

Textbook: Pages 18–20 ANSWER: E.

16. Gene-directed therapies are currently limited by:

A. Gene delivery *in vivo.*
B. Level and control of gene expression.
C. Persistence of gene expression.
D. Directed delivery into appropriate tissues.
E. All of the above.

DISCUSSION: In this era of molecular medicine, the genetic basis for an increasing number of inherited diseases, including many types of cancer, is being discovered. Gene therapy represents a new and exciting approach for the treatment of such diseases. In its conception, gene therapy seemed quite simple: To treat a genetic deficiency, give a functional copy of the defective gene to the cells of the deficient patient. To accomplish this in practice, most often a viral vector is used to transfer a cDNA copy of the wild-type gene, which is usually under the control of a heterologous promoter, to cells harboring a mutant version. If the human genome were simply a warehouse of information, this approach would probably be quite successful. Unfortunately for the gene therapist, the human genome appears to be extremely complicated and expression of the information contained within it is apparently highly regulated. This complexity may severely limit the utility of the simple gene "add-back" approach to gene therapy. Gene therapy is limited by *in vivo* delivery, control, level and persistence of expression, and directed delivery into appropriate tissue. Therefore, significant technical advances must be made if the simple gene add-back approach is to become useful for the treatment of genetic disorders associated with genes, which require regulated expression to function properly.

Textbook: Pages 34–35 ANSWER: E.

17. The current concept regarding the development of cancer in humans includes:

A. Alterations that activate proto-oncogenes are necessary and sufficient for the development of most common cancers in humans.
B. Alterations that inactivate tumor suppressor genes are necessary and sufficient for the development of most common cancers in humans.
C. Inherited traits that allow for higher frequencies of genetic mutations are necessary and sufficient for the development of most common cancers in humans.
D. The accumulation of alterations in oncogenes and tumor suppressor genes and/or acceleration of this accumulation owing to defects in DNA repair or environmental factors is likely to lead to most common forms of carcinogenesis.

DISCUSSION: Although the presence of an oncogene can cause a cell to become transformed, the development of a cancer is a complex and multistep process in which a series of progressive changes culminate in deregulation of cell proliferation. Therefore, the current understanding is that multiple steps are required for the development of cancer, and the contributions of oncogenes are linked to tumor suppressor genes. The best-characterized model of stepwise carcinogenesis is colon cancer, which has been studied extensively by Vogelstein and colleagues. Carcinogenesis in the colon occurs through a series of pathologically recognizable steps, from hyperplastic epithelium, to adenomatous polyps, to invasive carcinoma. The first histologically recognized step in neoplasia is a shift in the normal epithelium to continuous proliferation, leading to the formation of an adenomatous polyp. With time, certain adenomas grow and undergo pathologic changes in their morphology. Several genetic abnormalities commonly occur during the genesis of colorectal carcinoma, and the cumulative total of genetic abnormalities appears to be more important than the order of appearance.
Textbook: Pages 30–31 ANSWER: D.

18. The number of important genes estimated to be present in the human genome is:

A. 1000 to 2000.
B. 10,000 to 20,000.
C. 100,000 to 200,000.
D. 1,000,000 to 2,000,000.

DISCUSSION: The genes of human cells are contained in the 23 paired chromosomes. Most earlier human genetics studies involved analysis of the presence or absence of these chromosomes by karyotype analysis. Such analysis was limited to detecting large fragments of the chromosome being deleted or transposed. More recent techniques allow for complete mapping and sequencing of the human genome. Current estimates of the human genome put it between 3 and 3.5×10^9 base pairs; however, it is apparent that more than half the genome consists of noncoding DNA of no known function, so-called *junk DNA.* It has been estimated that there may be somewhere between 50,000 and 200,000 important genes to be found and mapped.
Textbook: Page 16 ANSWER: C.

19. The advantages of polymerase chain reaction (PCR) analysis in the detection of malignant cells include:

A. PCR allows for detection of proteins in cells.
B. PCR allows for detection of mRNA sequences in cells.
C. PCR allows for detection of complex carbohydrate molecules on the surface of cells.
D. Amplification of small sequences of DNA can be performed, allowing very uncommon segments to be detected.

DISCUSSION: PCR analysis allows for amplification of DNA sequences. mRNA can be amplified by first transcribing cDNA using reverse transcriptase. PCR cannot amplify proteins or carbohydrates on cells.
Textbook: Pages 23, 24, 31–33 ANSWER: D.

20. The RET proto-oncogene is found expressed in:

A. Medullary thyroid cancers (MTC).
B. Pheochromocytomas.
C. Normal thyroid tissue.
D. All of the above.

DISCUSSION: Recent studies have identified mutations in the RET proto-oncogene (which resides in this region of chromosome 10) in affected persons in more than 90% of kindreds with multiple endocrine neoplasias (MEN) 2A and 2B, and approximately 70% of those with familial non-MEN medullary thyroid cancer (FMTC). RET is a tyrosine kinase receptor that is expressed in normal human thyroid tissue, medullary thyroid carcinoma, and pheochromocytoma.
Textbook: Page 33 ANSWER: D.

21. Detection of germline mutations in the RET proto-oncogene in family members of affected persons is clinically useful in diagnosis of:

A. Medullary thyroid cancers.
B. Pheochromocytomas.
C. Pituitary adenomas.
D. All of the above.

DISCUSSION: Relatives of patients with medullary thyroid carcinoma (MTC) in whom a mutation in the RET proto-oncogene has been detected are all screened for the RET mutation. Asymptomatic family members who carry the RET mutation are then offered prophylactic thyroidectomy. Thyroidectomy in children identified to be carriers of the RET mutation is recommended at age 5 years or any time thereafter once the diagnosis is established. Those who by mutational analysis are negative for the RET mutation are considered to have essentially the same risk as the general population for MTC and thus warrant no further evaluation.
Textbook: Page 33 ANSWER: A.

22. Which of the following molecules is/are involved in signal transduction?

A. Receptor, such as tyrosine kinase growth factor receptor.
B. Receptor ligand, such as a growth factor.
C. Coupler proteins, such as G proteins.
D. None of the above.
E. All of the above.

DISCUSSION: After the ligand binds to a specific cell surface receptor, the consequent conformational change, usually dimerization in the receptor, causes it to become activated. Receptors then associate with a coupler protein, usually a G protein, that in turn binds to an effector. Effectors catalyze the production of small molecules that act as second messengers in the cell. These molecules bind to intracellular proteins that directly affect processes such as the opening of a channel that, for example, results in the flow of ions. The net effect is a physiologic process such as muscle contraction, secretion, or cell growth. Some processes are evoked promptly. Others, such as cell division, require new protein synthesis, and the transcription factors involved are also considered part of signal transduction.

Textbook: Pages 20–23 ANSWER: E.

NOTES

NOTES

CHAPTER 2

HOMEOSTASIS, SHOCK, FLUID AND ELECTROLYTE MANAGEMENT, PREOPERATIVE PREPARATION, BLOOD TRANSFUSIONS

1. Skeletal muscle breakdown produces predominantly liberation of which two amino acids?

A. Lysine.
B. Tyrosine.
C. Alanine.
D. Glutamine.
E. Arginine.

DISCUSSION: Alanine is released from skeletal muscle and extracted by the liver, where it is converted to new glucose. Glutamine is also released from muscle and participates in renal acid-base homeostasis and serves as fuel for rapidly growing cells such as enterocytes, stimulated macrophages, and fibroblasts. Together, these two amino acids account for approximately two thirds of the nitrogen released from skeletal muscle.

Textbook: Page 65 ANSWER: C, D.

2. In "catabolic" surgical patients, which of the following changes in body composition do not occur?

A. Lean body mass increases.
B. Total body water increases.
C. Adipose tissue decreases.
D. Body weight decreases.

DISCUSSION: Lean body mass represents the body compartment that contains protein. Because critical illness stimulates proteolysis and increased excretion of body nitrogen, this compartment is consistently reduced, not increased. The change in body composition is associated with a loss of body weight, an increase in total body water, and a decrease in body fat.

Textbook: Page 57 ANSWER: A.

3. The hormonal alterations that follow operation and injury favor accelerated gluconeogenesis. This new glucose is consumed by which of the following tissues?

A. Central nervous system.
B. Skeletal muscle.
C. Bone.
D. Kidney.
E. Tissue in the healing wound.

DISCUSSION: Glucose is produced in increased amounts to satisfy the fuel requirements of the healing wound. In addition, nerve tissue and the renal medulla also utilize this substrate. Skeletal muscle primarily utilizes fatty acids, and bone utilizes mineral substrate.

Textbook: Pages 65–66 ANSWER: A, D, E.

4. Cytokines are endogenous signals that stimulate:

A. Local cell proliferation within the wound.
B. The central nervous system to initiate fever.
C. The production of "acute-phase proteins."
D. Hypoferremia.
E. Septic shock.

DISCUSSION: Although cytokines exert primarily autocrine and paracrine effects, they may also cause systemic effects.

Textbook: Page 59 ANSWER: A, B, C, D, E.

5. The characteristic changes that follow a major operation or moderate to severe injury do not include the following:

A. Hypermetabolism.
B. Fever.
C. Tachypnea.
D. Hyperphagia.
E. Negative nitrogen balance.

DISCUSSION: The characteristic metabolic response to injury includes hypermetabolism, fever, accelerated gluconeogenesis, and increased proteolysis (creating a negative nitrogen balance). Food intake is generally impossible because of abdominal injury or ileus. With time, food intake increases, but the patient generally experiences anorexia, not hyperphagia.

Textbook: Pages 62–63 ANSWER: D.

6. Shock can best be defined as:

A. Hypotension.
B. Hypoperfusion of tissues.
C. Hypoxemia.
D. All of the above.

DISCUSSION: Shock, no matter what the cause, is a syndrome associated with tissue hypoperfusion. Tissue hypoperfusion leads to tissue hypoxia, which may or may not be due to hypoxemia. Hypotension is a late sign of shock and, therefore, is not a good clinical indicator of the presence of tissue hypoperfusion.

Textbook: Page 69 ANSWER: B.

7. Which of the following statements about continuous cardiac output monitoring are true?

A. Continuous cardiac output monitoring may unmask events not detected by intermittent cardiac output measurements.
B. Continuous cardiac output monitoring by the thermodilution method requires continuous infusion of fluid injectate at a constant rate and temperature.
C. The major advantage of the Fick method over the thermodilution method of calculating cardiac output is that it is noninvasive, requiring only the determination of oxygen consumption by respiratory gas analysis.
D. The technique of thoracic electrical bioimpedance utilizes sensors to determine stroke volume by detecting changes in resistance to a small, applied alternating current.

DISCUSSION: Various techniques are available to measure cardiac output continuously. The advantages of continuous cardiac output monitoring, as compared with intermittent methods, are (1) previously undetected events may be unmasked; (2) more prompt recognition of adverse events may be achieved; and (3) earlier therapeutic intervention may be possible. Continuous cardiac output monitoring using the thermodilution method appears to be as accurate as the "standard" intermittent bolus method, but it does not require fluid injectates. In this method, a modified pulmonary artery catheter incorporating a thermal filament heats blood in the right ventricle at pulsed intervals, and a distal thermistor detects the temperature change, which can be related mathematically to cardiac output. The Fick method combines respiratory gas analysis with oximetery to determine oxygen consumption ($\dot{V}O_2$) and to estimate mixed venous and arterial oxygen content differences, respectively. Cardiac output (CO) is then determined from the formula: $CO = \dot{V}O_2 / \{C(a\text{-}v)O_2 \times 10\} \cong \dot{V}O_2 / \{SaO_2 - SvO_2) \times (Hb) \times (1.39) \times 10\}$. Thoracic electrical bioimpedance is a technique by which the resistance to a small-amplitude alternating current (i.e., the impedance) is measured using various electrodes. The impedance change induced by each cardiac ejection is a function of the stroke volume, which then can be used to calculate the cardiac output.

Textbook: Pages 72–74 ANSWER: A, D.

8. Which of the following statements regarding cytokines is incorrect?

A. Cytokines act directly on target cells and may potentiate the actions of one another.
B. Interleukin 1 (IL-1) is a major proinflammatory mediator with multiple effects, including regulation of skeletal muscle proteolysis in patients with sepsis or significant injury.
C. Platelet-activating factor (PAF) is a major cytokine that results in platelet aggregation, bronchoconstriction, and increased vascular permeability.
D. Tumor necrosis factor alpha (TNF-α), despite its short plasma half-life, appears to be a principal mediator in the evolution of sepsis and the multiple organ dysfunction syndrome because of its multiple actions and the secondary cascades that it stimulates.

DISCUSSION: Cytokines are soluble peptide molecules that are synthesized and secreted by a number of cell types in response to injury, inflammation, and infection. Cytokines, which include the interleukins, tumor necrosis factor, colony-stimulating factors, and the interferons, comprise only one category of inflammatory mediators involved in the host response. Endotoxin, complement fragments, eicosanoids, kinins, nitric oxide, oxidants, and PAF are noncytokine mediators that also have important roles in the systemic inflammatory response. IL-1 and TNF-α, like other cytokines, have multiple effects on target cells and potentiate the actions of other mediators to produce an amplified inflammatory response. TNF-α is thought to play a central role in the stress response, particularly in response to endotoxemia.

Textbook: Pages 80–81 ANSWER: C.

9. True statements concerning hypoadrenal shock include which of the following?

A. Adrenocortical insufficiency may manifest itself as severe shock refractory to volume and pressor therapy.
B. The presence of hyperglycemia and hypotension may suggest the diagnosis of shock due to adrenocortical insufficiency.
C. Hydrocortisone does not interfere with the serum cortisol assay and should be given to hemodynamically unstable patients suspected of having hypoadrenal shock.
D. The rapid adrenocorticotropic hormone (ACTH) stimulation test should be performed to help establish the diagnosis of acute adrenocortical insufficiency.

DISCUSSION: Shock due to acute adrenocortical insufficiency is relatively uncommon but must be considered when shock refractory to volume replacement and pressor therapy is present. Hypoglycemia may be present. Patients with high metabolic stress may exhibit adrenal insufficiency only under conditions of severe stress; thus, a history of adrenal insufficiency or steroid dependency need not be elicited. When adrenocortical insufficiency is suspected, the rapid ACTH (cosyntropin) stimulation test should be performed. Serum cortisol levels should be drawn before intravenous administration of 250 μg. of cosyntropin, and 30 and 60 minutes afterward. A peak cortisol level of less than 20 μg./100 ml. suggests abnormal adrenal function. In a hemodynamically unstable patient therapy should be instituted before the test results become available. Dexamethasone does not interfere with the cortisol assay, and it is the corticosteroid of choice while the ACTH stimulation test is being performed.

Textbook: Pages 86–87 ANSWER: A, D.

10. All of the following are true about neurogenic shock except:

A. There is a decrease in systemic vascular resistance and an increase in venous capacitance.
B. Tachycardia *or* bradycardia may be observed, along with hypotension.
C. The use of an alpha agonist such as phenylephrine is the mainstay of treatment.
D. Severe head injury, spinal cord injury, and high spinal anesthesia may all cause neurogenic shock.

DISCUSSION: Neurogenic shock occurs when severe head injury, spinal cord injury, or pharmacologic sympathetic blockade leads to sympathetic denervation and loss of vasomotor tone. Both arteriolar and venous vessels dilate, causing reduced systemic vascular resistance and a great increase in venous capacitance. The patient's extremities appear warm and dry, in contrast to those of a patient in cardiogenic or hypovolemic shock. Tachycardia is frequently observed, though the classic description of neurogenic shock includes bradycardia and hypotension. Volume administration to fill the expanded intravascular compartment is the mainstay of treatment. The use of alpha-adrenergic agonist is infrequently necessary to treat neurogenic shock.

Textbook: Pages 69–70, 86 ANSWER: C.

11. True statements regarding eicosanoids include which of the following?

A. Prostaglandins and thromboxanes are synthesized via the cyclo-oxygenase pathway.
B. The vasoconstricting, platelet-aggregating, and bronchoconstricting effects of thromboxane A_2 are balanced by the actions of prostacyclin, which produces the opposite effects.
C. Leukotriene synthesis is inhibited by the action of nonsteroidal anti-inflammatory drugs (NSAIDs).
D. The principal prostaglandins have a short circulation half-life and exert most of their effects locally.

DISCUSSION: The eicosanoids are a group of compounds arising from the metabolism of arachidonic acid. The prostaglandins and thromboxanes are synthesized via the cyclo-oxygenase pathway; thus, their synthesis is blocked by NSAIDs. Leukotrienes, on the other hand, are synthesized via the lipoxygenase pathway. Prostacyclin, produced largely by vascular endothelium, inhibits platelet aggregation and causes vasodilatation as well as bronchodilatation. Its effects are balanced by those of thromboxane A_2, which is produced by platelets and also local actions, including platelet aggregation, vasoconstriction, and bronchoconstriction. The leukotrienes also have pulmonary and hemodynamic effects and may be involved in the physiologic responses associated with anaphylactic and septic shock.

Textbook: Pages 79–80 ANSWER: A, B, D.

12. Which of the following statements about delivery-dependent oxygen consumption are true?

A. Below the critical oxygen delivery ($\dot{D}O_{2crit}$), one would expect to see a decrease in the lactate-pyruvate ratio.
B. $\dot{D}O_{2crit}$ may be increased in patients with sepsis.
C. A desirable goal in the treatment of shock is to achieve delivery-independent oxygen consumption.
D. The oxygen extraction ratio remains constant as long as oxygen delivery remains above $\dot{D}O_{2crit}$.

DISCUSSION: Oxygen consumption is said to be delivery dependent below a critical point, $\dot{D}O_{2crit}$, at which anaerobic metabolism supervenes. Above this point, oxygen consumption is relatively independent of oxygen delivery because the body's cells can compensate for falls in oxygen delivery by extracting more oxygen. In the delivery-dependent region, if cellular hypoxia is present, the lactate-pyruvate ratio rises, owing to the switch to anaerobic metabolism. Generally, it is desirable to achieve delivery-independent oxygen consumption, to avoid ongoing tissue hypoxia. There is considerable debate, however, about the nature of the oxygen consumption–oxygen delivery relationship in cases of established sepsis or multiple organ dysfunction syndrome. In such cases, $\dot{D}O_{2crit}$ may be increased, although the therapeutic benefit of trying to achieve "supranormal" oxygen delivery has not been firmly established.

Textbook: Pages 75–76 ANSWER: B, C.

13. All of the following may be useful in the treatment of cardiogenic shock *except*:

A. Dobutamine.
B. Sodium nitroprusside.

C. Pneumatic antishock garment.
D. Intra-aortic balloon pump.

DISCUSSION: Cardiogenic shock occurs when the heart fails to generate adequate cardiac output to maintain tissue perfusion. Intrinsic causes such as myocardial dysfunction secondary to coronary artery disease, or extrinsic causes such as pulmonary embolism, tension pneumothorax, and pericardial tamponade, may produce cardiogenic shock. Principles of treatment of cardiogenic shock are aimed at optimizing preload, cardiac contractility, and afterload. Preload is usually adequate or high in cardiogenic shock. Dobutamine is a useful inotropic agent, particularly when filling pressures are high, because of its mild vasodilatory effect, as well as its effect to enhance cardiac contractility. Afterload-reducing agents, such as sodium nitroprusside, may be beneficial in cardiogenic shock in the setting of elevated filling pressures, low cardiac output, and elevated systemic vascular resistance. Cardiac output may improve with use of afterload-reducing agents by decreasing myocardial wall tension and optimizing the myocardial oxygen supply-demand ratio. The intra-aortic balloon pump (IABP), by providing diastolic augmentation, reducing left ventricular afterload, and reducing myocardial oxygen consumption, is sometimes useful in the treatment of cardiogenic shock. The IABP is especially useful in low–cardiac output postcardiotomy patients, in patients awaiting revascularization, and in patients with acute myocardial infarction complicated by mitral insufficiency or ventricular septal defect. The pneumatic antishock garment (PASG), which causes an increase in systemic vascular resistance, is contraindicated in cardiogenic shock.

Textbook: Pages 85–86 ANSWER: C.

14. Which of the following statements concerning monitoring techniques in the intensive care unit are true?

A. Pulmonary artery and pulmonary capillary wedge pressure readings should be made at end inspiration, to minimize ventilatory artifacts.
B. Continuous SvO_2 monitoring based on the technique of reflectance spectrophotometry has been shown to be accurate and reliable.
C. Direct measurement of gastric intramucosal pH can be provided by gastrointestinal tonometry.
D. Hyperlactatemia may be seen in a number of clinical conditions not associated with tissue hypoxia, including liver disease and hypermetabolic states.

DISCUSSION: Many different monitoring techniques may be used to assess the adequacy of therapy for shock. The pulmonary artery catheter can provide important hemodynamic and oxygen transport data that are very useful in directing therapy aimed at optimizing cardiac function and oxygen delivery. Pulmonary artery and pulmonary capillary wedge pressure readings should be made at end-expiration to minimize ventilatory artifacts. Continuous SvO_2 monitoring, an accurate, reliable method that combines pulmonary artery catheterization with the technique of reflectance spectrophotometry, may provide early warning signs of hemodynamic compromise or inadequate oxygen delivery. Gastrointestinal tonometry provides information that allows one to infer the adequacy of splanchnic tissue perfusion. In this technique, intramucosal pH is calculated using the Henderson-Hasselbalch equation and measurements of gut intraluminal PCO_2 and arterial bicarbonate concentration. Serum lactate concentration may be monitored in shock to detect metabolic acidosis associated with anaerobic metabolism; however, mild to moderate hyperlactatemia may also be seen with liver disease, toxin ingestion, and hypermetabolic states not associated with shock.

Textbook: Pages 70–75 ANSWER: B, D.

15. An 18-year-old man shot once in the left chest has a blood pressure of 80/50 mm. Hg, a heart rate of 130 beats per minute, and distended neck veins. Immediate treatment might include:

A. Administration of one liter of Ringer's lactate solution.
B. Subxiphoid pericardiotomy.
C. Needle decompression of the left chest in the second intercostal space.
D. Emergency thoracotomy to cross-clamp the aorta.

DISCUSSION: The finding of distended neck veins in conjunction with hypotension should suggest tension pneumothorax or pericardial tamponade. Absent ipsilateral breath sounds and a trachea deviated to the contralateral side may provide additional evidence for a tension pneumothorax, the immediate treatment of which is needle decompression of the chest in the second or third intercostal space in the midclavicular line. Pericardial tamponade may initially respond to volume administration by enhancing preload. Pericardiocentesis may need to be performed emergently if hemodynamic instability persists after an initial fluid bolus when signs of compressive cardiogenic shock are present. Subxiphoid pericardiotomy should be performed only in the operating room by experienced persons who are trained to deal with penetrating cardiac injuries. There is no role for aortic cross-clamping in this scenario of cardiogenic shock.

Textbook: Pages 84–85 ANSWER: A, C.

16. Which of the following statements are true of the multiple organ dysfunction syndrome (MODS)?

A. The "two-hit" model proposes that secondary MODS may be produced when even a relatively minor second insult reactivates, in a more amplified form, the systemic inflammatory response that was primed by an initial insult to the host.
B. The systemic inflammatory response syndrome (SIRS), shock due to sepsis or SIRS, and

MODS may be regarded as a continuum of illness severity.

C. Prolonged stimulation or activation of Kupffer cells in the liver is thought to be a critical factor in the sustained, uncontrolled release of inflammatory mediators.

D. The incidence of MODS in intensive care units has decreased owing to increased awareness, prevention, and treatment of the syndrome.

DISCUSSION: MODS is part of a clinical continuum that begins with the systemic inflammatory response syndrome, which is the host's stress response to any major insult such as injury or infection. MODS may develop as a result of the initial insult, but more commonly, it develops following a second or subsequent insult to the host. The two-hit theory holds that the systemic inflammatory response is amplified following the second hit, such as nosocomial pneumonia, leading to exaggerated, persistent release of inflammatory mediators that contribute to the pathogenesis of MODS. The liver appears to be a pivotal organ in the progression and outcome of MODS, partly because of the activation and prolonged stimulation of the Kupffer cells, which comprise the majority of the body's macrophage population. Macrophages are known to play a critical role in the elaboration of numerous inflammatory mediators. Despite advances in critical care and in the understanding of the pathogenesis of MODS, the incidence of MODS continues to increase without a significant improvement in outcome.

Textbook: Pages 87–90 ANSWER: A, B, C.

17. All of the following statements about hemorrhagic shock are true *except*:

A. Following hemorrhagic shock, there is an initial interstitial fluid volume contraction.

B. Dopamine, or a similar inotropic agent, should be given immediately for resuscitation from hemorrhagic shock, to increase cardiac output and improve oxygen delivery to hypoperfused tissues.

C. The use of colloid solutions or hypertonic saline solutions is contraindicated for treatment of hemorrhagic shock.

D. In hemorrhagic shock, a narrowed pulse pressure is commonly seen before a fall in systolic blood pressure.

DISCUSSION: Hemorrhagic shock is associated with a contraction of the interstitial fluid compartment because of precapillary vasoconstriction and reabsorption of interstitial fluid into the vascular compartment along hydrostatic pressure gradients. Systolic hypotension may not be evident in hemorrhagic shock until at least 30% or more of blood volume is exsanguinated. A decrease in the pulse pressure (the difference between systolic and diastolic pressures) may be observed with losses of 15% to 30% of blood volume. Treatment of hemorrhagic shock includes intravascular fluid administration and definitive control of the source of the hemorrhage. Inotropic agents should not be started before volume resuscitation but may be added to improve oxygen delivery to hypoxic tissues if volume administration alone does not produce resuscitative goals. Colloid or hypertonic saline solutions are not contraindicated in the treatment of hemorrhagic shock; however, definitive evidence that such solutions are better than standard crystalloid solutions is lacking.

Textbook: Pages 81–84 ANSWER: B, C.

18. Which of the following statements about septic shock are true?

A. A circulating myocardial depressant factor may account for the cardiac dysfunction sometimes seen with shock due to sepsis or SIRS.

B. A cardiac index (CI) of 6 liters per minute per square meter of body surface, a pulmonary capillary wedge pressure of 15 mm. Hg, and a systemic vascular resistance index (SVRI) of 800 dynes-sec/(cm^5-m^2) is a hemodynamic profile consistent with septic shock.

C. An increase in Svo_2 in septic patients may be explained by the finding of anatomic arteriovenous shunts.

D. Results of human trials employing antimediator therapy, such as antiendotoxin antibodies, IL-1 receptor antagonist, and tumor necrosis factor (TNF) antibodies, have confirmed animal studies that demonstrate a significant improvement in survival with the use of such agents.

DISCUSSION: Shock due to sepsis or SIRS frequently manifests as a hyperdynamic cardiovascular response, consisting of an elevated CI and a decreased SVR or SVRI. Occasionally, myocardial depression may be seen, characterized by increased ventricular volumes and decreased ejection fractions. A circulating myocardial depressant factor, possibly TNF, may be responsible for the cardiac dysfunction in such instances. The cause of the increased Svo_2 frequently observed in septic patients is unclear, but it may be secondary to bioenergetic failure, metabolic downregulation, or microcirculatory maldistribution leading to physiologic shunting. True anatomic arteriovenous shunting has not been demonstrated in humans in septic shock. Treatment of septic shock consists of appropriate antibiotic use and supportive therapy. Experimental antimediator therapies have not been encouraging thus far in human clinical trials, despite the promising results from many animal studies.

Textbook: Pages 87–90 ANSWER: A, B.

19. Which of the following statements are true of oxidants?

A. In addition to their pathophysiologic roles in inflammation, injury, and infection, oxidants also have physiologic roles.

B. Oxidants may be generated from activated neutrophils and during reperfusion following a period of ischemia.

C. The deleterious effects of oxidants include lipid peroxidation and cell membrane damage, oxidative damage to DNA, and inhibition of adenosine triphosphate (ATP) synthesis.
D. The mechanism of ischemia-reperfusion injury involved the catalytic production of superoxide anion ($O_2\cdot$) by the enzyme xanthine oxidase.

DISCUSSION: Oxidants are reactive oxygen metabolites that have both physiologic and pathophysiologic roles. As potent oxidizing agents, oxidants are involved in cytochrome P_{450}–mediated oxidations, for example. In pathophysiologic processes associated with inflammation, injury, and infection, oxidants may be generated by activated neutrophils and in ischemia-reperfusion injury. During ischemia, the enzyme xanthine oxidase accumulates. When oxygen availability increases during reperfusion, $O_2\cdot$ is formed in a reaction catalyzed by xanthine oxidase. Further oxidant formation ensues, causing the production of H_2O_2 and the extremely reactive hydroxyl ion (OH·). Oxidants may cause direct cell damage by the mechanisms of lipid peroxidation and cell membrane disruption, inhibition of ATP synthesis, reduction of cellular nicotinamide adenine dinucleotide (NAD), and oxidative damage to DNA and amino acids. In addition, oxidants may have a chemotactic role, leading to leukocyte infiltration and activation, causing further tissue damage by the release of cytotoxic proteases.

Textbook: Page 81 ANSWER: A, B, C, D.

20. Which of the following statements about the role of the gut in shock and sepsis are true?

A. Selective decontamination of the digestive tract with the use of oral antibiotics has been shown to reduce nosocomial pneumonias and to improve mortality rates.
B. Enteral nutrition, as compared with parenteral nutrition, preserves the villus architecture of the gut.
C. Gut dysfunction may be an effect of shock, but it may also contribute to the development of MODS by the mechanism of bacterial translocation.
D. As compared with parenteral nutrition, enteral nutrition is associated with a reduction in septic morbidity.

DISCUSSION: The gut has a vital role in the pathophysiology of shock. The splanchnic circulation is very vulnerable to the circulatory redistribution that occurs in shock, thus, gut ischemia may occur early in the various shock syndromes. Gut injury, as a result of ischemia or reperfusion injury, leads to disruption in the intestinal mucosal barrier and increased gut permeability. Translocation of enteric flora or bacterial toxins across the gut wall may then occur, resulting in amplification of the systemic inflammatory response and the development of multiple organ dysfunction. Gut dysfunction, therefore, may perpetuate the inflammatory process. Various methods have been tried to modulate the deleterious effects of gut dysfunction. Selective decontamination of the digestive tract by oral antibiotics has been shown to reduce the incidence of nosocomial pneumonias, but no improvement in mortality has been demonstrated thus far with this controversial technique. Early enteral nutrition probably has the biggest impact on the preservation of gut architecture and function. When compared to parenteral nutrition, enteral feeding is more cost effective and is associated with a lower rate of septic morbidity.

Textbook: Pages 88, 90 ANSWER: B, C, D.

21. Which of the following statements about head injury and concomitant hyponatremia are true?

A. There are no primary alterations in cardiovascular signs.
B. Signs of increased intracranial pressure may be masked by the hyponatremia.
C. Oliguric renal failure is an unlikely complication.
D. Rapid correction of the hyponatremia may prevent central pontine injury.
E. This patient is best treated by restriction of water intake.

DISCUSSION: Acute symptomatic hyponatremia is characterized by central nervous system signs of increased intracranial pressure. Changes in blood pressure and pulse are secondary to increased intracranial pressure. In the absence of hypovolemia, asymptomatic patients may be treated by restriction of water intake; however, in such patients, hyponatremia should be partially corrected by parenteral sodium administration. Rapid correction, particularly to hypernatremia, may lead to central pontine myelinolysis. Oliguric renal failure may rapidly develop in severe hyponatremia.

Textbook: Page 90 ANSWER: A.

22. Which of the following statements about total body water composition are correct?

A. Females and obese persons have an increased percentage of body water.
B. Increased muscle mass is associated with decreased total body water.
C. Newborn infants have the greatest proportion of total body water.
D. Total body water decreases steadily with age.
E. Any person's percentage of body water is subject to wide physiologic variation.

DISCUSSION: Since fat contains little water, lean persons with a proportionately greater muscle mass have a greater than expected volume of total body water. Likewise, the female body habitus and obesity contribute to decreased total body water percentage. The highest proportion of total body water is found in newborn infants, and total body water decreases steadily and significantly with age. The actual figure for a healthy person is remarkably constant.

Textbook: Page 92 ANSWER: C, D.

23. Which of the following statements about extracellular fluid are true?

A. The total extracellular fluid volume represents 40% of the body weight.
B. The plasma volume constitutes one fourth of the total extracellular fluid volume.
C. Potassium is the principal cation in extracellular fluid.
D. The protein content of the plasma produces a lower concentration of cations than in the interstitial fluid.
E. The interstitial fluid equilibrates slowly with the other body compartments.

DISCUSSION: The total extracellular fluid volume represents 20% of body weight. The plasma volume is approximately 5% of body weight. Sodium is the principal cation. The Gibbs-Donan equilibrium equation explains the higher total concentration of cations in plasma. Except for joint fluid and cerebrospinal fluid, the majority of the interstitial fluid exists as a rapidly equilibrating component.

Textbook: Pages 92–93 ANSWER: B.

24. Which of the following statements are true of a patient with hyperglycemia and hyponatremia?

A. The sodium concentration must be corrected by 5 mEq. per 100 mg. per 100 ml. elevation in blood glucose.
B. With normal renal function, this patient is likely to be volume overloaded.
C. Proper fluid therapy would be unlikely to include potassium administration.
D. Insulin administration will increase the potassium content of cells.
E. Early in treatment adequate urine output is a reliable measure of adequate volume resuscitation.

DISCUSSION: Each 100-mg. per 100 ml. elevation in blood glucose causes a fall in serum sodium concentration of approximately 2 mEq. per liter. Excess serum glucose acts as an osmotic diuretic, producing increased urine flow, which can lead to volume depletion. Insulin therapy and the correction of the patient's associated acidosis produce movement of potassium ions into the intracellular compartment.

Textbook: Page 109 ANSWER: D.

25. Which of the following statements about respiratory acidosis are true?

A. Compensation occurs by a shift of chloride out of the red blood cells.
B. Renal compensation occurs rapidly.
C. Retention of bicarbonate and increased ammonia formation are normal compensatory mechanisms.
D. Narcotic administration is an unusual cause of respiratory acidosis.
E. The ratio of bicarbonate to carbonic acid is less than 20:1.

DISCUSSION: Renal compensation for acute hypoventilation is relatively slow. Depression of the respiratory center by morphine can lead to respiratory acidosis. Renal retention of bicarbonate, ammonia formation, and shift of chloride into red cells combine to increase the ratio of bicarbonate to carbonic acid to 20:1.

Textbook: Pages 98–99 ANSWER: C, E.

26. Which of the following statements are true of elevated–anion gap metabolic acidosis?

A. Hypoperfusion from the shock state rarely produces an elevated anion gap.
B. Retention of sulfuric and phosphoric acids may lead to this form of acidosis.
C. Copious diarrhea does not produce this condition.
D. Rapid volume expansion may produce this form of acidosis.
E. Use of lactated Ringer's solution is inappropriate in the treatment of lactic acidosis.

DISCUSSION: An elevated anion gap may be produced by lactic acidosis from shock or by retention of inorganic acids from uremia. Lactated Ringer's solution rapidly corrects the lactic acidosis from hypovolemia, as lactate is converted to bicarbonate with hepatic reperfusion. Bicarbonate loss from diarrhea and "dilutional acidosis" are non–anion gap types of metabolic acidosis.

Textbook: Pages 99–100 ANSWER: B, C.

27. Which of the following is true of loss of gastrointestinal secretions?

A. Gastric losses are best replaced with a balanced salt solution.
B. Potassium supplementation is unnecessary in replacement of gastric secretions.
C. Bicarbonate wasting is an unusual complication of a high-volume pancreatic fistula.
D. Balanced salt solution is a reasonable replacement fluid for a small bowel fistula.
E. A patient with persistent vomiting usually requires hyperchloremic replacement fluids.

DISCUSSION: Gastric secretions are relatively high in chloride and potassium. Other than an isolated pancreatic fistula, gastrointestinal tract losses below the pylorus are best replaced by a balanced salt solution. Although potassium concentrations are low, copious losses require potassium supplementation to prevent hypokalemia.

Textbook: Pages 101–102 ANSWER: D, E.

28. Which of the following statements regarding hypercalcemia are true?

A. The symptoms of hypercalcemia may mimic some symptoms of hyperglycemia.
B. Metastatic breast cancer is an unusual cause of hypercalcemia.

C. Calcitonin is a satisfactory long-term therapy for hypercalcemia.
D. Severely hypercalcemic patients exhibit the signs of extracellular fluid volume deficit.
E. Urinary calcium excretion may be increased by vigorous volume repletion.

DISCUSSION: Markedly elevated serum calcium levels produce polydipsia, polyuria, and thirst. Vigorous volume repletion and saline diuresis correct the extracellular fluid volume deficit and promote the urinary excretion of calcium. Metastatic breast cancer is the most common cause of hypercalcemia, from bony metastasis. The calcitonin effect on calcium is diminished with repeat administrations.

Textbook: Pages 102–103 ANSWER: A, D, E.

29. Which of the following statements about normal salt and water balance are true?

A. The products of catabolism may be excreted by as little as 300 ml. of urine per day.
B. The lungs represent the primary source of insensible water loss.
C. The normal daily insensible water loss is 600 to 900 ml.
D. Excessive cell catabolism causes significant loss of total body water.
E. In normal humans, urine represents the greatest source of daily water loss.

DISCUSSION: The skin is the primary source of insensible water loss. Including losses from the lungs, this averages 600 to 900 ml. per day. Catabolism liberates "water of solution." In normal humans, urine represents the greatest source of water loss. The patient deprived of external access to water must still excrete a minimum of 500 to 800 ml. of urine per day to expel the products of catabolism.

Textbook: Pages 104–105 ANSWER: C, E.

30. Which of the following is/are *not* associated with increased likelihood of infection after major elective surgery?

A. Age over 70 years.
B. Chronic malnutrition.
C. Controlled diabetes mellitus.
D. Long-term steroid use.
E. Infection at a remote body site.

DISCUSSION: Controlled diabetes mellitus has been shown repeatedly not to be associated with increased likelihood of incisional infection provided one avoids operations on body parts that may be ischemic or neuropathic. Uncontrolled diabetes mellitus, such as ketoacidosis, is associated with a dramatic increase in surgical infection. The other parameters noted—age over 70, chronic malnutrition, regular steroid use, and an infection at a remote body site—are well-recognized adverse predictive factors and are identified in tables within the chapter.

Textbook: Page 112 ANSWER: C.

31. Which of the following *are not* determinants of a postoperative cardiac complication?

A. Myocardial infarct 4 months previously.
B. Clinical evidence of congestive heart failure in a patient with 8.5 gm. per dl. hemoglobin.
C. Premature atrial or ventricular contractions on electrocardiogram.
D. A harsh aortic systolic murmur.
E. Age over 70 years.

DISCUSSION: Clinical evidence of congestive heart failure in a patient with 8.5 gm. per dl. hemoglobin concentration is a misleading sign. Evidence of congestive failure is ordinarily a major risk factor, but in this particular patient the anemia lends itself to correction by preoperative transfusion with packed red blood cells, and often it is found that congestive failure and the associated increased risks disappear when the hemoglobin concentration is returned to the 12 gm. per dl. or higher ratio. All other factors are overt signs of increased likelihood of a postoperative cardiac event, the most ominous being a myocardial infarction 4 months preoperatively or the presence of a harsh aortic systolic murmur suggesting the presence of aortic stenosis. Age over 70 years and the presence of premature atrial or ventricular contractions on the electrocardiogram are less strong determinants of a postoperative cardiac complication.

Textbook: Pages 114–115 ANSWER: B.

32. Rank the clinical scenarios in order of greatest likelihood of serious postoperative pulmonary complications.

A. Transabdominal hysterectomy in an obese woman that requires 3 hours of anesthesia time.
B. Right middle lobectomy for bronchogenic cancer in a 65-year-old smoker.
C. Vagotomy and pyloroplasty for chronic duodenal ulcer disease in a 50-year-old who had chest film findings of old, healed tuberculosis.
D. Right hemicolectomy in an obese 60-year-old smoker.
E. Modified radical mastectomy in a 58-year-old woman who is obese.

DISCUSSION: If one considers the constellation of risk factors for pulmonary complications that is provided in tabular form in the accompanying chapter, one should readily recognize *B*, right middle lobectomy for bronchogenic cancer in a 65-year-old smoker, as the highest risk of a clinical situation for the likelihood of serious pulmonary complications. The next in rank may be properly debated between answer *D* and answer *C*. *D*, right hemicolectomy, is judged to have somewhat greater likelihood of complications since the patient is older, smokes, and is obese, although the procedure may be done through a transverse or lower abdominal incision. *C*, vagotomy and pyloroplasty, is viewed as being somewhat less serious since it is an upper abdominal operation on an elective basis in a 50-year-old whose only abnormalities include old, healed tuberculosis on a chest film. A very low risk of pulmonary complication should follow a transabdominal hysterectomy done through a lower abdominal incision in a woman whose only risk factors are obesity and a 3-hour anesthesia time. The lowest risk probably resides with the younger patient undergoing modified radical mastectomy, whose only risk factor is obesity. This is particularly true since this operation is conducted on the surface of the body, is associated with relatively little postoperative pain, and provides free and unrestricted respiratory function.

Textbook: Page 115 ANSWER: In order—B, D, C, A, E.

33. Rank the following laboratory tests and procedures in terms of their relative value to a 65-year-old woman who is to undergo elective resection of a sigmoid cancer.

A. Carcinoembryonic antigen (CEA).
B. Blood urea nitrogen (BUN).
C. Electrocardiogram (ECG).
D. Hemoglobin concentration (Hgb).
E. Serum creatinine (Cr).
F. Arterial blood oxygen tension (PaO_2) on room air.
G. Serum sodium concentration (Na^+).

DISCUSSION: The most important test by far is the electrocardiogram, with its capacity to indicate signs of occult heart disease. The second most important evaluation is the hemoglobin concentration, which in this patient may show an anemia related to chronic alimentary tract blood loss that would require correction prior to safe induction of a general anesthetic. Arterial blood gases vary from individual to individual depending primarily on smoking habits and age. Accordingly, each older person should have a resting baseline determination prior to operation. Serum creatinine may show evidence of occult renal disease and is substantially more useful than blood urea nitrogen, which is more vulnerable to transient volume changes. Carcinoembryonic antigen is important to know in many patients with cancer with respect to postoperative follow-up since in some cases it may be an early herald of recurrent disease. However, it has little to do with the patient's preoperative assessment in terms of risk and preparation for an elective operation. The presence of liver metastases, for example, can be discovered with significant accuracy by palpation at the time of operation, and an elevated carcinoembryonic antigen in no set of circumstances would lead one to withhold colon resection with its relief of potential obstruction and bleeding. Finally, serum sodium concentration in a 65-year-old woman who is admitted electively for resection of the colon is always normal and would be of least value among these tests.

Textbook: Pages 112–116 ANSWER: In order—C, D, F, E, B, A, G.

34. Which of the following statements regarding whole blood transfusion is/are correct?

A. Whole blood is the most commonly used red cell preparation for transfusion in the United States.
B. Whole blood is effective in the replacement of acute blood loss.
C. Most blood banks in the United States have large supplies of whole blood available.
D. The use of whole blood produces higher rates of disease transmission than the use of individual component therapies.

DISCUSSION: Whole blood is effective as a replacement fluid for acute blood loss because it provides both volume and oxygen-carrying capacity (red blood cells). It is rarely used in the United States nowadays, and most blood banks do not provide whole blood transfusions. It is significantly more efficient to separate donated blood into its components. In this manner, the red blood cell mass can be used to provide oxygen-carrying capacity, the plasma can be used for factor replacement, and the platelets and white cells can be used for patients deficient in these components. The use of whole blood to replace acute blood loss is associated with lower disease transmission rates than the use of packed red blood cells, fresh frozen plasma, and platelets, each from a different donor.

Textbook: Page 120 ANSWER: B.

35. Which of the following statements about the preparation and storage of blood components is/are true?

A. Solutions containing citrate prevent coagulation by binding calcium.
B. The shelf life of packed red blood cells preserved with CPDA-1 is approximately 35 days at 1° to 6° C.
C. There are normal numbers of platelets in packed red blood cells stored at 1° to 6° C for more than 2 days.
D. The storage lesion affecting refrigerated packed red blood cells includes development of acidosis, hyperkalemia, and decreased intracellular 2,3DPG (diphosphoglycerate).

DISCUSSION: After blood has been collected from a donor, it is anticoagulated with a solution containing citrate, which acts by binding calcium. Blood is then separated into its components. Packed red blood cells stored at 1° to 6° C using CPDA-1 preservative have a shelf life of 35 days. There are essentially no functional platelets in refrigerated blood stored at 1° to 6° C after approximately 48 hours in storage. Refrigerated packed red blood cells undergo progressive changes termed a *storage lesion.* Such changes include acidosis, hyperkalemia, and decreased levels of 2,3-DPG, which are reversed after transfusion or produce effects other than those predicted based on the content of the unit of blood.

Textbook: Pages 118–120 ANSWER: A, B, D.

36. Which of the following is/are acceptable reasons for the transfusion of red blood cells based on currently available data?

A. Rapid, acute blood loss with unstable vital signs but no available hematocrit or hemoglobin determination.
B. Symptomatic anemia: orthostatic hypotension, severe tachycardia (greater than 120 beats per minute), evidence of myocardial ischemia, including angina.
C. To increase wound healing.
D. A hematocrit of 26% in an otherwise stable, asymptomatic patient.

DISCUSSION: Currently accepted guidelines for the transfusion of packed red blood cells include acute ongoing blood loss, as might occur in an injured patient, and the development of symptomatic anemia with manifestations of decreased tissue perfusion related to decreased oxygen-carrying capacity of the blood. This includes situations in which the patient is unable to compensate for a decreased oxygen-carrying capacity by the usual mechanisms, such as increased cardiac output. Such patients develop myocardial dysfunction if an excessive demand is placed on the heart. The patient should be transfused with packed red blood cells, which afford added oxygen-carrying capacity. This decreases the workload on the myocardium while providing the necessary oxygen-delivery capability. The use of packed red blood cells to improve wound healing or to improve the patient's sense of well-being is highly questionable. No data support such a practice. In general, the use of a transfusion trigger such as a hematocrit of 30% or hemoglobin of 10 gm. per dl. constitutes a questionable indication for transfusion. If a patient is asymptomatic and stable and has no risk of myocardial ischemia, packed red blood cell transfusion should not be given based solely or predominantly on a numerical value such as a hematocrit of 28%.

Textbook: Pages 120–121 ANSWER: A, B.

37. The transfusion of fresh frozen plasma (FFP) is indicated for which of the following reasons?

A. Volume replacement.
B. As a nutritional supplement.
C. Specific coagulation factor deficiency with an abnormal prothrombin time (PT) and/or an abnormal activated partial thromboplastin time (APTT).
D. For the correction of abnormal PT secondary to warfarin therapy, vitamin K deficiency, or liver disease.

DISCUSSION: The use of FFP as a volume expander is not indicated. There are currently several preparations (both crystalloid and colloid) that are equally effective and do not carry the infectious and other risks associated with the use of FFP. The use of FFP as a "nutritional" supplement is to be condemned. Patients with specific deficiencies of coagulation factors generally benefit greatly from the infusion of FFP. In cases of specific factor deficiency, other preparations may be more appropriate, but FFP is generally immediately available and is effective in most patients. Patients receiving warfarin therapy, those who have vitamin K deficiency, and those with liver dysfunction have abnormalities of the vitamin K–dependent factors II, VII, IX, and X, as well as protein C and protein S.

Textbook: Page 122 ANSWER: C, D.

38. In patients receiving massive blood transfusion for acute blood loss, which of the following is/are correct?

A. Packed red blood cells and crystalloid solution should be infused to restore oxygen-carrying capacity and intravascular volume.
B. Two units of FFP should be given with every 5 units of packed red blood cells in most cases.
C. A "six pack" of platelets should be administered with every 10 units of packed red blood cells in most cases.
D. One to two ampules of sodium bicarbonate should be administered with every 5 units of packed red blood cells to avoid acidosis.
E. One ampule of calcium chloride should be administered with every 5 units of packed red blood cells to avoid hypocalcemia.

DISCUSSION: Patients who are suffering from acute blood loss require crystalloid resuscitation as the initial maneuver to restore intravascular volume and re-establish vital signs. If 2 to 3 liters of crystalloid solution is inadequate to restore intravascular volume status, packed red blood cells should be infused as soon as possible. There is no role for "prophylactic infusion" of FFP, platelets, bicarbonate, or calcium to patients receiving massive blood transfusion. If specific indications exist patients should receive these supplemental components. In particular, patients who have abnormal coagulation tests and have ongoing bleeding should receive FFP. Patients who have depressed platelet counts along with clinical evidence of oozing (microvascular bleeding) benefit from platelet infusion. Sodium bicarbonate is not necessary, since most patients who receive blood transfusion ultimately develop alkalosis from the citrate contained in stored red blood cells. The use of calcium chloride is usually unnecessary unless the patient has depressed liver function, ongoing prolonged shock associated with hypothermia, or, rarely, when the infusion of blood proceeds at a rate exceeding 1 to 2 units every 5 minutes.

Textbook: Pages 123–124 ANSWER: A.

39. Hemostasis and the cessation of bleeding require which of the following processes?

A. Adherence of platelets to exposed subendothelial glycoproteins and collagen with subsequent aggregation of platelets and formation of a hemostatic plug.
B. Interaction of tissue factor with factor VII circulating in the plasma.

C. The production of thrombin via the coagulation cascade with conversion of fibrinogen to fibrin.
D. Cross-linking of fibrin by factor XIII.

DISCUSSION: Hemostasis requires the interaction of platelets with the exposed subendothelial structures at the site of injury followed by aggregation of more platelets in that area. Interactions between endothelial cell and subendothelial tissue factor with factor VII activate the coagulation cascade. The end product is large amounts of thrombin that catalyze the conversion of fibrinogen into fibrin. Fibrin thus formed is cross-linked by factor XIII to form a stable clot that incorporates the platelet plug and fibrin thrombus into a stable clot.

Textbook: Pages 126–127 ANSWER: A, B, C, D.

40. Which of the statements listed below about bleeding disorders is/are correct?

A. Acquired bleeding disorders are more common than congenital defects.
B. Deficiencies of vitamin K decrease production of factors II, VII, IX, and X, protein C, and protein S.
C. Hypothermia below 32°C rarely causes a bleeding disorder.
D. Von Willebrand's disease is a very uncommon congenital bleeding disorder.

DISCUSSION: Acquired bleeding disorders are significantly more common than congenital bleeding defects. Vitamin K deficiency may be related to malnutrition or competitive inhibition of the production of the vitamin K–dependent factors II, VII, IX, X, protein C, and protein S by warfarin (Coumadin). Hypothermia causes significant platelet dysfunction with a significant bleeding disorder in many patients. It is among the least recognized causes of altered coagulation in surgical patients. Von Willebrand's disease is a relatively common disorder of bleeding and is generally undetectable by routine screening methods.

Textbook: Pages 131–135 ANSWER: A, B.

41. The evaluation of a patient scheduled for elective surgery should *always* include the following as tests of hemostasis and coagulation:

A. History and physical examination.
B. Complete blood count (CBC), including platelet count.
C. Prothrombin time (PT) and activated partial thromboplastin time (APTT).
D. Studies of platelet aggregation with adenosine diphosphate (ADP) and epinephrine.

DISCUSSION: The evaluation of most patients scheduled for elective surgery who do not have a history of significant bleeding disorders is somewhat controversial. An adequate history and physical examination screen out most patients with bleeding problems. For patients who are scheduled to undergo a major surgical procedure, it is advisable to obtain a CBC and platelet count, as well as a PT and APTT level. This detects a large number of bleeding disorders but does not rule out all possible causes of perioperative bleeding. Studies of platelet aggregation are indicated only for patients who are suspected of having qualitative defects of platelet function (e.g., von Willebrand's disease).

Textbook: Pages 130–131 ANSWER: A.

42. Which of the following statements regarding the transmission of infectious agents through blood transfusions is/are true?

A. The transmission rates for human immunodeficiency virus (HIV) have been decreasing progressively since the early 1980s.
B. The transmission rates of hepatitis have been decreasing steadily since the 1980s.
C. Cytomegalovirus (CMV) is the infectious agent most commonly transmitted in blood.
D. Severely immunocompromised patients (such as patients undergoing transplantation) should receive specially screened blood products.

DISCUSSION: The incidence of both HIV and hepatitis transmitted via blood transfusions has been steadily decreasing since the 1980s. This is related to improved methods for detection and increased awareness of surrogate markers of disease. The currently available techniques for the detection of HIV are highly effective, provided the donor is not in the "window" before the formation of specific antibody. The surrogate markers for hepatitis C, as well as the specific assays for the organism, are now sufficiently refined to allow the detection of a large percentage of hepatitis C infection in donated blood. Screening for hepatitis B surface antigen has effectively eliminated the transmission of hepatitis B through blood products in most cases. CMV is the most commonly transmitted infectious agent in blood. Since a large percentage of the population carry the virus, routine screening is not performed for this organism; however, severely compromised patients such as those undergoing transplantation should receive CMV-negative blood products.

Textbook: Pages 124–125 ANSWER: A, B, C, D.

43. The most common cause of fatal transfusion reactions is:

A. An allergic reaction.
B. An anaphylactoid reaction.
C. A clerical error.
D. An acute bacterial infection transmitted in blood.

DISCUSSION: The most common cause of fatalities related to transfusion reactions result from ABO-incompatible transfusion related to clerical error. Most such reactions occur if a type O person receives type A red cells owing to a clerical error that occurs either at the time the blood sample was drawn, during processing in the laboratory, or at the time a unit is administered.

The importance of extremely careful labeling, transfer, and handling of specimens and of cross-matched blood products cannot be overemphasized. Allergic and other reactions are common but rarely fatal. The transmission of bacterial organisms (e.g., *Staphylococcus aureus*) has been reported especially with platelet concentrates maintained at or near room temperature. Fortunately, such reactions are rare.

Textbook: Page 124 ANSWER: C.

44. Which of the following statements about the coagulation cascade is/are true?

A. The intrinsic pathway of coagulation is the predominant pathway *in vivo* for hemostasis and coagulation.
B. The intrinsic pathway beginning with the activation of factor XII is the predominant *in vivo* mechanism for activation of the coagulation cascade.
C. Deficiencies of factor VIII and IX cause highly significant coagulation abnormalities.
D. Deficiencies of factor XII cause severe clinical bleeding syndromes.

DISCUSSION: Although it was previously held that two somewhat distinct pathways existed for the activation of the coagulation cascade, it is now recognized that the predominant mechanism for coagulation *in vivo* is the "extrinsic pathway." Tissue factor is exposed in the subendothelial tissues when endothelial cell injury occurs. Tissue factor then tightly binds factor VII circulating in the plasma and activates the coagulation cascade. Factor VIII and factor IX deficiency cause the clinical syndromes of hemophilia A and hemophilia B, respectively. Both of these disorders involve very severe clinical bleeding disorders, whereas deficiencies of factor XII do not generally cause clinically significant bleeding. This further emphasizes the secondary role that the "intrinsic pathway" plays in coagulation.

Textbook: Pages 128–130 ANSWER: A, C.

NOTES

NOTES

CHAPTER 3

METABOLISM, DIABETES MELLITUS, ANESTHESIA, WOUND HEALING, BURNS

1. A major problem in nutritional support is identifying patients at risk. Recent studies suggest that these patients can be identified. Which of the following findings identify the patient at risk?

A. Weight loss of greater than 10% over 2 to 4 months.
B. Serum albumin of less than 3 gm. per 100 ml. in the hydrated state.
C. Malnutrition as identified by global assessment.
D. Serum transferrin of less than 220 mg. per 100 ml.
E. Functional impairment by history.

DISCUSSION: All of these are at least partially correct. It is not clear whether weight loss of 10% or 15% is the required threshold, but it certainly is close. Serum albumin of less than 3 gm per 100 ml. remains the most constant identifier of patients at risk in the literature and has been so for years. Global assessment in the hands of an experienced investigator is quite efficacious at identifying persons at risk. Serum transferrin is certainly a confirmatory identifier of patients with malnutrition—and may be even a primary one. Graham Hill and his co-workers have pioneered the concept of global assessment using functional parameters, and in the hands of an experienced observer is quite a reasonable way of approaching and identifying patients at risk.

Textbook: Page 147 ANSWER: A, B, C, D, E.

2. Essential fatty acid deficiency may complicate total parenteral nutrition (TPN). Which of the following statements are true?

A. Essential fatty acid deficiency may be prevented by the administration of 1% to 2% of total calories as fat emulsion.
B. Fat-free parenteral nutrition results in the appearance of plasma abnormalities, indicating essential fatty acid deficiency, within 7 to 10 days of initiation.
C. An abnormal plasma eicosatrienoic-arachidonic acid ratio is always associated with essential fatty acid deficiency.
D. Following initiation of fat-free parenteral nutrition, dry, scaly skin associated with a maculopapular rash indicates essential fatty acid deficiency.

DISCUSSION: Biochemical evidence of essential fatty acid deficiency may occur as early as 7 to 10 days following initiation of fat-free parenteral nutrition. The decrease in arachidonic acid in plasma and the appearance of the abnormal eicosatrienoic acid may yield the earliest indication of prostaglandin deficiency; it is not absolute. Decreased intraocular pressure, another early indication of prostaglandin deficiency, may appear as soon as 7 days following initiation of fat-free parenteral nutrition. While my current practice is to give at least 500 ml. of 10% lipid emulsion daily to provide 20% to 25% of total calories to support hepatic protein synthesis, as little as 4% to 6% of total daily calories as fat prevents essential fatty acid deficiency. Practically, this may be undertaken by the administration of 500 ml. of 10% lipid three times weekly. The appearance of eicosatrienoic acid and a decrease in arachidonic acid, and a change in ratio, is not essential to the diagnosis of essential fatty acid deficiency, but this plasma abnormality is often present.

Textbook: Pages 164–165 ANSWER: B, D.

3. It is stated that enteral nutrition is safer than parenteral nutrition. Which of the following may be complications of enteral nutrition?

A. Hyperosmolar, nonketotic coma.
B. Vomiting and aspiration.
C. Pneumatosis cystoides intestinalis.
D. Perforation and peritonitis.

DISCUSSION: It is not necessarily true that enteral nutrition is safer than parenteral nutrition, and it may in fact be associated with a higher risk of death than parenteral nutrition. Specifically, a well-run parenteral nutrition service should not be associated with significant mortality, except for the occasional death due to undetected yeast infection. On the other hand, enteral nutrition, especially if not carried out safely, can result in significant mortality. The most common of the severe complications of enteral nutrition result from the gastrostomy, or tube feedings into the stomach. Sudden changes in gastric motility, such as those associated with sepsis, may result in aspiration. Nasoenteric or nasoduodenal tubes help prevent this complication, as does shutting off enteral feedings between the hours of 11 P.M. and 7 A.M. It is also essential to keep the patient's head elevated 30 degrees. Also necessary is the use of extreme care when initiating enteral nutrition. If hypertonic material is given into the stomach, one can increase osmolality followed by an increase in volume. If, however, the material is given into the small bowel, volume must be increased first and then tonicity, with the expectation that osmolality greater than 400 or 500 mOsm per liter may never be achieved without provoking severe diarrhea. If care is not taken with the initiation of enteral nutrition, massive diarrhea may result, including fluid loss, the absorption of enormous amounts of carbohydrate into the circulation with inadequate fluid to support it, and the development of hyperosmolar, nonketotic coma. Alternatively, severe unremitting diarrhea may result in necrosis of the intestinal wall, the appearance of pneumatosis cystoides intestinalis, and, finally, perforation and death. All of these complications may be prevented by judicious use of enteral nutrition with the same care one uses for parenteral nutrition.

Textbook: Pages 149–150 ANSWER: A, B, C, D.

4. It has been suggested that enterocyte-specific fuels be utilized for all patients receiving parenteral nutrition. Theoretically, the benefits of such fuels include:

A. Glutamine increases gut mucosal protein content and wall thickness.
B. Butyrate increases jejunal mucosal protein content and wall thickness.
C. The short-chain fatty acids—butyrate, propionate, and acetate—are useful in supporting ileal mucosal protein content and thickness.
D. The use of glutamine-enriched solutions for parenteral nutrition for patients with chemotherapy toxicity or radiation enteritis is without hazards.

DISCUSSION: The use of enterocyte-specific fuels is part of a new and potentially exciting phase of "nutritional pharmacology" in parenteral nutrition; however, exciting as the research may be, the use of such fuels is by no means acceptable for indiscriminate use at present. Though some studies have shown that the provision of glutamine in amounts up to 2% in standard parenteral nutrition solutions increases both jejunal and ileal mucosal protein content, cell wall thickness, and DNA content, this has not been the case in all studies, and this reported effect seems very dependent on experimental design. In many of the studies that have shown such an effect, 2% glutamine has been used to replace virtually all nonessential amino acids, probably initiating a deficiency state. The beneficial effects seen with glutamine are far less impressive than those seen with epidermal growth factor, for example, and disappear entirely when a different experimental design is used in which 2% glutamine is added to an adequate amino acid formulation in which glutamine does not replace nonessential amino acids but is added to them. Nonetheless, the use of enterocyte-specific fuels, specifically glutamine, is potentially exciting and should be carefully investigated. More striking are the results that follow massive bowel resection, radiation enteritis, and chemotherapy toxicity. Glutamine may help the small bowel regenerate more quickly, enabling more rapid use of the small bowel for nutrition. It should be pointed out, however, that glutamine is a fuel utilized by many tumors and, thus, one runs the risk of stimulating the growth of the tumor with excessive glutamine. The short-chain fatty acids, produced from bacterial fermentation of soluble pectin, may be useful in both the maintenance of colonocyte-specific nutrition and, in the case of butyrate, ileal enterocyte nutrition.

Textbook: Pages 148–149 ANSWER: None is entirely true.

5. Essential amino acids have been advocated as standard therapy for renal failure. Which of the following statements are true?

A. Increased survival from acute renal failure has been reported with both essential and nonessential amino acid therapy of patients in renal failure.
B. Essential amino acids retard the rise of blood urea nitrogen (BUN) secondary to decreased urea appearance.
C. Essential amino acids and hypertonic dextrose are a convenient form of therapy for hyperkalemia.
D. Essential amino acids decrease BUN and creatinine to the same degree as solutions containing excessive nonessential amino acids.

DISCUSSION: Essential amino acids and hypertonic dextrose, as opposed to hypertonic dextrose alone, was reported by Abel and co-workers to be associated with a decreased mortality rate in mostly surgical patients with acute tubular necrosis. The most significant improvement in mortality, as compared with the control group receiving hypertonic dextrose, was among patients who required dialysis (i.e., the more severely affected patients). Another group responding favorably to treatment includes patients with nonoliguric renal failure whose need for dialysis is not clearly established. The effect of essential amino acids in preventing a rise in BUN, as well as its beneficial effect in preventing hyperkalemia, may obviate dialysis in such patients. With increasing amounts of nonessential amino acids, BUN increases, and thus, dialysis is required. Prospective randomized studies comparing the use of essential versus nonessential amino acids in patients with acute renal failure have not been carried out in sufficient numbers to yield answers to this question.

Textbook: Pages 159–160 ANSWER: B, C.

6. A modified amino acid solution with increased equimolar branched-chain amino acids and decreased aromatic amino acids has been proposed for patients with hepatic insufficiency. Which of the following statements is/are true?

A. This formulation is proposed for the use of patients with fulminant hepatitis.
B. Nitrogen balance is achieved in such patients with amounts of 40 gm. of amino acids per 24 hours.
C. The use of 80 to 100 gm. of such solutions is associated with hepatic encephalopathy.
D. In some studies of surgical patients, improvements in mortality have been reported.

DISCUSSION: The use of modified amino acid solutions is based on the false neurotransmitter hypothesis of the cause of hepatic coma. According to this hypothesis, the imbalance between aromatic and branched-chain amino acids in the plasma results in abnormally high levels of the toxic aromatic amino acids in the brain, thus provoking hepatic encephalopathy. The use of modified amino acid mixtures, with glucose as the calorie base, has been associated in a number of studies with improvement in encephalopathy. Meta-analysis has concluded that the use of such solutions is indicated as therapy for hepatic encephalopathy but has been proposed only for hepatic encephalopathy complicating acute exacerbation of chronic liver disease. Although there are a few anecdotal reports of beneficial effects on hepatic encephalopathy of acute fulminant hepatitis, the use of such a solution has not been advocated, but such a modified solution is tolerated better than standard amino acid mixtures in patients requiring TPN. In some studies, particularly in complicated surgical cases, the use of a high–branched-chain, low–aromatic amino acid solution has been associated with lower mortality. These statements are true only for studies in which the modified solutions are given with hypertonic glucose as a calorie base. Studies in which lipid was the principal calorie source have not revealed such improvements in mortality. In recent studies, giving an aromatic amino acid–deficient, branched-chain amino acid–enriched solution to patients about to undergo resection of the liver has proved particularly efficacious in a group of patients with cirrhosis, decreasing morbidity and showing a trend toward decreased mortality.

Textbook: Page 160 ANSWER: D.

7. In the nutritional support of patients with cancer, which of the following statements is/are true?

A. Nutritional support benefits the patient's lean body mass but does not enable the tumor to grow.
B. In experimental animals, the growth of implanted tumors is directly proportional to the amount of calories and protein supplied.
C. Prospective randomized trials of nutritional support utilizing chemotherapy and radiation therapy have revealed benefits to patients receiving total parenteral nutrition.
D. Studies of nutritional support for patients with cancer about to undergo surgery revealed decreased morbidity and mortality, especially morbidity from sepsis.

DISCUSSION: The problem with the patient with cancer is a very vexing one. Clearly, one of the metabolic effects of cancer, cachexia, affects patients in the last quartile of their disease and makes such patients intolerant of chemotherapy, radiation therapy, and, in many cases, operative procedures. Total parenteral nutrition (TPN) has been proposed as a means of reversing cachexia and enabling patients to better tolerate surgery, chemotherapy, and radiation therapy. In experimental animals, it is clear that the provision of calories and protein, especially in excessive amounts, is associated with the more rapid growth of tumors and decreased survival, especially in the group that is overfed in the extreme. There is also evidence suggesting that overfeeding, or at least TPN, may result in increased growth (or at least change cell kinetics) in patients who are overnourished with TPN. Of the randomized prospective trials that have been carried out, no trial utilizing chemotherapy or radiation therapy has revealed a survival advantage for patients receiving TPN. Indeed, in Shamberger's study, there is a suggestion that the tumor-free interval following treatment of lymphoma may be shorter in patients receiving TPN. In patients undergoing surgery, however, especially those who are severely malnourished (as recently revealed in the VA study) or in patients with major procedures such as esophagogastrectomy (as in Muller's study), evidence suggests that TPN is beneficial. In a late follow-up in Muller's study, there was no apparent increase in recurrence, and the survival rate was the same, despite much higher mortality in the non-TPN group. This suggests that any improved survival following operation may have been offset by an increased late recurrence rate, although it is difficult to reach this conclusion. In summary, for patients with cancer TPN probably nourishes the tumor as well as the host. Nonetheless, in severely malnourished patients provision of TPN from 5 to 10 days preoperatively may increase survival and decrease morbidity. Overfeeding must be avoided. Future studies will undoubtedly reveal that there are certain nutrients that tumors require, which probably should be best avoided.

Textbook: Pages 161–163 ANSWER: B.

8. Glucose overload results in increased CO_2 production. Which of the following statements are true?

A. In patients with respiratory insufficiency, administration of glucose as a principal calorie source is contraindicated.
B. In patients with pulmonary infection and sepsis, calorie support should consist of 95% fat and 5% glucose.
C. In Askanazi's study, increased CO_2 production

and difficulty in weaning was associated only with pronounced overfeeding.

D. CO_2 production should be measured in most patients who are supported by respirators in intensive care units and are receiving nutritional support.

DISCUSSION: Few papers have excited as much interest as that by Askanazi, Kinney, and co-workers, which demonstrated that glucose calories given to patients with severe respiratory impairment may result in difficulty in weaning from a respirator. Subsequent research has suggested, however, that this occurs only with severe overfeeding, when the respiratory quotient is greater than 1 and calories are excessive. If one examines the conditions under which Askanazi's patients were studied, these were a group of septic, depleted patients who were taken from almost no nutritional support to a caloric supply of 2.25 times their caloric requirement, most of the calories consisting of glucose. Suffice it to say that, in patients with impaired respiratory function, one should measure V_{CO_2} and, when V_{CO_2} is significantly elevated and appears to interfere with weaning, decrease the amount of glucose calories and increase the amount of fat. If one measures or estimates calorie requirements and does not overfeed, lipid can be utilized for 25% of the caloric requirement and glucose for the remainder, without much fear of excessive CO_2 production.

Textbook: Pages 142, 162 ANSWER: C.

9. Hepatic abnormalities have been noted in adults since the beginning of hyperalimentation. Which of the following statements are true?

A. Hepatic steatosis appears to be associated with an overload of glucose.
B. Hepatic steatosis is usually associated with abnormalities in hepatic enzymes.
C. Hyperbilirubinemia is inevitably associated with hepatic steatosis.
D. Abnormalities in the portal insulin-glucagon ratio are thought to be causative of hepatic steatosis in experimental animals.

DISCUSSION: The most common metabolic complication of TPN in adults is hepatic steatosis. Unlike the hepatic abnormalities in children, which may progress to cholestasis, liver damage, and in some cases death, hepatic steatosis, or fatty infiltration of the liver with triglycerides, appears to be a rather benign complication. It may be, but is not necessarily, associated with hepatic enzymatic abnormalities, which usually occur in the first week, peak at the third week, and generally disappear by the sixth week of parenteral nutrition. Abnormalities in the transaminases are most common, with alkaline phosphatase also being elevated, but there is no correlation between the degree of fatty infiltration and enzymatic abnormalities. Fatty infiltration appears to be largely vacuolization with increased storage of triglycerides. Hepatic steatosis is almost always associated with an overload of glucose. Recent studies in experimental animals have suggested that the portal insulin-glucagon ratio, which is elevated under these circumstances, may be causally related to hepatic steatosis. Insulin is the leading storage enzyme and is responsible for lipogenesis. The presence of insulin inhibits lipolysis. Glucagon, on the other hand, results in the mobilization of hepatic lipid. The liver "sees" the portal vein insulin-glucagon ratio. Excesses of insulin elicited by hypertonic dextrose increase lipid deposition in the liver, whereas glucagon, which is elicited by certain amino acids, results in the mobilization of hepatic lipid.

Textbook: Page 165 ANSWER: A, D.

10. Which of the following statements about the presence of gallstones in diabetes patients is/are correct?

A. Gallstones occur with the same frequency in diabetes patients as in the healthy population.
B. The presence of gallstones, regardless of the presence of symptoms, is an indication for cholecystectomy in a diabetes patient.
C. Diabetes patients with gallstones and chronic biliary pain should be managed nonoperatively with chemical dissolution and/or lithotripsy because of severe complicating medical conditions and a high operative risk.
D. The presence of diabetes and gallstones places the patient at high risk for pancreatic cancer.
E. Diabetes patients with symptomatic gallstones should have prompt elective cholecystectomy, to avoid the complications of acute cholecystitis and gallbladder necrosis.

DISCUSSION: Gallstones have been found to be very prevalent in patients with type II (non–insulin-dependent) diabetes mellitus, perhaps related to the dyslipoproteinemia in such patients. Although the complications of acute cholecystitis (infection, sepsis, gangrene of the gallbladder) are more common in diabetics, a decision-analysis study has shown that prophylactic cholecystectomy cannot be justified since the risk of morbidity and/or mortality from the cholecystectomy procedure is as great as that of complications or death from acute cholecystitis. Patients who become symptomatic should be promptly prepared and should undergo elective cholecystectomy, because an emergency operation in these patients with comorbid conditions, especially coronary artery disease, has substantial added mortality associated with it. There is no causal relationship between diabetes and pancreatic cancer.

Textbook: Page 179 ANSWER: E.

11. Intensive insulin therapy:

A. Prevents the aggressive development of atherosclerosis in diabetic patients.
B. Is not associated with unawareness of hypoglycemia.
C. Improves peripheral neuropathy.
D. Improves established retinopathy and nephropathy.

E. Is indicated in all patients with non–insulin-dependent diabetes mellitus (NIDDM).

DISCUSSION: Intensive insulin therapy is indicated in patients with IDDM who can actively participate in their own management and the attainment of the goals set for their blood glucose and glycosylated hemoglobin ($HgA1_c$) levels. Because the main complication of intensive therapy is iatrogenic hypoglycemia, this mode of treatment is not indicated for patients with NIDDM, who often have coexisting medical conditions such as coronary artery disease and who tolerate hypoglycemia poorly. There is little or no evidence that macrovascular disease is affected by intensive insulin therapy, and the added weight gain and hyperinsulinemia associated with the therapy may worsen atherosclerosis. Unawareness of hypoglycemia is directly related to a recent hypoglycemia episode, so patients treated intensively are often unaware of the problem. Intensive therapy does not improve established retinopathy or nephropathy but slows or prevents progression of these complications; however, better glucose control may improve peripheral neuropathy.

Textbook: Pages 180–181 ANSWER: C.

12. Which of the following statements about hypertension in diabetes patients is/are correct?

A. Hypertension worsens the macrovascular disease of diabetes patients.
B. Hypertension accelerates the progression of diabetic nephropathy.
C. Hypertension is associated with sodium retention in diabetes patients.
D. Angiotensin-converting enzyme (ACE) inhibitors should be used in all patients with chronic hyperglycemia, regardless of the presence of hypertension.
E. Diuretics, as single-drug therapy, are not indicated in the treatment of hypertension in diabetes patients.

DISCUSSION: All of the answers listed are correct. By damaging endothelial cells, hypertension worsens macrovascular disease in all patients but especially in diabetics. Hypertension dramatically accelerates the onset and progression of diabetic renal disease and proteinuria, and this phenomenon can be slowed or prevented by a combination of treatment modalities, including ACE inhibitors, which dilate efferent glomerular vessels and lower intraglomerular pressure. Despite sodium retention in diabetes patients, single-drug therapy with a diuretic is not indicated because the chronic state of dehydration in such patients may become worse.

Textbook: Pages 180, 182 ANSWER: A, B, C, D, E.

13. What is the major determinant in an individual patient's risk for perioperative complications?

A. The surgical procedure.
B. The length of the surgical procedure.
C. The anesthetic technique (e.g., general, regional).
D. The length of anesthesia.
E. All of the above.

DISCUSSION: The planned surgical procedure is the major determining factor in assessing an individual patient's risk for perioperative complications and in deciding which anesthetic technique will be most appropriate. Good communication between the surgeon and the anesthesiologist is vital, as the surgeon knows better than anyone else the extent of the operation and the length of time it will require.

Textbook: Page 187 ANSWER: A.

14. Which of the following are considered routine intraoperative monitors?

A. Temperature probe.
B. Electrocardiogram.
C. Capnograph.
D. Blood pressure cuff.
E. Foley catheter.

DISCUSSION: The American Society of Anesthesiologists requires that the patient's ventilation, circulation, oxygenation, and temperature be continually monitored during all anesthetics. Routine monitors are considered to be a temperature probe, electrocardiogram, pulse oximetry, and blood pressure cuff.

Textbook: Page 188 ANSWER: A, B, D.

15. Muscle relaxants can be used for which of the following?

A. To facilitate intubation.
B. To provide optimal surgical conditions.
C. To optimize ventilator support.
D. To provide sedation.

DISCUSSION: Muscle relaxants are administered to facilitate endotracheal intubation, to provide the surgeon with optimal working conditions during anesthesia, and to optimize mechanical ventilator support in some patients. They do not produce analgesia, sedation, or amnesia. Therefore, muscle paralysis should not be performed without sedation or general anesthesia.

Textbook: Pages 189–190 ANSWER: A, B, C.

16. Local anesthetics:

A. Inhibit transmission of nerve impulses by increasing sodium membrane permeability and the displacement of ionized calcium.
B. Are classified as amides or esters.
C. Produce peripheral vasodilation.
D. Are weak acids.

DISCUSSION: Local anesthetics act within the nerve membrane, where they inhibit transmission of nerve impulses by *reducing* sodium membrane permeability and the displacement of ionized calcium. All local anesthetics consist of a hydrophilic region and a hydrophobic region separated by an alkyl chain. The bond of the alkyl chain is either an ester or an amide, and these drugs are classified based on this bond. All local anesthetics except cocaine produce vasodilatation and are weak bases.

Textbook: Page 192 ANSWER: B, C.

17. Absolute indications for a double-lumen endotracheal tube during thoracic surgery are:

A. Massive hemorrhage from one lung.
B. Unilateral lung infection.
C. Facilitation of surgical exposure.
D. Unilateral bronchopulmonary lavage.
E. All of the above.

DISCUSSION: The absolute indications for a double-lumen tube are for the purposes of protecting one lung from the other. These indications include ventilation with a bronchopleural fistula, massive hemorrhage from one lung, pulmonary air cyst resection, unilateral lung infection, and unilateral bronchopulmonary lavage. Relative indications include facilitation of surgical exposure, for pneumonectomy, upper lobectomy, and thoracic aneurysm repair.

Textbook: Pages 194–195 ANSWER: A, B, D.

18. Determinants of cerebral blood flow include:

A. Preoperative neurologic dysfunction.
B. Arterial CO_2 tension.
C. Arterial O_2 tension.
D. Systemic arterial pressure.
E. All of the above.

DISCUSSION: Determinants of cerebral blood flow include arterial CO_2 and O_2 tensions, systemic arterial pressure, and temperature. Other factors that may affect cerebral blood flow and intracranial pressure are head position, jugular venous obstruction, and positive end-expiratory pressure.

Textbook: Page 196 ANSWER: B, C, D.

19. Discharge criteria following ambulatory surgery include:

A. Ability to eat solid food.
B. Stable vital signs.
C. Ability to ambulate.
D. Ability to have protective airway reflexes.

DISCUSSION: Discharge criteria following ambulatory surgery include the patient's being fully awake and oriented, the ability to have protective airway reflexes, stable vital signs, adequate hydration with the ability to hold down oral intake, the ability to ambulate, and adequate pain control. All patients must have a competent person with them to transport them—and ideally to stay with them on the first postoperative night.

Textbook: Page 198 ANSWER: B, C, D.

20. Advantages of patient-controlled analgesia (PCA) include:

A. Immediate medication delivery.
B. Less contact with nursing staff.
C. Rapid onset of analgesia.
D. Patient control over pain medication.
E. All of the above.

DISCUSSION: Advantages of PCA are immediate medication delivery, rapid onset of analgesia, and patient control over pain medication. Disadvantages of PCA are less contact with nursing staff and patients' fears that they could inadvertently administer an overdose or possibly become addicted to the opioid.

Textbook: Page 199 ANSWER: A, C, D.

21. Advantages of epidural analgesia include:

A. Earlier mobilization after surgery.
B. Earlier return of bowel function.
C. Shorter hospitalizations.
D. Decreased stress response to surgery.
E. All of the above.

DISCUSSION: Epidural analgesia include excellent pain relief, decreased sedation with more rapid recovery to presurgical levels of consciousness, earlier mobilization after surgery with increased ability to co-operate with respiratory therapy and physical therapy. Following vascular surgery epidural analgesia may also improve graft flow through mild sympathetic blockade. Earlier return of bowel function, decreased stress response, shorter hospitalizations, and decreased morbidity have all been associated with epidural analgesia.

Textbook: Page 201 ANSWER: E.

22. Ketorolac:

A. Is a nonsteroidal anti-inflammatory drug (NSAID) approved for intravenous, intramuscular, and oral administration.
B. Can be used indefinitely for postoperative analgesia.
C. Can cause renal dysfunction.
D. May decrease surgical blood loss.

DISCUSSION: Ketorolac tromethamine, an NSAID, is approved by the FDA for intravenous, intramuscular, and oral administration. The agent is an effective analgesic with minimal side effects; however, ketorolac, like all NSAIDs, can enhance surgical bleeding and cause renal and platelet dysfunction. Additionally, it is recommended that ketorolac should not be used for more than 5 consecutive days.

Textbook: Page 204 ANSWER: A, C.

23. Factors that decrease collagen synthesis include all of the following *except*:

A. Protein depletion.
B. Infection.
C. Anemia.
D. Advanced age.
E. Hypoxia.

DISCUSSION: Collagen synthesis, an integral part of wound healing, is affected by many local and systemic factors. Protein depletion impairs fibroplasia. Hypoproteinemia leads to diminution of fibroblast proliferation, proteoglycan and collagen synthesis, angiogenesis, and wound remodeling. Although anemia was once believed to be a significant cause of wound disruption, studies have shown that, in the absence of malnutrition or hypovolemia, anemia with a hematocrit greater than 15% does not interfere with wound healing. In contrast, molecular oxygen is critical for collagen synthesis because it is one of the factors required for the hydroxylation of lysine and proline. Also, hypoxia favors wound infection. The role of age in collagen synthesis is not clear, but the incidence of wound failure and incisional hernias is greater in patients older than 60. Fibroplasia occurs at a slower rate in older animals. Perhaps more than any other factor, wound infection is associated with the risk of wound failure.

Textbook: Pages 214–215 ANSWER: C.

24. Wound contraction and ultimate contracture may be controlled by which of the following drugs?

A. Colchicine.
B. D-Penicillamine.
C. Thiphenamil (Trocinate).
D. Glucocorticoids.
E. Ibuprofen (Motrin).

DISCUSSION: Wound contraction is carried out by highly specialized cells called myofibroblasts, which, as their name implies, have histologic characteristics of fibroblasts and smooth muscle cells. The activity of these cells, and therefore wound contraction, can be influenced by topical application of smooth muscle inhibitors such as thiphenamil. Inhibitors of microtubule formation in myofibroblasts, such as colchicine and vinblastine, also inhibit wound contraction under experimental conditions. Glucocorticoids and NSAIDs do not affect the wound contraction process.

Textbook: Pages 209–210 ANSWER: A, C.

25. Which of the following is/are true of the actions of transforming growth factor beta (TGF-β) during wound repair?

A. Increased matrix and proteoglycan synthesis.
B. Inhibition of proteases.
C. Stimulation of plasminogen inhibitor.
D. Chemotaxis for fibroblasts and macrophages.
E. Autoinduction of TGF-β.

DISCUSSION: Through autocrine and paracrine mechanisms TGF-β stimulates the deposition of collagen and other matrix components by fibroblasts, inhibits proteases, blocks plasminogen inhibitor, enhances angiogenesis, and is chemotactic for fibroblasts, monocytes, and macrophages. TGF-β modulates the expression of cell-surface integrins in a manner that enhances cell-matrix interaction and matrix assembly. TGF-β also induces cell production by cells, thus amplifying its biologic effects. The sustained production of TGF-β at the wound site leads to tissue fibrosis.

Textbook: Pages 210–212 ANSWER: A, B, D, E.

26. In contrast to adult wound healing with scar formation, which of the following are characteristic of scarless fetal skin repair?

A. Matrix rich in hyaluronic acid.
B. Increased inflammatory response.
C. Increased production of TGF-β.
D. No collagen deposition.
E. Minimal angiogenesis.

DISCUSSION: The ability of a fetus to heal without scar formation depends on its gestational age at the time of injury and the size of the wound defect. In general, linear incisions heal without scar until late in gestation, whereas excisional wounds heal with scar at an earlier gestational age. The profiles of fetal proteoglycans, collagens, and growth factors are different from those in adult wounds. The less differentiated state of fetal skin is probably an important characteristic responsible for scarless repair. There is minimal inflammation and angiogenesis in fetal wounds. Fetal wounds are characterized by high levels of hyaluronic acid and its stimulator(s) with more rapid, highly organized collagen deposition. The roles of peptide growth factors such as TGF-β and basic fibroblast growth factor are less prominent in fetal than in adult wound healing. An understanding of scarless tissue repair has possible clinical applications in the modulation of adult fibrotic diseases and abnormal scar-forming conditions.

Textbook: Pages 216–218 ANSWER: A, E.

27. Which of the following cell types are not crucial for healing a clean, incisional wound?

A. Macrophage.
B. Platelet.
C. Fibroblast.
D. Polymorphonuclear leukocyte.
E. Myofibroblast.

DISCUSSION: Experimental studies have shown that healing may progress normally in the absence of polymorphonuclear leukocytes in an uninfected wound. In contrast, depletion of monocytes and macrophages causes a severe alteration in wound healing with poor débridement, delayed fibroblast proliferation, and inadequate angiogenesis. Platelets carry a cadre of biologically active substances that are important for wound repair, including peptide growth factors like platelet-derived growth factor (PDGF) and TGF-β. Fibroblasts are the principal cell for matrix synthesis and deposition. Myofibroblasts are important for wound contraction in open defects but have little if any role in clean, incisional wounds.

Textbook: Pages 208–210 ANSWER: D, E.

28. Which of the following is/are not a substrate or cofactor for prolyl hydroxylase?

A. Alpha-ketoglutarate.
B. Ascorbate.
C. Biotin.
D. Oxygen.
E. Copper.

DISCUSSION: Prolyl hydroxylase is one of the rate-limiting enzymes in collagen synthesis. Substrates and cofactors such as iron, alpha-ketoglutarate, ascorbate, and oxygen are important participants in this process. If insufficient prolines are hydroxylated, then the alpha-peptide collagen chains cannot assume a stable triple helix, the collagen cannot be exported from the fibroblasts, and the incomplete, unassociated alpha chains are broken down. Thus, ascorbate deficiency (scurvy) and hypoxia have similar effects on collagen synthesis.

Textbook: Page 212 ANSWER: C, E.

29. Which of the following is an adhesion glycoprotein?

A. Fibronectin.
B. Tenascin.
C. Laminin.
D. Hyaluronic acid.
E. Collagen type IV.

DISCUSSION: Cell adhesion glycoproteins such as fibronectin, vitronectin, laminin, and tenascin provide a "railroad track" to facilitate epithelial and mesenchymal cell migration over the wound matrix. Hyaluronic acid is a glycosaminoglycan, and collagen type IV is a protein that is a crucial component of basement membrane.

Textbook: Pages 213–214 ANSWER: A, B, C.

30. Which of the following is/are true concerning wound fibroblasts?

A. Fibroblasts synthesize and secrete collagen molecules.
B. Wound fibroblasts are derived from blood-borne precursor cells.
C. Fibroblasts migrate to a wound along fibrin strands, which are used as a scaffold.
D. Large amounts of fibrin or blood clot can act as a physical barrier to fibroblast penetration, which delays normal wound healing.

DISCUSSION: Fibroblasts appear in the wound on about the third day of healing and begin to synthesize and secrete collagen molecules. Wound fibroblasts arrive from cells surrounding the wound (e.g., the adventitia of blood vessels), change their phenotype(s), and become mobile during the process of replication. Fibroblasts migrate into a wound using the provisional fibronectin and fibrin matrix as a scaffold. Fibroblasts do not have fibrinolytic enzymes, and large amounts of fibrin and blood clot prevent fibroblasts from entering the wound.

Textbook: Page 208 ANSWER: A, C, D.

31. Which of the following is/are true?

A. Because of its thickness, the tensile strength of a healing wound on the eyelid is much less than one on the thick skin of the back.
B. By 2 days, the experimental burst strength of skin is minimal since collagen has been formed in the wound but has not yet cross-linked.
C. Wound strength reaches a plateau by 3 weeks.
D. Wounds rarely, if ever, regain the strength of intact tissues.

DISCUSSION: Tensile strength measures load per cross-section area at rupture, whereas burst strength measures load required to break a wound, regardless of dimension. Therefore, skin wounds have comparable tensile strength, regardless of thickness. Collagen appears in the wound by 3 to 4 days. Minimal wound strength on day 2 is due to fibrin polymerization and adhesion of globular proteins. Wounds rapidly gain strength for about 4 months and then continue to gain strength at a slower rate for more than a year. Wounds do not regain the strength of normal tissue.

Textbook: Page 209 ANSWER: B, D.

32. Which of the following interfere with normal collagen formation or cross-linking?

A. Beta-aminopropionitrile.
B. Iron chelators.
C. Vitamin C depletion.
D. Proline analogs (e.g., *cis*-hydroxyproline).
E. D-Penicillamine.

DISCUSSION: Intramolecular and intermolecular cross-links are crucial for collagen structural stability. Formation of cross-links can be inhibited by two pharmacologic agents: beta-aminopropionitrile inhibits the enzyme lysyl oxidase, and D-penicillamine binds to collagen substrate directly to prevent collagen cross-link formation. Iron is a cofactor for prolyl hydroxylase, which is important for collagen synthesis. In high enough concentration, proline analogs prevent collagen formation with minimal effects on noncollagenase protein synthesis.

Textbook: Page 212 ANSWER: A, B, C, D, E.

33. The intravenous fluid that a 60 kg., 30-year-old woman with an 80% burn should be given in the first 24 hours following burn injury is:

A. 19.2 liters of 5% glucose in lactated Ringer's.
B. 14.4 liters of lactated Ringer's.
C. 9.6 liters of hypertonic salt solution (sodium concentration 200 mEq. per liter).
D. 7.2 liters of 5% albumin solution.
E. 5.5 liters of the pentafraction component of hydroxyethyl starch.

DISCUSSION: The consensus range for estimating fluid needs of burn patients in the first 24 hours is 2 to 4 ml. of a physiologic crystalloid solution per kilogram body weight per percent of body surface burned. In this patient that would be 9.6 to 19.2 liters of lactated Ringer's solution. The early elevation of circulating levels of catecholamines and glucocorticoids following burn injury induces glycogenolysis, which results in elevated circulating blood glucose levels. Glucose should not be administered in the resuscitation fluids, since the resulting exaggeration of hyperglycemia could induce osmotic diuresis. In the first 24 hours colloid-containing solution is not commonly used, but if it is used even the Evans formula recommends only

1 ml. per kg. body weight per percent of body surface burned. Moreover, patients in one study who received colloid-containing fluids continued to gain weight during the first 3 postinjury days, retained more sodium, and had less urine output than patients who received only crystalloid fluids in the first 24 hours. Hypertonic salt solution is also not commonly used for burn patient resuscitation because of the recently described and surprisingly frequent occurrence of acute renal failure and increased mortality associated with its use. If hypertonic salt is used, the amount infused should be less than 9 liters, to avoid excessive elevation of the serum sodium concentration (i.e., above 160 mEq. per liter). The recommended limit of hydroxyethyl starch infusion is currently 1500 ml. per day. Although a 10% pentastarch form of hydroxyethyl starch has been used to expand the plasma volume of burn patients at the end of the first 24 hours, even as little as 500 ml. of that solution has been reported to prolong both prothrombin and plasma thromboplastin time.

Textbook: Pages 227–229 ANSWER: B.

34. Indications for escharotomy of a circumferentially burned right lower limb include all of the following *except*:

A. Progressively severe deep tissue pain.
B. Coolness of the unburned skin of the toes of the right foot.
C. A pressure of 40 mm. Hg in the anterior compartment of the distal right leg.
D. Edema of the unburned skin of the right foot.
E. Absence of pulsatile flow in the posterior tibial artery.

DISCUSSION: The blood flow to distal and underlying unburned tissue in a limb can be compromised by vascular compression due to edema formation beneath the unyielding eschar of a full-thickness circumferential burn. The most reliably noninvasive means of monitoring adequacy of the circulation in a circumferentially burned limb is serial examination using the ultrasonic flowmeter. The absence or progressive diminution of pulsatile flow in the posterior tibial artery in the lower limb or the palmar arch arteries in the upper limb indicates a need for escharotomy. Delayed capillary refilling, cyanosis of the digits, and progressively severe paresthesias, particularly deep tissue pain, are all clinical signs that may indicate vascular compromise and should be monitored if an ultrasonic flowmeter is not available. Persistent deep tissue pain and progressively severe paresthesias are the most reliable of the nonspecific clinical signs. A muscle compartment pressure that exceeds 30 mm. Hg, which is greater than normal capillary pressure, has also been used as an indication for escharotomy in burn patients. Edema and coolness to the touch of distal unburned tissue commonly accompany thermal injury and are not useful in assessing the need for escharotomy.

Textbook: Pages 229–230 ANSWER: B, D.

35. Which of the following is/are true about inhalation injury in burn patients?

A. A chest x-ray obtained within 24 hours of injury is an accurate means of diagnosis.
B. Its presence characteristically necessitates administration of resuscitation fluids in excess of estimated volume.
C. When moderate or severe, it exerts a comorbid effect that is related to both extent of burn and the age of the patient.
D. It increases the prevalence of bronchopneumonia.
E. Prophylactic high-frequency ventilation reduces the occurrence of pneumonia and the mortality in burn patients with inhalation injury.

DISCUSSION: Extensive inflammatory changes are evoked in the airway following the inhalation of smoke and other irritating products of incomplete combustion. Clinical signs are nonspecific and may be delayed. Chest x-rays are also unreliable in detecting even severe inhalation injury. Chest x-rays taken within 24 hours of injury were found to be falsely negative in 92% of 106 patients with inhalation injury. Fiberoptic bronchoscopic examination is the most reliable single means of diagnosing inhalation injury of the large airways, but in patients who inhaled finely particulate smoke the large airways may show little if any inflammatory change. The distance smoke particles travel before deposition in the airways is inversely related to particle size. When the smoke particle mass median diameter is less than 0.5 μm., deposition occurs in the terminal bronchioles and alveoli. In such patients, inhalation injury is best identified by prolonged retention of xenon 133 as assessed by a ventilation perfusion lung scan.

Historically, fluid restriction was recommended for patients with inhalation injury, but in recent years it has become obvious that such patients typically require more resuscitation fluid than the volume estimated by commonly used formulas. Edema of the small airways and occlusion due to endobronchial sloughing and inspissation predispose burn patients to develop pneumonia. In one study, 46% of burn patients with inhalation injury developed pneumonia and 69% of the pneumonias occurred in the first postburn week. The comorbid effect of moderate to severe inhalation injury is related to both age and burn size and increases mortality by a maximum of 20% above that predicted on the basis of age and burn size in patients whose burn injury alone would be associated with a 75% likelihood of death. In patients with only mild inhalation injury there is little if any increase in mortality above that predicted on the basis of age and burn size alone. Prophylactic use of high-frequency percussive ventilation minimizes airway collapse and atelectatic changes, as a consequence of which the incidence of pneumonia is reduced and survival is significantly increased.

Textbook: Pages 230–232 ANSWER: B, C, D, E.

36. Adequacy of fluid resuscitation in burn patients is indicated by which of the following?

A. Urine output of 45 ml. per hr. in a 70-kg. 30-year-old man with flame burns involving 55% of the total body surface.
B. Hourly urine output of 7 ml. in a 7-kg. 15-month-old child with burns involving 40% of the total body surface.
C. A pulmonary capillary wedge pressure of 17 to 20 mm. Hg.
D. Hourly output of 40 ml. of port wine–colored urine in an 80-kg. male who has severe high-voltage electric injury of the right arm and left leg.
E. A urinary sodium concentration of 4 mEq. per liter.

DISCUSSION: The goal of burn patient resuscitation is the maintenance of vital organ function at the least immediate or delayed physiologic cost. Fluid resuscitation of burn patients does not need to be a test of maximum renal function. Adequacy of volume replacement and of renal blood flow are indicated by an hourly urine output of 30 to 50 ml. in adults and 1 ml. per kg. per hr. in children weighing less than 30 kg. In patients with extensive muscle damage caused by high-voltage electric injury, heavy loads of hemochromagens give the urine the appearance of port wine. Such patients are prone to develop acute renal failure unless brisk urine output is maintained until the pigment concentration is reduced to insignificant levels. Fluid should be infused into such patients at the rate needed to achieve an hourly urine output of 75 to 100 ml., but if the patient does not respond to increased fluid input with an increase in urine volume and clearing of the heme pigments, a diuretic should be given. A pulmonary capillary wedge pressure of 17 to 20 mm. Hg is indicative of an adequate circulating blood volume, but a urinary sodium concentration of less than 20 mEq. per liter is consistent with an intravascular volume deficit.

Textbook: Pages 228–229 ANSWER: A, B, C.

37. Common electrolyte changes during and after resuscitation in a patient with a burn of 65% of the total body surface include:

A. A serum sodium concentration of 128 mEq. per liter following 48 hours of resuscitation fluid therapy.
B. A serum sodium concentration of 152 mEq. per liter on the fifth postburn day in a 75-kg. male with a 75% burn who has received only calculated maintenance fluids each day following successful resuscitation.
C. A serum potassium concentration of 5.7 mEq. per liter as a consequence of the destruction of red cells and other tissues in a patient with high-voltage electrical injury.
D. Hypokalemia due to the kaliuretic effect of 0.5% silver nitrate soaks.
E. Hypocalcemia with a low ionized calcium level on the third postburn day as a consequence of dilution and hypoalbuminemia.

DISCUSSION: At the end of the first 48 hours of resuscitation, when lactated Ringer's solution is used in the first 24 hours and colloid-containing fluid and electrolyte-free fluid in the second 24 hours, modest hyponatremia (serum sodium concentration of 128 to 130 mEq. per liter) is commonly observed but requires no treatment. The total body salt load is actually increased, and appropriate fluid management permits the increased evaporative water loss to correct that imbalance. The most common postresuscitation fluid and electrolyte disturbance is hypernatremia associated with dehydration due to inadequate replacement of insensible water loss. The hourly insensible water loss, which far exceeds maintenance fluid requirements in uninjured patients, can be calculated thus:

Insensible water loss (in ml./hr.) = (25 + % of body surface burned) × total body surface area (sq. m.)

The release of potassium from red cells and other tissues injured by the burn or by electrical current can cause usually modest hyperkalemia. If acidosis occurs, the hyperkalemia may be exaggerated to symptomatic levels that require treatment. Hypokalemia can be induced following resuscitation by the kaliuretic effect of sulfamylon burn cream, but the hypokalemia associated with 0.5% silver nitrate soak treatment is due to transeschar leaching of potassium. Hypocalcemia is frequently associated with hypoalbuminemia as a consequence of hemodilution by the resuscitation fluid and the cytokine-induced reprogramming of hepatic protein synthesis. In such cases ionized calcium levels are commonly normal.

Textbook: Pages 227–228, 232–233 ANSWER: A, B, C.

38. The clinical and histologic signs of invasive burn wound infection include which of the following?

A. Focal dark red or dark brown discoloration of the eschar.
B. Delayed separation of the eschar.
C. Conversion of an area of partial-thickness burn to full-thickness necrosis.
D. The presence of micro-organisms in the unburned subcutaneous tissue in a burn wound biopsy specimen.
E. Perineural and perivascular microbial migration through the eschar with proliferation of micro-organisms in the subeschar space.

DISCUSSION: It is essential to examine the entire burn wound at the time of the daily cleansing to identify invasive burn wound infection at the earliest possible time. The appearance of focal areas of dark red or dark brown discoloration are the most common changes indicative of burn wound infection, but similar changes may be caused by hemorrhage due to local trauma or maceration. Accelerated separation of the eschar is often produced by burn wound infections, but delayed separation of the eschar is indicative of effective control of the microbial population in the burn wound. Conversion of an area of partial-thickness burn to full-thickness necrosis is the most reliable clinical sign of invasive burn wound infection. Identification of such a change mandates histologic examination of a burn wound biopsy, which is the only reliable means of differentiating the colonization of nonviable tissue from the invasion of viable tissue. Identification of micro-organisms in the unburned viable tissue of a burn wound biopsy confirms the diagnosis of invasive burn wound infection. Microbial migration along the skin appendages, terminal nerve radicles, and thrombosed capillaries in the eschar and heavy growth of micro-organisms in the subeschar space are manifestations of the colonization of nonviable tissue and represent the mechanisms by which eschar separation occurs.

Textbook: Pages 241–243 ANSWER: A, C, D.

39. The treatment of invasive burn wound infection may include which of the following?

A. Subeschar infusion of half the daily dose of a broad-spectrum penicillin suspended in 1 liter of normal saline.
B. Use of 0.5% silver nitrate soaks for topical therapy.
C. Specific systemic antibiotic therapy.
D. Excision and immediate autografting.
E. Amputation when the infection has extended to involve underlying muscle.

DISCUSSION: The *Pseudomonas* organisms that most commonly cause invasive bacterial burn wound infection are typically sensitive to high concentrations of broad-spectrum penicillins. When the diagnosis of invasive *Pseudomonas* burn wound infection has been made, one half of the daily dose of a broad-spectrum penicillin, typically piperacillin, suspended in 1 liter of normal saline, should be infused into the subeschar tissues beneath the infected wound. A number 20 spinal needle should be used for the infusion, to minimize the number of injection sites. Following a second subeschar infusion of the broad-spectrum penicillin just prior to operation, the infected tissue should be excised. The excised wounds should not be autografted but covered with a biologic dressing or a dressing soaked with an antimicrobial solution such as 5% mafenide acetate. The patient is returned to the operating room in 24 to 48 hours to examine the excised wound and assess the adequacy of the débridement. The frequency of perilymphatic and perivascular proliferation of invading *Pseudomonas* organisms is associated with a risk of metastatic spread to remote organs or tissues. Consequently, systemic antimicrobial therapy should be instituted based on the sensitivity patterns of the resident microbial flora and adjusted as necessary on the basis of the patient's culture and sensitivity results. Amputation is frequently necessary to control invasive burn wound infection when a phycomycotic infection on a limb has traversed the investing fascia and involves significant amounts of the subfascial tissue.

Textbook: Pages 241–243 ANSWER: A, C, E.

40. The treatment of patients with high-voltage electric injury differs from that of patients with conventional thermal injury with respect to the need for:

A. Fasciotomy.
B. Hemodialysis.
C. Amputation.
D. Pulse oximetry.
E. Prehospital cardiopulmonary resuscitation.

DISCUSSION: Both lightning injury and contact with electric current can induce cardiopulmonary arrest due to either asystole or fibrillation. Cardiopulmonary resuscitation must be initiated at the site of injury if cardiac arrest is present. Cardiac arrhythmias may also occur following resuscitation, necessitating electrocardiographic (ECG) monitoring for at least 48 hours following injury in patients with a history of loss of consciousness or an abnormal ECG. Tissue damage and tissue destruction beneath the investing fascia can result in the formation of edema that increases muscle compartment pressure to a level that necessitates fasciotomy (> 30 mm. Hg). The current flow in a limb in contact with high-voltage current can be so great as to damage even the periosseous muscles and make amputation necessary. Liberation of hemochromogens as a consequence of deep tissue injury is associated with an increased incidence of acute renal failure necessitating hemodialysis. Electric injury does not influence the need for monitoring by pulse oximetry, and in fact the destruction of deep tissue in a limb may preclude application of the pulse oximeter to that extremity.

Textbook: Pages 237–238 ANSWER: A, B, C, E.

41. Therapeutic interventions needed for specific chemical agents include which of the following?

A. Prolonged saline irrigation of eyes injured by concentrated sodium hydroxide using a scleral lens with an irrigating sidearm.
B. Administration of an emetic agent as immediate treatment following lye ingestion.
C. Intra-arterial infusion of calcium gluconate for relief of refractory deep tissue pain due to hydrofluoric acid injury.
D. Use of propylene glycol to remove residual phenol following water lavage.
E. Application of 5% copper sulfate solution soaks to areas of embedded particles of white phosphorus.

DISCUSSION: An eye injured by a strong chemical agent must be irrigated immediately at the site of the accident to minimize corneal damage. Prolonged irrigation for 12 to 72 hours is recommended for eyes injured by a strong alkali solution. Irrigation is difficult because of blepharospasm unless a modified scleral contact lens with an irrigating sidearm is used. Emetics should be avoided in the early treatment of patients following chemical ingestion since additional injury of the esophagus, oropharynx, and upper airway may be caused as the chemical is regurgitated.

The intra-arterial infusion of calcium gluconate has been reported to limit tissue damage and relieve pain, but local excision of the involved tissue may be necessary for definitive control of pain and removal of the injured tissue.

Even though phenol is only slightly soluble in water, initial water lavage of burns caused by phenol should be carried out. Following that initial lavage, the involved area should be washed with a lipophilic solvent such as polyethylene glycol, propylene glycol, or glycerol to remove the residual phenol. A dilute 0.5% to 1% solution of copper sulfate can be used as a wash to facilitate identification and impede the ignition of embedded phosphorus particles. If excessive amounts of copper sulfate are absorbed through the injured tissues, intravascular hemolysis can occur and may cause renal failure. Consequently, one should avoid the use of more concentrated solutions of copper sulfate and should never apply the copper sulfate solution as a soak. The important principle of treatment is to prevent ignition of the particles by preventing their exposure to air, and that can be done most safely by applying an occlusive dressing soaked with saline or water.

Textbook: Pages 238–239 ANSWER: A, C, D.

42. Characteristics of the hypermetabolic response to burn injury include:

A. Elevation of core temperature, skin temperature, and core-to-skin heat transfer.
B. Ambient temperature dependency of metabolic rate.
C. A marked increase of blood flow to the burn wound.
D. A curvilinear relationship to the extent of burn.
E. Oxidation of stored lipid as the major source of metabolic energy.

DISCUSSION: At thermal neutral and higher temperatures, the core temperature, skin temperature, and core-to-skin heat transfer in burn patients remain elevated, but metabolic rate can be diminished in patients with burns of more than 50% of the body surface by maintaining the ambient temperature above 30° C. Blocking evaporative water loss by application of an impermeable membrane is not attended by a consistent diminution in metabolic rate, indicating that the burn patient is not externally cold but is internally warm. The hypermetabolism in burn patients is temperature sensitive but not temperature dependent. Even though earlier measurements described a curvilinear relationship between metabolic rate and extent of burn, recent measurements have shown that metabolic rate increases in linear fashion and rises to levels of twice normal in patients with burns of 75% and more of the total body surface. Lipid stores are the major source of metabolic fuel that is oxidized for energy, and not lean body mass, which undergoes proteolysis to provide the amino acids necessary for protein synthesis and wound healing as well as gluconeogenic processes that provide fuel for tissues requiring glucose. Blood flow to a burned limb is markedly increased as compared with flow in an unburned limb of the same patient, and the flow increase is directed to the wound per se, not the underlying muscles.

Textbook: Pages 239–241 ANSWER: A, C, E.

43. A 32-year-old mountain climber who struck his head in a fall lay in the snow overnight before he could be rescued and brought to the hospital. Upon admission he is semicomatose and not shivering, with a pulse rate of 48 beats per minute and a blood pressure of 80/50 mm. Hg. His rectal temperature as measured by a standard thermometer is reported as 34° C. All the digits on both feet appear to be frozen. Treatment for this patient should include:

A. Administration of inotropic and chronotropic vasoactive agents.
B. Intra-arterial infusion of vasodilating agents.
C. Infusion of lactated Ringer's solution warmed to 40° C.
D. Immersion in a circulating water bath heated to 40° C.
E. Excision of damaged tissue within 48 hours after thawing.

DISCUSSION: A standard clinical thermometer will not measure body temperatures below 34° C. This patient's clinical condition—depressed mental status, bradycardia, and hypotension—indicates that the patient is likely suffering from severe hypothermia and, so, requires prompt active rewarming by immersion in a water bath at 40° C. or the use of partial cardiopulmonary bypass, if available, and the administration of resuscitation fluid warmed to 40° C. Vasoactive agents do not treat the basic pathology in hypothermic patients and are typically ineffective. Vasodilating agents will be of little if any value in the treatment of the frozen tissue in the feet since histologic studies have indicated that the vasculature in freeze-injured tissue is dilated, not constricted. Since assessment of tissue viability immediately after thawing is difficult and often erroneous, one should await clear demarcation of dead tissue before undertaking surgical excision of damaged tissue.

Textbook: Pages 249–250 ANSWER: C, D.

NOTES

NOTES

CHAPTER 4

PRINCIPLES OF OPERATIVE SURGERY, SURGICAL INFECTIONS AND CHOICE OF ANTIBOTICS, SURGICAL ASPECTS OF THE ACQUIRED IMMUNODEFICIENCY SYNDROME, AND BITES AND STINGS

1. For a given closing force, perpendicular interrupted sutures exert:

A. The least amount of tension.
B. No tension.
C. Tension leading to ischemia.
D. More tension than continuous running sutures.
E. Tension leading to "railroad tracks."

DISCUSSION: Perpendicular interrupted sutures exert the least amount of tension. Symmetrical continuous sutures require great tension. Continuous closure is achieved at the expense of increased tension.
Textbook: Page 256 ANSWER: A.

2. Electrosurgical injuries in laparoscopy are *not* caused by:

A. Inadvertent touching or grasping of tissue during current application.
B. Direct coupling between a portion of intestine and a metal probe that is touching the activated probe.
C. Insulation breaks in the electrodes.
D. Direct sparking to the intestine from the diathermy probe.
E. Bipolar diathermy in most injuries.

DISCUSSION: Bipolar diathermy is safer and should be used in preference to monopolar diathermy, especially in anatomically crowded areas. Most injuries, not surprisingly, are caused by monopolar diathermy. The main causes of electrosurgical injuries in laparoscopy are inadvertent touching or grasping of tissue during current application, direct coupling between a portion of intestine and a metal probe that is touching the activated probe, insulation breaks in the electrodes; direct sparking to the intestine from the diathermy probe, and current passage to the intestine from recently coagulated, electrically isolated tissue. An all-metal cannula around the laparoscope seems prudent.
Textbook: Page 257 ANSWER: E.

3. Closures with skin staples are associated with:

A. Considerable damage to wound defenses.
B. More necrosis than suturing methods.
C. Less necrosis than suturing methods.
D. Significant increase in operative time.
E. Myocutaneous flap necrosis.

DISCUSSION: Numerous studies have confirmed the speed and efficacy of stapling as compared with suture repair of wounds, primarily in a postoperative environment. Staple closure has been found to cause considerably less damage to wound defenses than closure with the least reactive nonabsorbable suture. In myocutaneous flaps suturing caused significantly more necrosis than stapling.
Textbook: Page 260 ANSWER: C.

4. For closure of skin wounds plain catgut is:

A. Contraindicated.
B. Extremely helpful in children.
C. Inferior to nonabsorbable sutures.

D. A cause of permanent stitch marks.
E. Responsible for allergic reactions.

DISCUSSION: Plain catgut is superior to nonabsorbable sutures for elective surgical wound repair to prevent patient discomfort with suture removal, to spare time for the surgeon and staff when absorbable suture material is selected, and to lower the incidence of stitch marks. Repair with plain catgut is extremely helpful in children, who are frightened by the prospect of suture removal and often expect the same discomfort that occurred with suture placement. There is no evidence that catgut can produce an allergic response.
Textbook: Page 259 ANSWER: B.

5. Which of the following statements about the use of latex gloves during an operation is/are correct?
A. The incidence of puncture holes may be as high as 90%.
B. The incidence of puncture holes is not related to the duration of surgery.
C. The right hand is the most common site of perforation.
D. The left (nondominant) index finger is the most common site of perforation.
E. Approximately 40,000 organisms may pass through a glove pinhole in a 20-minute period.

DISCUSSION: Gloves are commonly made of latex and are disposable. Gloves perform two functions: They protect the patient from the hands of the surgeon and protect the surgeon from potentially contaminated blood. The incidence of puncture holes developing may be as high as 50% to 70%, and as many as 40,000 organisms pass through a glove pinhole in a 20-minute period. Most perforations in gloves (90.6%) are found after surgeries that last longer than 2 hours. The left (nondominant) index finger is the most common site of perforation (44%).
Textbook: Page 254 ANSWER: D, E.

6. All of the following situations are known to increase the risk of infection of the surgical site following elective hernia repair *except*:
A. Shaving the operative site before taking the patient to the operating room.
B. Placing a drain in the wound.
C. Failing to continue prophylactic antibiotics for 24 hours after the end of the operation.
D. Getting a hematoma in the wound.
E. Tying the skin sutures very tightly.

DISCUSSION: There is no evidence for any operation that continuing prophylactic antibiotics beyond the end of the procedure increases efficacy or reduces infection. A single dose of prophylactic antibiotic reduces infection following hernia repair, but controversy remains about whether the magnitude of reduction in this procedure, which already should have a low infection rate, is worthwhile. Shaving the operative site before the procedure increases the rate of infection. Placing a drain in a clean wound increases the rate of infection. A hematoma in an operative wound increases the rate of infection. Tying sutures too tightly increases the rate of infection.
Textbook: Pages 254, 255, 256, 257, 262 ANSWER: C.

7. The most common source of bacteria that cause postoperative surgical infections following procedures other than elective clean operations is:
A. The hands of the operating team.
B. The nasopharynx of a member of the operating team.
C. The patient's endogenous bacteria.
D. Airborne bacteria from the operating room environment.
E. Contamination from improperly cleaned surgical instruments.

DISCUSSION: In carefully controlled circumstances and with sensitive culture techniques, bacteria often gain access to a clean operative wound from the hands and nasopharynges of operating room personnel as well as from bacteria in the air. Improperly cleaned surgical instruments can contaminate the surgical wound, but with proper care and procedures in the operating room there should almost never be improperly cleaned instruments. Infections that follow clean contaminated and contaminated operations are almost always from the patient's endogenous flora, usually from the gastrointestinal tract.
Textbook: Pages 253–255 ANSWER: C.

8. A 62-year-old man cuts his hand on a broken soft-drink bottle at a family picnic. He has a history of a full tetanus immunization as a child, and his last tetanus toxoid booster was 14 years ago. The proper treatment for him is appropriate local wound care and:
A. Tetanus and diphtheria toxoid (Td) injection.
B. Tetanus immune globulin (TIG) infiltrated into the tissues around the wound and Td.
C. Td and scheduling for additional boosters 1 and 6 months later.
D. Prophylactic antibiotics started immediately and Td.
E. Prophylactic antibiotics started immediately, Td, and TIG injected into the other arm from that used to give Td.

DISCUSSION: TIG is needed only for dirty wounds in patients who have not previously been vaccinated against tetanus. A patient who has had a full initial series needs only to have Td given if the last booster was more than 5 years previously. All adults should have a booster every 10 years, whether or not they suffer an injury. An adult who has not had a full initial series should receive the booster and then be scheduled to complete the series.
Textbook: Pages 267, 331–332 ANSWER: A.

9. Preoperative prophylactic antibiotics are recommended for an operation on the stomach in all of the following circumstances except:

A. Gastric outlet obstruction.
B. Gastric cancer.
C. Nissen fundoplication.
D. Gastric ulcer.
E. Gastric restriction procedure for treatment of morbid obesity.

DISCUSSION: Antibiotics are not indicated for a Nissen fundoplication, because they do not enter the lumen of the stomach and thus do not expose the wound to a high risk of bacterial contamination. Even when the stomach is entered, if the patient has normal or increased acid production bacterial counts are very low and prophylactic antibiotics are not required. With obstruction, gastric cancer, and gastric ulcer, gastric bacterial counts are increased and antibiotics are recommended. Although bacterial counts may or may not be elevated in patients with morbid obesity, excessive weight increases the risk of infection and a controlled trial has shown that prophylactic antibiotics lower the rate of postoperative infection.

Textbook: Pages 267–269 ANSWER: C.

10. All of the following are accepted principles for the effective use of prophylactic antibiotics to prevent postoperative infection at the surgical site except:

A. Antibiotics should be administered before the operation is initiated.
B. Antibiotics should be given to maintain therapeutic levels in tissues for the duration of the operation.
C. Cefazolin is the prophylactic antibiotic of choice for an appendectomy.
D. Prophylactic antibiotics should be discontinued within 12 hours after the operation, and in many cases at the end of the procedure.
E. The dose of prophylactic antibiotic used should always be at least as high as the usual therapeutic dose for the drug.

DISCUSSION: An appendectomy involves exposure to colonic bacteria with the probability that *Bacteroides fragilis* will be encountered. Cefazolin, which is appropriate for upper abdominal procedures and those that do not enter the gastrointestinal tract, does not have activity against *B. fragilis*. An appropriate antibiotic following appendectomy would be cefotetan or cefoxitin.

Textbook: Page 268 ANSWER: C.

11. Which one of the following statements regarding surgical infections is true?

A. A surgical infection always requires a procedure in the operating room for resolution.
B. A suspected intra-abdominal surgical infection should be treated as soon as possible by high-dose, broad-spectrum antibiotics until a definitive diagnosis can be made.
C. Usually *one* bacterial species is responsible for a serious surgical infection.
D. A postoperative surgical site (wound) infection requires a procedure to achieve resolution.
E. The bacteria responsible for surgical infections usually cause the infection because of special virulence characteristics that allow them to invade the tissues and proliferate.

DISCUSSION: A wound infection needs to be opened for resolution. This may be done in the operating room but is usually accomplished by simply removing the skin sutures or staples and allowing the wound to open and then pursuing a regimen of dressing changes. *A* is incorrect because not all surgical infections need to be opened in the operating room, as explained in *D*. *B* is incorrect because giving antibiotics before making the diagnosis risks delaying the diagnosis and does not cure the infection unless the appropriate procedure is also performed. *C* is incorrect because most surgical infections are mixed and derive from the endogenous flora where the procedure was performed. *E* is incorrect because the bacteria that cause surgical infections usually do not possess special virulence. Instead, they gain access to the site of infection because of injury to an epithelial surface by trauma, operation, or disease.

Textbook: Pages 264, 269, 270–271 ANSWER: D.

12. Signs found in a soft tissue infection that indicate that operative exploration and débridement are needed include all except:

A. Very high fever and white blood cell count.
B. Skin necrosis.
C. Crepitus.
D. Bullae.
E. Edema in excess of local signs of infection.

DISCUSSION: Many nonsurgical soft-tissue infections are accompanied by a high fever and white blood cell count, although also common in surgical infections. The four other signs listed commonly denote a necrotizing soft-tissue infection that requires operative débridement.

Textbook: Pages 269–270 ANSWER: A.

13. Which two of the following statements about intra-abdominal infection are *not* true?

A. Bacterial flora are usually mixed, including both aerobic and anaerobic species.
B. Laparotomy is required for effective treatment in all cases.
C. Approximately one case in four requires a second procedure to ensure resolution of the procedure.
D. Antibiotic therapy must be continued for 10 days to resolve the infection.
E. Initially the choice of antibiotic must be empirical.

DISCUSSION: Many intra-abdominal abscesses can be treated by radiologically guided placement of percutaneous drains instead of laparotomy, and antibiotics need be continued only until the patient has demonstrated a favorable clinical response and has maintained a normal temperature for 24 to 48 hours. Statements *A, C,* and *E* are true.

Textbook: Pages 270–271 ANSWER: B, D.

14. Abdominal pain in persons infected with human immunodeficiency virus type 1 (HIV-1):

A. Is more common in late-stage disease (acquired immunodeficiency syndrome [AIDS]).
B. Is associated with reduced patient survival.
C. Frequently requires surgical intervention.
D. Usually can be categorized into one of four discrete clinical syndromes.
E. Is seen in approximately 15% of infected persons at some time in the course of the disease.

DISCUSSION: Abdominal pain in HIV-1–infected persons is a relatively common problem, affecting 15% of patients at some time during the course of their disease. It is more common in late-stage disease (AIDS) and is associated with decreased patient survival. Four discrete clinical syndromes have been described: (1) epigastric pain, with or without esophageal symptoms; (2) right upper quadrant pain, with or without jaundice; (3) right iliac fossa pain; and (4) diffuse abdominal pain. Surgical treatment is rarely needed for patients with abdominal pain and is usually reserved for cases of bleeding, obstruction, or perforation.

Textbook: Pages 283–284 ANSWER: A, B, D, E.

15. Gastrointestinal bleeding in HIV-1 infected persons:

A. Is usually related to complications of HIV-1 infection.
B. Should be evaluated aggressively in patients who are not terminally ill, as specific therapy exists for 75% of precipitating lesions.
C. Is a common problem seen in most patients at some time during the course of their disease.
D. Is evaluated with endoscopy in stable patients.
E. Is most commonly related to lymphomas of the gastrointestinal system.

DISCUSSION: Gastrointestinal bleeding is an uncommon problem in HIV-1 infected persons. The etiology of the bleeding is usually varied but most of the time is related to HIV-1 infection. Evaluation should be undertaken aggressively except in terminally ill persons, as specific therapy exists for 75% of precipitating lesions. Work-up in stable patients should begin with either upper or lower endoscopy. Gastrointestinal lymphoma is an uncommon cause of bleeding.

Textbook: Pages 284–285 ANSWER: A, B, D.

16. Which of the following statements about papillary stenosis of the ampulla of Vater are true?

A. Papillary stenosis occurs with surprising frequency in association with HIV-1 infection.
B. Jaundice is the most common presenting symptom.
C. Endoscopic retrograde cholangiopancreatography (ERCP) plus sphincterotomy can provide prompt relief of abdominal pain associated with this process.
D. The etiology appears to be related to cytomegalovirus (CMV) infection or cryptosporidiosis.
E. Alkaline phosphatase levels return to normal shortly after successful papillary sphincterotomy.

DISCUSSION: Papillary stenosis and sclerosing cholangitis are both observed with surprising frequency in HIV-1–infected persons. The cause appears related to either CMV infection or cryptosporidiosis. Abdominal pain in the right upper quadrant is the most common presenting symptom. Jaundice is uncommon, as biliary obstruction is rarely complete. ERCP allows one to make the diagnosis, and sphincterotomy usually leads to prompt relief of the abdominal pain. Serum alkaline phosphatase levels frequently stay the same or increase, presumably owing to ongoing intrahepatic duct disease or parenchymal infiltration of the liver.

Textbook: Page 281 ANSWER: A, C, D.

17. Which are true statements about anorectal problems in HIV-1–infected persons?

A. There is an increased incidence of anal cancer in this patient population.
B. Anal ulceration is frequently secondary to an infection and responds quickly to topical antibiotics.
C. Patients with asymptomatic HIV-1 infection can have serious healing problems after anorectal surgery.
D. Abdominoperineal resection is the treatment of choice for squamous cell carcinoma (SCC) of the anus in HIV-1–infected patients.
E. Perirectal abscesses should be treated initially with antibiotics in HIV-1–infected patients.

DISCUSSION: Anorectal disease is a common and serious problem for HIV-1–infected persons. There is an increased incidence of anal and rectal cancers in the HIV-1–infected patient population, especially those who engage in anal intercourse. While surgical therapy is usually required for patients with rectal cancer, HIV-1–positive patients who develop SCC of the anus are treated initially with chemotherapy and radiation therapy. In general, patients with asymptomatic HIV-1 infection tolerate anorectal operations well and have no increased risk of wound complications. Patients with AIDS tend to have a significantly higher incidence of wound problems. Regardless of disease stage, a perirectal abscess requires immediate surgical drainage. Antibiotics are used in conjunction with operation, not instead of it. Finally, in AIDS patients anal ulcers frequently have an infectious cause, but they can be very difficult to treat. Ulcers are often resistant to appropriate therapy but sometimes respond to intralesional steroid injections or surgical excision.

Textbook: Page 283 ANSWER: A.

18. Optimal treatment of rattlesnake bites includes which of the following?

A. Ice should be applied to the wound as soon as it is available.
B. The extremity should be immobilized.
C. A fasciotomy should be performed to prevent development of compartment syndrome.
D. Arterial occlusive tourniquets should be applied proximal to the bite site.
E. Tetanus prophylaxis should be administered if indicated.

DISCUSSION: Field treatment of a rattlesnake bite victim includes moving the patient away from the snake and immobilizing the extremity. Cryotherapy, incision and suction, tourniquets, and electric shock are potentially harmful and are not recommended. Application of a lymphatic constriction band is recommended by some experts. Antivenin is administered to patients with mild to severe envenomation. Broad-spectrum antibiotics should be given. Tetanus prophylaxis should be administered. Routine fasciotomies have not proved beneficial.

Textbook: Pages 287–288 ANSWER: B, E.

19. Which of the following is/are correct statements about animal bites?

A. *Pasteurella multocida* is a common organism cultured from cat bites.
B. Prophylactic antibiotics should be administered for all animal bites.
C. Human bites to the hand rarely become infected. Therefore, primary closure is recommended.
D. Administration of prophylactic antibiotics is recommended for high-risk bites such as puncture wounds.
E. In the United States, dogs are the primary source of rabies.

DISCUSSION: *P. multocida* is a common pathogen isolated from infected cat bites. Bites to the hand are at high risk of developing infection; therefore, primary closure is not recommended. Prophylactic antibiotics should be administered to persons with "high-risk bites" such as hand bites and puncture wounds. Dogs are the primary source of rabies worldwide; however, skunks account for most cases seen in the United States.

Textbook: Pages 288–290 ANSWER: A, D.

20. Which of the following statements about spider bites is/are correct?

A. Ice should be applied to the affected area.
B. The venom produced by a brown recluse can cause severe abdominal wall muscle spasm, occasionally mimicking acute abdomen.
C. Mild envenomation from black widow spider bites should be treated with calcium gluconate and antivenin.
D. Patients bitten by black widow spiders typically present with severe local manifestations.
E. Cutaneous necrosis is usually produced by a bite from a brown recluse spider.

DISCUSSION: Envenomation by a brown recluse spider principally produces necrosis at the bite site. Systemic complaints are unusual. Black widow spider bites cause neuromuscular symptoms, with abdominal wall rigidity occasionally mimicking acute abdomen. Local manifestations are atypical. Ice therapy is recommended for spider bites. Patients with mild envenomation from black widow spider bites need local wound care only, consisting of ice application and administration of tetanus toxoid. The role of calcium gluconate administration for severe black widow envenomation is controversial.

Textbook: Pages 290–292 ANSWER: A, E.

NOTES

NOTES

NOTES

CHAPTER 5

TRAUMA: MANAGEMENT OF THE ACUTELY INJURED PATIENT

1. Nasotracheal intubation:

A. Is preferred for the unconscious patient without cervical spine injury.
B. Is preferred for patients with suspected cervical spine injury.
C. Maximizes neck manipulation.
D. Is contraindicated in the patient who is breathing spontaneously.

DISCUSSION: The first principle in the management of any injured patient is to secure an adequate airway. This can be particularly difficult in the presence of facial or laryngeal trauma, or in the unconscious patient with a suspected cervical spine injury. The mechanical removal of oral debris followed by the "chin lift" or "jaw thrust" maneuvers to relieve soft tissue obstruction of the pharynx are the first steps. However, when there is any question regarding the adequacy of the airway, or in the presence of severe head injury, or when the patient is in profound shock, more definitive airway control is required. In most patients this involves oral endotracheal intubation. However, the insertion of an oral endotracheal tube often involves hyperextension of the neck with the potential for aggravating cervical spine ligamentous or bony injury. Nasotracheal intubation is the preferred option for the patient with suspected cervical spine ligamentous or bony injury since the head and neck can be maintained in the neutral position with minimal manipulation. This technique requires a breathing patient, as the passage of air must be heard through the nasotracheal tube prior to its insertion through the larynx into the trachea. Nasotracheal intubation is contraindicated in the presence of mid-face fractures. In this situation, a surgical airway (cricothyroidotomy, tracheostomy, or needle cricothyroidotomy) is the preferred option.

Textbook: Page 296 ANSWER: B.

2. Cardiac contusions caused by blunt chest trauma:

A. Are fairly easy to diagnose.
B. Occur in up to 20% to 40% of patients with major blunt thoracic trauma.
C. Do not usually cause right ventricular dysfunction.
D. Demonstrate arrhythmia as the most common complication.

DISCUSSION: Cardiac contusions are often difficult to diagnose, but have been estimated to occur in 5% of major trauma patients, and up to 20% to 40% of patients with severe blunt chest injury. The difficulty in diagnosing cardiac contusions is that they remain a pathologic diagnosis, confirmed only at autopsy or on direct cardiac examination. The injury may vary from superficial epicardial petechiae to complete transmural damage. Although significant myocardial injuries, such as ventricular rupture, coronary vessel thrombosis, and valvular disruption, have been reported, the most common clinically significant result of cardiac contusion is the occurrence of arrhythmias. Hence, an initial electrocardiogram (ECG) and subsequent continuous cardiac monitoring for at least 24 hours is generally recommended. Alternative methods of diagnosing myocardial contusion include creatine phosphokinase cardiac isoenzymes (CPK-MB), two-dimensional echocardiography, gated ventricular scintigraphic angiography (GVA), radioactive thallous chloride (^{201}Tl) uptake, and right ventricular monitoring. Unfortunately, none of these tests is adequately sensitive or specific in the diagnosis of cardiac contusion, and their correlation with the presence of arrhythmias or ECG changes is also imprecise.

Textbook: Pages 309–310 ANSWER: B and D.

3. According to the recommendations of the American College of Surgeons Committee on Trauma, which of the following patients should be transported to a trauma center?

A. Fifty-year-old female who fell 8 feet from a step ladder, with isolated hip fracture and normal vital signs.
B. Fifteen-year-old bicyclist with closed head injury and Glasgow Coma Scale score of 12.
C. Twenty-three-year-old male assault victim with stab wound to the back, normal vital signs, and respiratory distress.

D. Three-year-old infant passenger (restrained) in motor vehicle accident with normal vital signs and no apparent injuries except abdominal wall contusion.

DISCUSSION: The American College of Surgeons Committee on Trauma has developed a field triage decision scheme to help identify trauma victims with a significant risk of dying as a result of their injuries. This classification is based on four factors: (1) abnormal physiologic signs, (2) anatomic area of injury, (3) mechanism of injury, and (4) concurrent or co-morbid disease states. Major *physiologic abnormalities* include a Glasgow Coma Scale score of less than 13, systolic blood pressure less than 90 mm. Hg, respiratory rate less than 10 or greater than 29 per minute, or a Revised Trauma Score of less than 11 or a Pediatric Trauma Score of less than 9. Significant *anatomic considerations* include penetrating injuries to the torso, head and neck, and proximal extremities, flail chest, combination of trauma with burns to greater than 10% of body surface area, two or more proximal long bone fractures, pelvic fractures, paralysis, or traumatic amputation above the wrist or ankle. Significant *mechanisms of injury* include a death in the same passenger compartment or ejection from the automobile, high-impact (greater than 5 miles per hour) auto-pedestrian injuries, or a pedestrian thrown or run over. The *co-morbid factors* include pediatric or elderly (<5 or >55) patients or known history of insulin-dependent diabetes or cardiac, respiratory, or psychotic disorders. These criteria should serve as guidelines for medical control and the pre-hospital care providers. Such triage guidelines have been shown to produce the triage of only a small fraction (5% to 10%) of all injured patients to Level I or Level II trauma centers.

Textbook: Pages 334–335 ANSWER: B, C, D.

4. Which of the following statements about head injuries is/are *false*?

A. The majority of deaths from auto accidents are due to head injuries.
B. Head injury alone often produces shock.
C. A rapid and complete neurologic examination is part of the initial evaluation of the trauma patient.
D. Optimizing arterial oxygenation is part of initial therapy.

DISCUSSION: Head injuries cause the majority of deaths following automobile accidents, with rupture of the thoracic aorta the second most common cause of fatality. Head injury itself rarely produces hypotensive shock. It is only in the terminal phases of brain death that hypotension may be attributable to head injury alone. Therefore, hypotension in trauma patients must be assumed to be secondary to volume depletion or ongoing hemorrhage. An occult site of hemorrhage (chest, abdomen, pelvis, retroperitoneum, or extremities) must be strongly suspected and dealt with accordingly. A rapid and complete neurologic assessment is a crucial part of the initial assessment of all trauma patients. This initial exam gives an excellent indication of injury severity and prognosis. Since the ultimate outcome of a brain injury is dependent on adequate cerebral perfusion and oxygenation, adequate airway control, ventilation, hemorrhage control, volume restitution, and arterial oxygenation are crucial factors in the early management of head injuries.

Textbook: Pages 297–298 ANSWER: B.

5. Which of the following statements about maxillofacial trauma is/are *false*?

A. Asphyxia due to upper airway obstruction is the major cause of death from facial injuries.
B. The mandible is the most common site of facial fracture.
C. The Le Fort II fracture includes a horizontal fracture of the maxilla along with nasal bone fracture.
D. Loss of upward gaze may indicate either an orbital floor or orbital roof fracture.

DISCUSSION: Maxillofacial injuries generally do not cause life-threatening injuries, with the exception of those that occlude the airway. Therefore, the first priority in assessing and managing the patient with maxillofacial trauma is to assess and assure the adequacy of the airway. The face is typically divided into thirds when defining injuries. Injuries to the upper third of the face are often accompanied by ocular or central nervous system complications as well as facial deformities. Fractures of the orbital roof are frequently associated with frontal sinus and nasal ethmoid fractures, and are accompanied by a loss of upward gaze due to involvement of the superior rectus muscle. However, the most common cause of loss of upward gaze is orbital floor injury and associated entrapment of the globe or injury to the inferior rectus muscle. Middle third of facial structures include the maxilla, zygoma, orbits, and nose. The Le Fort classifications of facial fractures are commonly employed to describe these complex fracture lines. In a Le Fort II fracture, the superior fracture line is transverse through the nasal bones or through the articulation of the maxillary and nasal bones with the frontal bones. This is also known as the "pyramidal" fracture of the mid-face. The diagnosis is established by digital manipulation of the anterior maxilla and observation for mobility of the central triangle (the maxilla and nose). The lower third of the face contains a single facial bone, the mandible. After the nasal bones, the mandible is the second most commonly fractured facial bone.

Textbook: Pages 303–306 ANSWER: B.

6. What percentage of patients with thoracic trauma require thoracotomy?

A. 10%–15%.
B. 20%–25%.
C. 30%–40%.
D. 45%–50%.

DISCUSSION: Twenty-five per cent of civilian trauma deaths are caused by thoracic trauma, and two thirds of these deaths occur after the patient reaches the hospital. Mortality of hospitalized patients with isolated chest injury ranges from 4% to 8% and increases to 35% when multiple additional organ systems are involved. Despite high mortality, only 10% to 15% of thoracic injuries require thoracotomy. Most injuries are successfully managed by the rather simple lifesaving maneuvers of airway control and tube thoracotomy. Unrelenting hemorrhage following either penetrating or blunt thoracic trauma is a primary indication for immediate thoracotomy. An initial thoracic blood loss of greater than 1500 ml. (30% of blood volume) or an ongoing loss of 250 ml. for 3 consecutive hours serves only as a practical guideline. The patient's hemodynamic status and overall condition should be the most influential factors.

Textbook: Pages 306, 312 ANSWER: A.

7. The radiographic findings indicating a torn thoracic aorta include:

A. Widened mediastinum.
B. Presence of an apical "pleural cap."
C. First rib fractures.
D. Tracheal deviation to the right.
E. Left hemothorax.

DISCUSSION: All of the listed radiographic findings should arouse suspicion of a possible torn thoracic aorta. The most common abnormality noted is a widening of the mediastinal shadow, although only 20% to 40% of patients with a wide mediastinum have aortic injury. In addition to the radiographic signs listed, other findings that may alert the physician to the possibility of an aortic tear include loss of aortic contour, elevation of the left mainstem bronchus, depression of the right mainstem bronchus, shift of the nasogastric tube to the left, and the presence of retrocardiac density. Aortography remains the "gold standard" diagnostic modality and is indicated if aortic injury is suspected on the basis of mechanism of injury and any of these suggested findings.

Textbook: Pages 310–312 ANSWER: A, B, C, D, E.

8. Which of the following statements about diagnostic peritoneal lavage (DPL) is/are *false*?

A. DPL is the diagnostic procedure of choice for gunshot wounds to the abdomen with no obvious intra-abdominal injuries.
B. The average reported incidence of false-positive DPL in patients with significant pelvic fractures is 20% to 30%.
C. Accuracy rates for DPL have generally been reported between 95% and 97%.
D. DPL has been entirely replaced by computed tomography as the diagnostic procedure of choice following blunt abdominal trauma.

DISCUSSION: DPL remains the most sensitive and specific indicator of intra-abdominal injury in the trauma patient. The accuracy rates for DPL in several large collective series reveal an overall sensitivity of 95%, specificity of 98% to 99%, and overall accuracy of 97%. As result, DPL remains the mainstay for diagnosis of intraperitoneal injury in the trauma patient; however, not every trauma patient requires DPL. In the awake, alert, and responsive patient with isolated abdominal injuries, the physical examination and history are very helpful in predicting the presence of significant injury. In the patient with lower torso (nipples to pubis) or back or flank gunshot wounds, the incidence of intra-abdominal injury is so high that exploratory laparotomy without further diagnostic modalities is generally advocated. In addition, DPL is generally inaccurate in the diagnosis of retroperitoneal injuries (duodenum, renal, pancreas), and significant retroperitoneal hemorrhage in association with pelvic fractures produces a false-positive DPL rate of up to 30%. Computed tomography (CT) scans have proved extremely valuable in these situations. General recommendations for the use of abdominal CT scans in trauma victims include patients who are hemodynamically stable (normal) with (1) equivocal abdominal examination, (2) closed head injury, (3) spinal cord injury, (4) hematuria, and (5) pelvic fractures with significant bleeding. These five indications are appropriate if the patient is truly hemodynamically stable and the time required to perform CT does not delay any surgical procedures.

Textbook: Page 313 ANSWER: A, D.

9. A 28-year-old male was injured in a motorcycle accident in which he was not wearing a helmet. On admission to the emergency room he was in severe respiratory distress and hypotensive (blood pressure 80/40 mm. Hg), and appeared cyanotic. He was bleeding profusely from the nose and had an obviously open femur fracture with exposed bone. Breath sounds were decreased on the right side of the chest. The initial management priority should be:

A. Control of hemorrhage with anterior and posterior nasal packing.
B. Tube thoracostomy in the right hemithorax.
C. Endotracheal intubation with in-line cervical traction.
D. Obtain intravenous access and begin emergency type O blood transfusions.
E. Obtain cross-table cervical spine film and chest film.

DISCUSSION: Airway remains the first priority in the management of any patient with multiple injuries. Control of the airway in a patient with head, face, and neck injury can be extremely challenging. In the patient presented, the best option given for control of the airway is endotracheal intubation with in-line cervical traction. This requires at least two persons, one to maintain the head in the neutral position and one to insert the endotracheal tube under direct vision. An alternative in this case would be emergency cricothyroidotomy, tracheostomy, or needle-jet insufflation. Nasotracheal intubation is not an option in the presence of a mid-face fracture and a nasal hemorrhage. Clearly, attention must also be directed at assuring adequacy of ventilation (potential right pneumothorax), assessing and treating obvious hemorrhage, determining if there is occult intra-abdominal or thoracic hemorrhage, and determining the patient's neurologic status. While management of these other issues can occur simultaneously, they do not take priority over securing an adequate airway. In this patient the airway is so tenuous that time should not be spent obtaining a cross-table cervical spine film and chest film prior to definitive control of the airway.

Textbook: Pages 296–297 ANSWER: C.

10. True or False?

A. Trauma is second only to congenital heart disease as the leading cause of death in children.
B. Each year in the United States, approximately 50,000 people die from injuries.
C. Motor vehicle accidents (MVAs) involving intoxicated drivers are responsible for 50% of all MVA fatalities.
D. Active prevention strategies (e.g., seat belts, helmets) have not proved effective in reducing injuries and fatalities.
E. Falls and diving accidents comprise approximately 30% to 40% of cervical spine injuries.

DISCUSSION: The statistics on injuries highlight trauma as "the principal public health problem in America today." Trauma remains the leading cause of death in children and adults up to the age of 44 years, and injuries kill more Americans age 1 to 34 years than all diseases combined. Each year more than 140,000 Americans die of injuries, 50,000 due to motor vehicle accidents. Just over 50% of motor vehicle injuries involve intoxicated drivers. Injury prevention would be the most cost-effective method of dealing with this major social and economic burden. Active injury prevention strategies are those that require active continued cooperation on the part of the individual, such as wearing a helmet when driving a motorcycle or wearing seat belts in automobiles. Passive approaches such as fitting all motor vehicles with driver air bags require little or no individual cooperation and have clearly proved the more effective option, but active prevention strategies have repeatedly been demonstrated to reduce injury fatalities. States with seat belt and child restraining laws show an increase in seat belt use of more than 60% with a concurrent 9% to 12% reduction in occupant fatalities. Motor vehicle accidents are responsible for approximately 60% of spinal cord injuries, falls for 20% to 30%, and diving accidents for an addition 5% to 10%. Spinal cord injury acute care and rehabilitation represent some of the most expensive medical treatment, with an average *hospital* charge of $50,000 in 1988 for a quadriplegic survivor.

Textbook: Pages 298, 333–334 ANSWER: True, C, E; False, A, B, D.

11. Regarding the diagnosis and treatment of cardiac tamponade, which of the following statements is/are *true*?

A. Accumulation of greater than 250 ml. of blood in the pericardial sac is necessary to impair cardiac output.
B. Beck's classic triad of signs of cardiac tamponade include distended neck veins, pulsus paradoxicus, and hypotension.
C. Approximately 15% of needle pericardiocenteses give a false-negative result.
D. Cardiopulmonary bypass is required to repair most penetrating cardiac injuries.

DISCUSSION: Cardiac tamponade is most frequently caused by penetrating thoracic injury, but may occasionally be observed following blunt thoracic trauma from cardiac chamber rupture, coronary artery laceration, or ascending dissection of an aortic tear. Accumulation of as little as 150 ml. of blood in the pericardium will sufficiently decrease diastolic filling to produce distended neck veins, cyanosis, and decreased cardiac output. Beck's classic triad of distended neck veins, muffled heart sounds, and hypotension is present in only one third of patients with tamponade. Pulsus paradoxicus is even less frequently discernible. Immediate temporary treatment consists of pericardiocentesis, which also provides a diagnosis. However, approximately 15% of pericardiocenteses give false-negative results because of a clotted hemopericardium. Therefore, echocardiography prior to needle aspiration is generally advisable if promptly available. In the patient *in extremis,* emergency thoracotomy with pericardiotomy and cardiac repair should be performed. Most patients with penetrating cardiac wounds do not require cardiopulmonary bypass to repair their injuries.

Textbook: Pages 310–311 ANSWER: C.

12. Which of the following statements or descriptions typically characterizes the syndrome of overwhelming postsplenectomy sepsis?

A. A syndrome of fulminant gram-negative bacteremia and septicemia in asplenic individuals, characterized by the presence of as many as 10^6 bacterial organisms per cu. mm. circulating in the bloodstream.
B. A syndrome caused primarily by impaired host ability to mount an effective humoral (immunoglobulin) response to infection.
C. A syndrome that occurs in 5% to 7% of patients following traumatic splenectomy.
D. A syndrome of rapidly appearing septic shock unresponsive to antibiotic therapy, with an average mortality of 50%.
E. The syndrome may be prevented by preserving as little as 15% of splenic mass in adult trauma victims.

DISCUSSION: In 1952 King and Schumaker suggested that children who had undergone splenectomy were at risk for the development of bacterial infections, and the syndrome of overwhelming postsplenectomy sepsis (OPSS) was suggested by Diamond in 1969. The syndrome is unlike fulminating bacteremias and septicemia in individuals with normal splenic function. The onset is sudden, with nausea, vomiting, headache, and confusion leading to coma. The new infecting organism is a gram-*positive* organism in over half the cases, primarily *Streptoccoccus pneumoniae.* Blood cultures may occasionally demonstrate up to as many as 10^6 bacterial organisms per cu. mm. circulating in the bloodstream. Disseminated intravascular coagulation is common along with hypoglycemia, electrolyte imbalance, and shock unresponsive to antibiotics and fluid or pharmacologic support. Mortality has generally been reported as high as 50% and even up to 80% for pneumococcal infections. The true incidence of overwhelming postsplenectomy sepsis following a splenectomy from trauma is not well defined. Green and colleagues suggested that the risk of OPSS is 166 times the rate expected for the general population. Eraklis and Filler suggested that the incident rate of mortality from sepsis and OPSS is 78 times greater than that expected for the general population. Despite this increased frequency, overwhelming postsplenectomy sepsis remains a rare event. Singer's large review of 688 children who had undergone splenectomy for trauma demonstrated only a 1.45% incidence of postsplenectomy sepsis, but a 40% mortality. The occurrence of OPSS appears to be less following splenectomy for trauma when compared with splenectomy for congenital hematologic disorders. Nonetheless, the recognition of the severe nature of this entity has prompted many trauma surgeons to more aggressively attempt splenic salvage. Animal laboratory evidence suggests that at least 50% of the splenic tissue mass must be preserved to prevent overwhelming postsplenectomy sepsis. The immunologic function of the spleen that appears to be most beneficial in preventing OPSS is the spleen's capacity for clearance of blood-borne particles and the provision of circulating opsins, which assist in cell-mediated immunologic functions.

Textbook: Pages 320–321 ANSWER: D.

NOTES

NOTES

NOTES

CHAPTER 6

SURGICAL COMPLICATIONS AND ACUTE RENAL FAILURE IN SURGICAL PATIENTS

1. The earliest sign of hypovolemia in a postoperative patient is:

A. Hypotension.
B. Tachycardia.
C. Dry mucous membranes.
D. Pale and cold skin.

DISCUSSION: Tachycardia is the earliest sign of hypovolemia, followed by hypotension when compensatory mechanisms are overwhelmed. The mucous membranes are dry, and there is loss of cutaneous elasticity. The skin is pale, cold, and sweaty in response to catecholamine release. The respiratory rate increases in response to catecholamine release, baroreceptor reflexes, tissue hypoxia, and metabolic acidosis.

Textbook: Page 349 ANSWER: B.

2. The most common site of intra-abdominal abscess formation is:

A. Right iliac fossa.
B. Pouch of Douglas.
C. Beneath the diaphragm.
D. Left iliac fossa.

DISCUSSION: The most common site of intra-abdominal abscess formation is beneath the diaphragm. Unfortunately, a large collection of pus may exist in either the right or left subphrenic space with few localizing symptoms. However, when intraperitoneal soiling is followed by a septic course, and especially after pulmonary infection or pelvic abscess has been excluded, the subphrenic space should always be suspected.

Textbook: Page 351 ANSWER: C.

3. The incidence of anastomotic leakage is greatest in:

A. Large bowel anastomoses.
B. Gastrojejunal anastomoses.
C. Ileoileal anastomoses.

DISCUSSION: Because of their more tenuous blood supply, large bowel anastomoses are at greatest risk of leakage; and because of the associated contamination, initial surgical management involves exteriorizing both ends of the anastomosis. Leaks from more proximal gastrointestinal anastomoses are less common.

Textbook: Page 356 ANSWER: A.

4. The pathogenic organism responsible for pseudomembranous colitis in a postoperative patient is:

A. *Shigella* or *Salmonella.*
B. *Campylobacter.*
C. *Clostridium difficile.*
D. *Staphylococcus.*

DISCUSSION: Pseudomembranous colitis is associated with *Clostridium difficile,* an anaerobic bacterium that releases a toxin. The condition can be induced by a variety of antibiotics, especially clindamycin and lincomycin. *Shigella, Salmonella,* and *Campylobacter* are associated with persistent postoperative diarrhea and should be identified from a fecal specimen.

Textbook: Page 356 ANSWER: C.

5. In the treatment of adult respiratory distress syndrome (ARDS), which of the following has the highest risk of pneumothorax?

A. Intermittent mechanical ventilation (IMV).
B. Positive end-expiratory pressure (PEEP).
C. Continuous positive airway pressure (CPAP).
D. Continuous mechanical ventilation (CMV).

DISCUSSION: Occasional complications of PEEP therapy include alveolar rupture with the development of tension pneumothorax. CPAP has the advantage over PEEP because peak inspiratory pressures are lower, reducing the risk of pneumothorax. The rationale for IMV is to provide an intermediate support between 100% mechanical ventilation and spontaneous respiration that is tailored to the individual patient's requirement.

Textbook: Pages 347–348 ANSWER: B.

6. Match the following with the best answers:

A. Pasteur.
B. Lister.
C. Semmelweis.

(1) Physician-patient pathogen transfer.
(2) Bacterial identification in human infection.
(3) Importance of asepsis.

DISCUSSION: Since the mid-nineteenth century, a host of independent observations and studies have broadened understanding of the process of infection. Semmelweis noted that contagion that passed from the physician to the patient was responsible for the dreaded childhood fever and for subsequent septic deaths of postpartum patients. Pasteur and Koch recognized bacteria as pathogens in human infection. Lister demonstrated the usefulness of antisepsis, which caused the evolution of asepsis and emphasized the need for even more sophisticated efforts to control infection, which remains the most persistent enemy of the surgeon.

Textbook: Page 341 ANSWER: A-2, B-3, C-1.

7. All the following impair healing in the surgical patient except:

A. Malnutrition.
B. Sepsis.
C. Anemia.
D. Jaundice.

DISCUSSION: Factors that appear to interfere with wound healing include malnutrition, sepsis, anemia, uremia, liver failure, diabetes, and corticosteroid therapy. Jaundice by itself is not proven to impair healing.

Textbook: Page 344 ANSWER: D.

8. The most frequent cause of postoperative pulmonary edema is:

A. Atrial fibrillation.
B. Direct toxic effect of anesthetic gases.
C. Overload of infused fluid.
D. Inadequate analgesia that prevents patient coughing.
E. Pulmonary hypertension secondary to peripheral shutdown.

DISCUSSION: Pulmonary edema in the postoperative patient may be due to left ventricular failure following cardiac complications or to injury to the alveolar membrane as a result of sepsis or oxygen toxicity, but is generally the result of circulatory overload following excessive administration of intravenous fluids.

Textbook: Page 347 ANSWER: C.

9. The prevalence of abdominal hernia in an infected wound is approximately:

A. 1%.
B. 10%.
C. 30%.
D. 50%.

DISCUSSION: Hernia formation is a relatively common complication of abdominal and flank wounds. Its incidence after primary healing is approximately 1%, rising to 10% for infected wounds and 30% after dehiscence and reclosure.

Textbook: Page 345 ANSWER: B.

10. Acute renal failure is conveniently classified according to its cause as prerenal, renal, or postrenal. Prerenal conditions that may impair renal function and that must be considered in the differential diagnosis of postoperative acute renal failure are:

A. Hypotension.
B. Hypovolemia.
C. Aminoglycoside toxicity.
D. Radiographic contrast toxicity.
E. Cardiac failure.

DISCUSSION: Common prerenal causes of surgical acute renal failure are hypotension, hypovolemia, arterial occlusion, arterial stenosis, and cardiac failure. Although some toxins may have systemic effects that cause hypotension or hypovolemia, their common effects are upon the kidney itself. Renal toxins include radiographic contrast and endotoxin. Certain drugs such as aminoglycosides, cyclosporine, amphotericin B, and nonsteroidal anti-inflammatory drugs are intrarenal toxins. Pigment nephropathy due to myoglobin or hemoglobin is another intrarenal cause of acute renal failure.

Textbook: Pages 360–361 ANSWER: A, B, E.

11. An important differential diagnosis for the postoperative patient with acute renal failure is to distinguish prerenal azotemia from renal tubular injury. Measurements of urine osmolality and sodium concentration aid in making the correct diagnosis. A patient with prerenal azotemia is likely to have:

	Osmolality (mOsm./L.)	*Sodium (mEq./L.)*
A.	>500	>40
B.	<350	>40
C.	>500	<20
D.	<350	<20
E.	350–500	20–40

DISCUSSION: The urine in acute tubular necrosis (ATN) is isosthenuric—that is, the urine osmolality is very close to that of plasma. Thus, oliguric patients with a urine osmolality near 300 mOsm./L. are likely to have ATN, whereas patients with prerenal azotemia are likely to have a more concentrated urine with osmolality greater than 500 mOsm./L. The hypoperfused kidney is sodium avid, and a low urinary sodium concentration is characteristic of prerenal azotemia. However, when actual tubular injury has occurred there is diminished renal sodium reabsorption. Thus, patients with established ATN or prolonged urinary obstruction usually have a higher urine sodium, specifically above 40 mEq./L. In actuality, many patients in either group have osmolality values between 300 and 500 mOsm./L. and urine sodium values between 20 and 40 mEq./L. Values within this range are nondiscriminating and may reflect evolving tubular injury from a prolonged prerenal state.

Textbook: Pages 371–372 ANSWER: C, E.

12. Absolute indications for dialysis of a postoperative patient with acute renal failure include:

A. Volume overload.
B. Blood urea nitrogen (BUN) greater than 100 mg. per 100 ml.
C. Hyperkalemia.
D. Need for multiple transfusions.
E. Acidosis.

DISCUSSION: Absolute indications for postoperative dialysis include volume overload, electrolyte abnormalities, acidosis, and uremic signs and symptoms. In the absence of such signs and symptoms BUN elevation by itself does not necessitate dialysis. Multiple transfusions may be given without dialysis, but careful monitoring is required to avoid volume overload and hyperkalemia, which would be indications for dialysis therapy.

Textbook: Pages 374–375 ANSWER: A, C, E.

13. The late complication of acute renal failure that most often causes patient death is:

A. Respiratory failure.
B. Cardiac failure.
C. Hemorrhage.
D. Infection.
E. Malnutrition.

DISCUSSION: When one examines the primary causes of death in patients with acute renal failure it is apparent that the evolution of complications during the course of renal failure has a dramatic impact on patient prognosis. More than 50% of patients who die in the setting of acute renal failure do so because of sepsis and pulmonary infections. Respiratory and cardiac failure comprises another 25%, and severe bleeding is responsible for 10 to 15% of patient deaths. Malnutrition is a frequent concomitant and is probably a primary permissive factor.

Textbook: Page 377 ANSWER: D.

14. Of all the electrolyte abnormalities encountered in postoperative acute renal failure, hyperkalemia (which may cause cardiac arrest) is the most serious. The early treatment with the most immediate beneficial effect on the diminished cardiac excitability and imminent cardiac standstill caused by hyperkalemia is:

A. Hemodialysis.
B. Glucose and insulin infusion.
C. Sodium bicarbonate infusion.
D. Calcium gluconate infusion.
E. Sodium polystyrene sulfonate (Kayexelate) administration.

DISCUSSION: The severity of hyperkalemia can be judged by the electrocardiographic changes, including peaked T waves, prolongation of P-R intervals, loss of P waves, and widening of the QRS complex. These changes indicate diminished cardiac excitability and imminent cardiac standstill. When significant electrocardiographic changes are apparent, emergent therapy is indicated. First, a calcium infusion with 1 to 3 ampules of 10% calcium gluconate should be given over 5 to 15 minutes to stabilize the cardiac membranes and reverse the toxic effects of hyperkalemia. This membrane-stabilizing action of calcium is immediate in onset but is relatively short lived. It is often life saving, but other therapy must be instituted to actually lower the serum potassium and remove the excess potassium from the body. Possible such therapies include all of the other answers listed.

Textbook: Page 373 ANSWER: D.

15. Renal replacement therapies for postoperative acute renal failure include the following modalities:

A. Cadaveric donor renal transplantation.
B. Hemodialysis.
C. Peritoneal dialysis.
D. Hemofiltration.
E. Living-related donor renal transplantation.

DISCUSSION: Hemodialysis, peritoneal dialysis, and hemofiltration are useful renal replacement therapies for postoperative acute renal failure. Hemodialysis is the most efficient of the three, but peritoneal dialysis and hemofiltration cause less cardiovascular strain. Renal transplantation is suitable therapy for chronic renal failure but is not appropriate treatment for acute renal failure because most patients who survive acute tubular necrosis will have sufficient functional recovery that dialysis is not required.

Textbook: Pages 374–377 ANSWER: B, C, D.

16. Acute renal failure is defined as an abrupt decline in renal function sufficient to cause:

A. Retention of nitrogenous waste.
B. Volume overload.
C. Anuria.
D. Oliguria.
E. Hyperkalemia.

DISCUSSION: Acute renal failure is defined as an abrupt decline in renal function sufficient to produce retention of nitrogenous waste. This definition of acute renal failure does not depend upon the urine output of the patient. The emphasis is on the quality of urine rather than the quantity since nonoliguric forms are apt to occur quite frequently. Whether or not oliguria is present, a progressive rise in blood urea nitrogen and serum creatinine concentration in the posttrauma or postoperative period should suggest the presence of acute renal failure. Hyperkalemia may be caused by excessive administration or excessive release of potassium as well as by renal insufficiency.

Textbook: Page 360 ANSWER: A.

17. Biochemical alterations in acute renal failure include:

A. Retention of nitrogenous wastes.
B. Metabolic acidosis.
C. Hyperkalemia.
D. Hypermagnesemia.
E. Hypercalcemia.

DISCUSSION: Biochemical alterations in acute renal failure include retention of nitrogenous wastes, which are largely the products of tissue catabolism and protein breakdown. In the acutely ill patient who is hypercatabolic because of recent surgical intervention, trauma, or burn injury, the plasma urea nitrogen concentration may increase by as much as 40 mg. per 100 ml. per day. Metabolic acidosis in postoperative patients with acute renal failure is due to increased cellular catabolism and release of fixed-acid equivalents and the inability of the kidneys to excrete the accumulating acid load and regenerate new bicarbonate as a chemical buffer. Electrolyte abnormalities include hyperkalemia, hyponatremia, hyperphosphatemia, and hypermagnesemia. Hypercalcemia is not ordinarily seen in acute renal failure. In fact, hypocalcemia is a common, untoward consequence of acute hyperphosphatemia, especially in cases of major rhabdomyolysis.

Textbook: Pages 363–365 ANSWER: A, B, C, D.

18. A 67-year-old patient is severely injured in an automobile accident. His pelvis is crushed and his right femur fractured by the dashboard of the car. Extraction from the vehicle is a long and difficult procedure. An intravenous infusion of lactated Ringer's solution is begun at the scene of the accident, and additional intravenous fluid is administered upon arrival in the emergency room to raise his central venous pressure (CVP) to 10 cm. H_2O is given. His blood pressure rises from 70/40 to 130/80 mm. Hg during the fluid resuscitation but no urine output is observed. The initial step to evaluate the patient's anuria should be:

A. Furosemide (Lasix), 100 mg. as an intravenous bolus.
B. Mannitol, 12.5 gm, as an intravenous bolus.
C. Lactated Ringer's solution as an intravenous bolus to raise the CVP to 15 cm. H_2O.
D. Computed tomography of the abdomen and pelvis with contrast.
E. Digital rectal exam.

DISCUSSION: Obstruction must be suspected any time *anuria* develops after surgical intervention or trauma to the pelvis or retroperitoneum. Total anuria is rarely seen in the intrinsic renal and prerenal forms of acute renal failure. In the case of acute postrenal failure following pelvic fracture in the male, rectal examination often reveals displacement of the prostate gland. The cystogram and urethrogram demonstrate traumatic rupture of the bladder and disruption of the urethra, respectively. Prompt recognition of the postrenal problem and surgical correction of the obstruction produce complete recovery, whereas delayed recognition causes acute renal failure.

Textbook: Pages 361, 365–366, 367 ANSWER: E.

19. Following surgical treatment, the patient described in Question 18 has a urine output of 300 ml. over the next 24 hours, with rising BUN and serum creatinine concentration, a urine sodium of 18 mEq. per liter, and urine osmolality of 550 mOsm. per liter. His renal failure is most appropriately characterized as:

A. Nonoliguric prerenal azotemia.
B. Oliguric prerenal azotemia.
C. Nonoliguric renal tubular injury.
D. Oliguric renal tubular injury.
E. Oliguric postrenal obstruction.

DISCUSSION: Although the patient has a history of trauma, hypotension, and surgical treatment that could produce acute tubular necrosis, his blood and urine indices suggest that a prerenal azotemia exists. Since the urine output is less than 400 ml. over 24 hours, oliguria is evident. The rising BUN and serum creatinine concentration confirm renal failure. The low urine sodium (less than 20 mEq. per liter) and high urine osmolality (greater than 500 mOsm. per liter) are characteristic of a prerenal cause, usually low intravascular volume. Tubular necrosis or obstruction produces urine with normal or high levels of sodium and normal or low osmolality.

Textbook: Pages 360, 371 ANSWER: B.

20. Among the continuous hemodialysis techniques, venovenous dialysis therapy has largely replaced arteriovenous therapy for renal replacement because:

A. No arterial line is required.
B. No blood pump is required.
C. Extracorporeal blood flow is not blood pressure dependent.
D. No artificial kidney is required.
E. No continuous anticoagulation is required.

DISCUSSION: Arteriovenous continuous therapy is a dialysis technique that uses the patient's own blood pressure to provide blood flow through a highly permeable artificial kidney. It requires a large-bore arterial line and is very blood pressure dependent, unlike venovenous continuous therapy. The venovenous technique uses a blood pump to maintain extracorporeal blood flow through an artificial kidney, so it is not blood pressure dependent. It is increasingly popular since it provides smooth, continuous therapy with minimal cardiovascular effects. It does, however, require some form of continuous anticoagulation.

Textbook: Page 377 ANSWER: A, C.

NOTES

NOTES

CHAPTER 7

TRANSPLANTATION

1. The "father of experimental surgery" who performed pioneering research, including several transplantation procedures, was:

A. Homer, the Greek who described the Chimaera in his *Iliad.*
B. Gasparo Tagliacozzi, the Italian who described a method of reconstructing the nose.
C. John Hunter, the Scot who performed autografts and xenografts.
D. Emrick Ullmann, the Austrian who performed the first successful renal allograft.
E. Alexis Carrel, the Franco-American who described a successful technique for vascular anastomosis.

DISCUSSION: All of the descriptions are correct and represent important contributions to the history of transplantation. However, the Scottish surgeon John Hunter (1728–1793), is rightfully known as the father of experimental surgery because of his pioneering research. Several of his experimental procedures involved transplantation, including autografting of a cock's spur to its comb and xenografting of a human tooth to the comb of a cock.

Textbook: Page 383 ANSWER: C.

2. Transplantation terminology contains terms to describe the relationship of the graft donor to the graft recipient. Historical terms such as "homograft" and "heterograft" have been replaced by less ambiguous terms. The correct modern terminology for a graft between genetically nonidentical members of the same species is:

A. Allogeneic graft.
B. Autogeneic graft.
C. Isogeneic graft.
D. Syngeneic graft.
E. Xenogeneic graft.

Textbook: Pages 383–384 ANSWER: A.

3. The modern era of clinical organ transplantation began with the advent of chemical immunosuppression. The important drug discovery that produced the initial success of cadaveric transplantation was:

A. Cyclophosphamide.
B. Azathioprine.
C. Cyclosporine.
D. Antilymphocyte serum.
E. Monoclonal antibody OKT3.

DISCUSSION: All of the listed drugs have immunosuppressive activity that has proved useful in transplant recipients. However, the discovery in 1959 by Schwartz and Dameshek that 6-mercaptopurine blocked antibody production and the subsequent creation by Hitchings in 1961 of its safe, convenient imidazole derivative named azathioprine produced the first consistently effective immunosuppression for successful cadaveric renal transplantation.

Textbook: Page 386 ANSWER: B.

4. Which of the following statements correctly characterize the genetic basis of histocompatibility?

A. Histocompatibility is determined by a series of genes inherited as a complex and subject to the mendelian rules that characterize recessive traits.
B. Histocompatibility depends in part on the inheritance of histocompatibility genes and in part on the inheritance of T-cell receptor genes.
C. Major histocompatibility genes are polymorphic.
D. Histocompatibility genes are independently segregating and co-dominant.
E. Histocompatibility is learned.

DISCUSSION: *Histocompatibility* refers to the genetic determinants of graft rejection. The determinants of overwhelming importance consist of a series of histocompatibility genes that segregate independently during meiosis. Each gene has multiple, dominant alleles. Histocompatibility genes and the proteins they encode are highly polymorphic (i.e., they exist in multiple forms).

Textbook: Pages 389–391, 395 ANSWER: C, D, E.

5. The major histocompatibility complex (MHC) includes genes that encode which of the following proteins?

A. HLA-A.
B. HLA-DR.
C. TAP-1.
D. 21-Hydroxylase.
E. HLA-L.

DISCUSSION: The major histocompatibility complex (MHC) includes genes encoding histocompatibility antigens, some other proteins, and a number of pseudogenes that do not encode proteins. The class I region encodes more than 15 genes, including the classical transplant genes A, B, and C as well as HLA-E, F, and G and four pseudogenes, H, J, K, and L. The class II region contains more than 25 genes, including those for the transplantation antigens HLA-DR, DQ, and DP. The region also includes two alpha genes, DMA and DNA, and two beta genes, DMB and DOB, genes for the low-molecular-weight proteins (LMPs) LMP2 and LMP3 and for the transporter molecules TAP1 and TAP2. The class III region, lying between class II and class I, contains more than 30 genes, among which are the genes encoding the complement components factor B, C2, and both C4 molecules, both tumor necrosis factor genes alpha and beta, and the heat shock proteins Hsp 1H and Hsp 70 2, and 21-hydroxylase.

Textbook: Page 396 ANSWER: A, B, C, D.

6. Which of the following distinguish MHC class I from MHC class II antigens?

A. MHC class I and class II antigens are encoded in different regions of the MHC complex.
B. MHC class I antigens are expressed on specialized antigen-presenting cells, whereas MHC class II antigens are expressed on all cells.
C. MHC class I and class II are members of different supergene families.
D. MHC class I are considered to be the major histocompatibility antigens and MHC class II the minor histocompatibility antigens.
E. MHC class I is recognized by the CD8 glycoprotein, whereas MHC class II is recognized by the CD4 glycoprotein.

DISCUSSION: MHC class I and class II antigens are encoded by genes in different regions of the MHC. The genes and the proteins they encode are homologous to immunoglobulins and thus are members of the immunoglobulin supergene family. MHC class I antigens are expressed on the surface of all cells, whereas MHC class II antigens are largely restricted in expression to antigen-presenting cells and endothelial cells. Both MHC class I and class II antigens are major histocompatibility antigens because their incompatibility in the donor and recipient can lead to very rapid and vigorous rejection of an allograft. The T cells that have antigen receptors specific for MHC class I plus peptide express CD8, a co-receptor that binds to the MHC class I molecules. The T cells that have antigen preceptors specific for MHC class II plus peptide express CD4, a co-receptor that binds to MHC class II molecules.

Textbook: Pages 396–397 ANSWER: A, E.

7. Which of the following characterize the role of the major histocompatibility antigens in immune responses?

A. The major histocompatibility antigens are critical in antigen processing and presentation.
B. Major histocompatibility antigens contribute to the maturation of T cells in the thymus.
C. T cells recognize only foreign antigens that are complexed with major histocompatibility antigens.
D. Expression of major histocompatibility antigens is increased in inflammation.
E. Recognition of major histocompatibility antigens is critical to the development of tolerance.

DISCUSSION: Once thought to be solely markers of individuality, MHC antigens are crucial to cell-mediated immune responses. Foreign antigens taken up by antigen-presenting cells are degraded and then become complexed with MHC molecules and expressed on the cell surface, and these events are enhanced in inflammation. Since T cells recognize only foreign antigens expressed as peptides in association with MHC antigens, the possibility for recognition is increased as a consequence of inflammation. Since T cells recognize only antigens expressed in association with MHC antigens, recognition of these antigens is critical to the development of tolerance to "self."

Textbook: Pages 395–396 ANSWER: A, B, C, D, E.

8. The unusual intensity of alloimmune responses reflects which of the following characteristics?

A. The presence of a peptide-binding groove in the MHC molecule.
B. Recognition of the native structure of allogeneic MHC molecules.
C. The high frequency of T cells able to recognize directly allogeneic MHC antigens.
D. Stimulation of many T-cell receptors during the interaction of a T cell with an antigen-presenting cell.
E. The high frequency of antigen-presenting cells able to be recognized by T cells.

DISCUSSION: Allotransplantation evokes an unusually intense and rapid cellular immune response. In contrast to conventional cellular immune responses, in which foreign antigens are recognized only as peptides in the groove of self MHC antigens, allogeneic MHC antigens are recognized directly as native proteins on the surface of allogeneic antigen-presenting cells. Thus, a large fraction of antigen-presenting cells is able to present alloantigen in this fashion, and a large fraction (up to 10%) of T cells is able to respond.

Textbook: Pages 395–396 ANSWER: B, C, D, E.

9. Which of the following statements correctly characterize the role of histocompatibility typing in transplantation?

A. Histocompatibility typing must be carried out before transplantation can safely be undertaken.
B. The "rules" of histocompatibility were established shortly after the advent of

immunosuppressive therapy made transplantation feasible.
C. Histocompatibility typing may involve serologic, cellular, and molecular procedures for typing.
D. The role of histocompatibility matching in transplantation is controversial.
E. The cross-match test is carried out to determine whether a potential graft recipient has antibodies against the donor.

DISCUSSION: The concept of histocompatibility and the rules governing the susceptibility to rejection were deduced early in this century by such investigators as Jensen, Little, and Tyzzer, who were interested in the inherited resistance or susceptibility to transplanted tumors. The application of histocompatibility to clinical transplantation, however, had to await the advent of immunosuppressive therapy. Despite the practice of organ transplantation for more than 30 years, the role of histocompatibility typing in transplantation is controversial. Although grafts between HLA-matched donors and recipients exhibit better survival than HLA-mismatched grafts, matching is not routinely performed before transplantation of the heart or liver, and the outcome of these grafts may be very good. Histocompatibility typing involves the use of a variety of techniques—serologic, cellular, and molecular—to identify the antigens carried by the donor and the recipient. In addition to formal typing, the recipient is tested via cross-match for antibodies against the donor.
Textbook: Pages 397–398 ANSWER: C, D, E.

10. Activation of T cells requires:
A. Stimulation of the antigen receptor.
B. Stimulation of the MHC antigen.
C. Co-stimulation.
D. Anergy.
E. CD3.

DISCUSSION: The activation of T cells generally involves the delivery of two types of signals. One signal is initiated when the T-cell antigen receptor binds in a cognate manner to an MHC antigen bearing an antigenic peptide expressed on the surface of an antigen-presenting cell. This interaction is enhanced by the coordinate binding of CD4 or CD8 to the MHC antigen complex. This interaction initiates signaling through CD3, as well as through CD4 or CD8, both of which are associated with tyrosine kinases. Full activation of the T cell also requires the delivery of "co-stimulatory" signals. These signals may arise through the interaction of CD28 expressed by the T cell with B7-1 or B7-2 expressed on antigen-presenting cells. If only the T-cell antigen receptor is stimulated (and co-stimulation is not provided) the T-cell becomes anergic, that is, resistant to further stimulation. Anergy may be an important mechanism contributing to tolerance.
Textbook: Pages 393–394 ANSWER: A, C, E.

11. Which of the following statements characterize the biology of allotransplantation?
A. The rejection response is systemic.
B. The rejection response is learned.
C. The rejection response involves a constellation of immunologic and environmental factors.
D. Allotransplantation evokes a cellular immune response.
E. Allotransplantation evokes a humoral immune response.

DISCUSSION: Medawar and Gibson elucidated some of the basic principles of transplantation biology. Rejection of a second skin graft from the donor of a first graft is very much hastened, indicating that the response is learned and that the second response evokes "memory." The second graft is rejected rapidly, regardless of its location, indicating that the response is systemic. The major immune reaction causing rejection of a first graft is a cellular immune response; however, the recipient exposed to allogeneic cells develops antibodies against alloantigens, indicating that a humoral response has also occurred.
Textbook: Pages 384, 400 ANSWER: A, B, D, E.

12. Allograft rejection may involve which of the following?
A. Helper T cells.
B. Veto cells.
C. Cytotoxicity.
D. Cytokines.
E. The Arthus reaction.

DISCUSSION: The effector mechanisms that underlie the pathogenesis of allograft rejection remain the subject of controversy. Rejection, like delayed-type hypersensitivity, may be mediated by helper T cells, which release cytokines that activate other cells such as macrophages and directly alter endothelial cell functions. On the other hand, rejection may be mediated by cytotoxic T cells, which kill or injure target cells through direct interactions. Both types of cells can be found in grafts undergoing rejection, and there is experimental evidence suggesting that both may be involved. Veto cells kill T cells, which recognize MHC antigens on the veto cell surface; this action is thought to contribute to tolerance and not to rejection. The Arthus reaction is an immune response that, in contrast to allograft rejection, is mediated primarily by antibodies and not by cells.
Textbook: Pages 401, 403–405 ANSWER: A, C, D.

13. Which of the following statements about allograft rejection are true?
A. In the absence of immunosuppression, the time and intensity of rejection of transplants between unrelated donors and recipients is highly variable.
B. Allograft rejection may be mediated by antibodies or by cells.
C. Allograft rejection is thought to be caused by Th2 cells.
D. Acute cellular rejection is the major cause for loss of clinical organ transplants.

E. An individual with "tolerance" is unable to reject an allograft.

DISCUSSION: In the absence of immunosuppression, allografts from randomly selected donors are always rejected, and the rate of rejection is rapid as compared with the rate of development of most immune responses. Although allograft rejection in naive recipients is mediated predominantly by cells, antidonor antibodies can cause very severe types of rejection, including hyperacute and acute vascular rejection. Antidonor antibodies or cellular responses may contribute to the development of chronic rejection, which is now the most common cause of graft loss. Recent studies demonstrate that helper T cells may differentiate along one of two pathways. The Th1 pathway leads to secretion of interferon-gamma and other cytokines and is associated with delayed-type hypersensitivity and allograft rejection. The Th2 pathway is associated with secretion of interleukin-10 (IL-10) and IL-4 and may actually inhibit alloimmune responses. The development of Th2 responses may thus contribute to tolerance. Like allograft rejection, tolerance is highly specific. Thus, a person who is tolerant to one antigen or one individual is still able to mount an immune response against other antigens and other individuals.

Textbook: Pages 403–405 ANSWER: B.

14. The presence of donor-reactive lymphocytotoxic antibodies in the serum of a potential kidney transplant recipient:

A. Can be detected by *in vitro* testing with recipient leukocytes and donor serum.
B. Is a contraindication to kidney transplantation.
C. Can be found in all male patients older than 20 years.

DISCUSSION: The presence of donor-reactive antibodies, detected by incubation of the recipient's serum with donor lymphocytes in the presence of complement, results in a "positive crossmatch," and is a contraindication to renal transplantation. They occur as a result of pregnancy, blood transfusions, or previous organ transplants.

Textbook: Pages 409–410 ANSWER: B.

15. Utilization of a living related donor instead of a cadaver donor is no longer an advantage in renal transplantation because:

A. Public recognition of transplantation as a successful therapy has facilitated obtaining family permission for recovery of transplantable organs. Thus, because sufficient kidneys are available from "brain-dead" accident victims, there is no need to use related donors.
B. Cyclosporine therapy after cadaveric renal transplants has improved their outcome, which is now comparable to related-donor transplants.
C. Modern preservation techniques can maintain viability of kidneys from cadaver donors for many hours, consistently allowing their early function to be as good as that of kidneys from living donors.
D. None of the above.

DISCUSSION: It is generally accepted that transplantation is a useful therapy; however, the number of recipients continues to greatly exceed the number of suitable cadaver donors whose families grant permission for organ recovery. Thus, availability of a living donor may shorten the waiting period for a transplant by several years. Cyclosporine has improved the short-term results of cadaveric transplantation, but the attrition of these grafts is greater than that for living-donor transplants, especially those with close histocompatibility. The predicted 10-year survival of grafts from HLA-identical siblings is 80%, whereas for cadaver grafts it is only 40%. Although preservation techniques can maintain viability of kidneys for 36 to 48 hours, cadaver kidneys suffer a much higher rate of posttransplant acute tubular necrosis than those from related donors. Acute tubular necrosis has been shown to have a definite detrimental effect on long-term graft survival.

Textbook: Pages 411–412 ANSWER: D.

16. Large volumes of urine in the early postoperative course of renal transplant patients:

A. Result from osmotic stimuli to diuresis.
B. May signify reversible polyuric acute tubular necrosis.
C. Should be replaced by administration of equal volumes of crystalloid.
D. Facilitate the diagnosis of rejection and obstruction of the renal artery and/or collecting system.

DISCUSSION: Factors responsible for the brisk diuresis following renal transplantation include osmotic stimuli secondary to high urea and/or glucose concentrations in the serum, and mild proximal tubular damage resulting from allograft ischemia. To avoid severe dehydration in the early postoperative period, an attempt should be made to replace urine losses with equal volumes of 0.45% NaCl solution to which 20 to 30 mEq. $NaHCO_3$ per liter may be added. The diagnosis of rejection and/or obstruction to urine flow is made easier when a transplanted kidney is undergoing voluminous diuresis rather than demonstrating oliguria or anuria secondary to severe acute tubular necrosis.

Textbook: Page 416 ANSWER: A, B, C, D.

17. As compared with the early immunosuppressive drugs (azathioprine, steroids, antilymphocyte serum) some newer agents have the following specific advantages:

A. Cyclosporine, which interferes with lymphokine production, exhibits neither bone marrow nor renal toxicity.

B. Monoclonal antibody (OKT3) is more available and has greater specificity and fewer side effects than antilymphocyte serum.
C. Tacrolimus (FK506) has properties similar to those of cyclosporine but is especially valuable for rescue of grafts that are failing on cyclosporine therapy.
D. None of the above.

DISCUSSION: Cyclosporine interferes with production of cytokines and lacks the bone marrow toxicity of azathioprine. Unfortunately its chief toxicity is renal. Although OKT3 is more available, more uniform, and more specific than antilymphocyte serum, some of its side effects are even greater, such as fever, chills, nausea, vomiting, diarrhea, and pulmonary edema. Tacrolimus has been used most extensively for liver grafts. It has been found especially valuable in reversing rejection of failing grafts.
Textbook: Pages 417–418 ANSWER: C.

18. Survival rates for patients on dialysis are better than those for patients receiving renal allografts in the following circumstances:
A. A living related donor is available.
B. A cadaver donor must be used.
C. The recipient's renal failure is secondary to diabetes.
D. None of the above.

DISCUSSION: Patients receiving chronic dialysis have a mortality rate of 6% to 20% per year, every year. The mortality rate is as high as 11% to 25% per year in diabetic dialysis patients. Patients undergoing renal transplantation have an operative mortality rate of less than 2%, and the 1-year survival for recipients of living related kidneys is better than 95%. Survival is greater than 90% for recipients of cadaver kidneys. The 5-year patient survivals are approximately 80% for nondiabetic recipients of living related and cadaver kidneys, and 60% to 70% for diabetic recipients. Thus, a well-functioning renal allograft provides a greater chance for a longer life than does chronic dialysis.
Textbook: Pages 408, 425–428 ANSWER: D.

19. Posttransplantation hypertension can be caused by:
A. Rejection.
B. Cyclosporine nephrotoxicity.
C. Renal transplant artery stenosis (RTAS).
D. Recurrent disease in the allograft.

DISCUSSION: Both acute and chronic rejection may result in hypertension. The former causes acute fluid retention and plugging of peritubular capillaries with inflammatory cells. This may progress to intimal swelling and medial necrosis and eventuate in ischemia secondary to endothelial proliferation and obliteration of small vessels. Chronic rejection, thought to be related to protracted humoral injury, results in obliteration of capillaries via the development of intimal hyperplasia. Cyclosporine has a vasoconstrictive effect which, through activation of the renin-angiotensin system, may lead to hypertension. RTAS is responsible for hypertension in 4% to 12% of renal allograft recipients. It responds well to percutaneous angioplasty. A careful trial of angiotensin-converting enzyme inhibitors may be diagnostic of RTAS. Recurrent disease such as membranoproliferative glomerulonephritis and focal glomerular sclerosis may result in significant hypertension in renal allograft recipients.
Textbook: Pages 421–422 ANSWER: A, B, C, D.

20. Which of the following statements about posttransplantation malignancy is correct?
A. Certain immunosuppressive agents increase the incidence of malignancy in transplant recipients, whereas others do not.
B. Those malignancies most commonly seen in the general population (breast, colon) are substantially more common in transplant recipients.
C. Lymphoproliferative states and B-cell lymphomas are associated with Epstein-Barr virus.
D. None of the above.

DISCUSSION: Both naturally occurring and iatrogenic states of immune deficiency are associated with an increased rate of *de novo* malignancy. Transplant recipients have a rate of malignancy approximately 100 times that of the normal population. The degree of immunosuppression, rather than a specific immunosuppressive agent, appears to be responsible. Squamous and basal cell carcinomas of the skin are most common; however other tumors that are common in the general population, such as breast and colon cancers, do not appear to be increased in incidence. Lymphomas, which occur at a rate that is 350 times normal, and the lymphoproliferative states that often precede them appear to be associated with Epstein-Barr virus. Possible explanations for these high malignancy rates include defective immunosurveillance, chronic stimulation of the reticuloendothelial system by the allograft, the carcinogenic effect of immunosuppressive drugs, and viral oncogenesis.
Textbook: Pages 424–425 ANSWER: C.

21. One week after receiving a cadaver renal allograft, the recipient remains oliguric and dialysis dependent. Ultrasonography reveals a larger perigraft fluid collection. Your next step in management includes:
A. No further investigations (since perigraft collections are fairly common after renal transplantation).
B. Aspiration of the perigraft fluid collection and instillation of a fibrosis-inducing agent to obliterate the dead space.
C. Angiography for localization of a bleeding site in the renal allograft.
D. Aspiration of the perigraft fluid collection for chemical analysis.

DISCUSSION: Urine leaks usually occur early after transplantation, and the most frequent site of leakage is from the ureteroneocystostomy or ischemic ureter. The clinical signs are pain, swelling, and deterioration of renal function before leakage from the wound is observed. Aspiration of the perigraft fluid collection for chemical analysis of blood urea nitrogen (BUN) and creatinine would aid the differentiating urinoma from lymphocele. The composition of urinoma reveals BUN and creatinine concentrations several orders of magnitude higher than those of a lymphocele, which are comparable to the values in blood.

Textbook: Pages 422–423 ANSWER: D.

22. Regarding access for hemodialysis, which of the following statements is/are incorrect?

A. Some patients are not candidates for hemodialysis.
B. Some complications can lead to exsanguination.
C. The best access to place for a patient beginning dialysis is a leg polytetrafluoroethylene (PTFE) graft from the femoral artery to the saphenous vein.
D. First of all one should attempt to create a Brescia-Cimino fistula.
E. The leading complication of PTFE grafts is infection.

DISCUSSION: Some patients do not tolerate hemodialysis because of cardiac difficulties or because they cannot be heparinized for hemodialysis. If a peripheral shunt becomes disconnected, the patient can exsanguinate. This can occur if a cap or clamp is inadvertently removed from a central dialysis catheter. The ideal location for a dialysis fistula or graft is in the upper extremity as far distal as possible, such as with a Brescia-Cimino fistula or a forearm loop graft. The leading complication of PTFE grafts is thrombosis caused by intimal hyperplasia in the venous limb. Infection is the second leading complication with these grafts.

Textbook: Pages 429, 431–434 ANSWER: C, E.

23. Access to the peritoneal cavity for peritoneal access can be gained:

A. Percutaneously.
B. Surgically.
C. Using laparoscopy.
D. Only using general anesthesia.

DISCUSSION: Chronic ambulatory peritoneal dialysis (CAPD) catheters may be placed at the bedside with a straight Tenckhoff catheter under local anesthesia. They can be placed laparoscopically or by making a small perimedian incision and placing the catheter through the rectus muscle. All of the techniques can be performed using local anesthesia; however, use of the laparoscopy commonly calls for general anesthesia.

Textbook: Pages 434–435 ANSWER: A, B, C.

24. Which of the following are true concerning immunosuppression?

A. Current immunosuppressive agents function in a nonspecific manner to suppress rejection.
B. The use of immunosuppressive agents is associated with an increased rate of opportunistic infections.
C. An increased rate of malignancy is *not* associated with the use of immunosuppressive agents.
D. In almost all cases, the graft is rejected if immunosuppression is discontinued.

DISCUSSION: At the present time, clinical immunosuppression involves the use of agents that function in a nonspecific manner to prevent rejection. These agents suppress almost all aspects of the immune response. Because of their mechanism of action, they have associated toxicities and side effects, such as an increased rate of opportunistic infections. An increase in certain malignancies is also associated with use of these agents. In almost all cases, the graft is rejected if the immunosuppression is discontinued. Therefore, immunosuppression must be continued for the life of the graft.

Textbook: Pages 439, 453 ANSWER: A, B, D.

25. Which of the following is true for hyperacute rejection?

A. It is mediated by preformed cytotoxic antibody.
B. It occurs late in the life of the graft.
C. It is usually reversible with a bolus of steroids.
D. None of the above.

DISCUSSION: Hyperacute rejection is mediated by preformed cytotoxic antibody. It can be screened for by cross-matching procedures. It usually occurs immediately after graft placement or within the first 24 to 48 hours after graft placement. It is almost never reversible.

Textbook: Pages 405, 443 ANSWER: A.

26. The major components of the immune system include which of the following?

A. T lymphocytes.
B. B lymphocytes.
C. Cytokines.
D. Macrophages.

DISCUSSION: The development of the lymphoid system begins with a pluripotent stem cell in the liver and bone marrow of the fetus. With maturation of the fetus toward term, the bone marrow becomes the primary site for lymphopoiesis. It produces the T lymphocytes, B lymphocytes, and macrophages that are critical to the immune response. These cells then produce cytokines or soluble growth factors, which amplify the immune response.

Textbook: Pages 437–440 ANSWER: A, B, C, D.

27. The most common types of immunosuppressive agents used clinically include which of the following?

A. Antimetabolites.
B. Alkylating agents.
C. Inhibitors of helper T-cell activation.
D. Irradiation.
E. Lymphocyte depletion compounds.

DISCUSSION: Much of the susceptibility of lymphocytes to immunosuppression is due to the vast cellular changes that follow immune stimulation. The biosynthetic events that take place make the lymphocytes vulnerable to inhibition at various stages of the cell cycle. Cyclosporine inhibits cytokine gene expression, whereas alkylating agents and radiation produce cross-linkages and breaks in DNA strands that interfere with cell differentiation and division. Agents that produce depletion of lymphocytes include antilymphocyte globulin (ALG) and monoclonal antibodies (OKT3).

Textbook: Pages 444–445, 448–449 ANSWER: A, B, C, D, E.

28. Which of the following is/are true of the antiproliferative agents?

A. They act by preventing the differentiation and division of the immunocompetent lymphocyte after it encounters antigen.
B. The antimetabolites in this group have a structural similarity to cell metabolites and either inhibit enzymes of a metabolic pathway or are incorporated during synthesis to produce faulty molecules.
C. The most frequently used antiproliferative agent is azathioprine.

DISCUSSION: Antiproliferative agents inhibit the full expression of the immune response by preventing the differentiation of the immunocompetent lymphocyte after it encounters antigen. They act in one of two ways: they either structurally resemble necessary metabolites, or they combine with certain cellular components, such as DNA, and thereby interfere with function. Until recently, azathioprine was the most widely used immunosuppressive drug in transplantation, and it still has a major clinical role in preventing rejection.

Textbook: Pages 446–447 ANSWER: A, B, C.

29. Which of the following is the one true statement about acute rejection.

A. Acute rejection is mediated by T lymphocytes.
B. Acute rejection is mediated by preformed cytotoxic antibody.
C. Acute rejection most frequently occurs over months.

DISCUSSION: Acute rejection is mediated primarily by T lymphocytes. It occurs over 1 to 3 weeks after placement of an allograft. Hyperacute rejection is mediated by preformed cytotoxic antibody. It occurs within 48 hours of placement of a graft. Chronic rejection is mediated by both T cells and B cells and occurs over months.

Textbook: Page 443 ANSWER: A.

30. Which of the following are true of cyclosporine?

A. It was the first immunosuppressive agent to be used clinically.
B. It acts selectively on T cells to suppress rejection.
C. Toxic effects include hirsutism, hypertension, nephrotoxicity, and increased risk of opportunistic infections.

DISCUSSION: Cyclosporine is a product of a fungus and was discovered in 1972. It has contributed very significantly to the development of the field of transplantation. The mechanism of action is relatively specific for T lymphocytes. Other inflammatory cells are much less sensitive to its immunosuppressive effects. It inhibits activated T lymphocytes and prevents the cells from manufacturing and releasing interleukin 2 (IL-2). Toxicities include hirsutism, hypertension, nephrotoxicity, and increased risk of opportunistic infections (because it still functions as a nonspecific immunosuppressive agent).

Textbook: Pages 447–448 ANSWER: B, C.

31. Which of the following are true of OKT3?

A. It is not a monoclonal antibody.
B. It binds to the T-cell receptor and inactivates T-cell function.
C. It is the monoclonal antibody most frequently used in clinical transplantation.

DISCUSSION: OKT3 is a monoclonal antibody produced in limitless supply by a hybridoma. It binds to a site associated with the T-cell receptor complex to inactivate the T cell. It is the most widely used monoclonal antibody in clinical transplantation.

Textbook: Pages 449–450 ANSWER: B, C.

32. Hypothermia (0° to 4° C) is a critical component of successful organ cold storage because:

A. Oxygen is more soluble in cold solutions and provides a continual supply for energy metabolism.
B. There is no way to suppress microbial growth except by cooling and slowing the growth rate.
C. Hypothermia diminishes energy requirements and allows the limited energy reserve to keep the organ alive.
D. It slows metabolism and the enzymic processes that would destroy the cell.

DISCUSSION: Hypothermia in simple organ cold storage serves one primary function but secondary ones as well. The primary function is to slow metabolism. Metabolic rates decrease about twofold for every 10° C drop in temperature. Cooling an organ from 37° to 0° to 4° C drops metabolism about 12- to 13-fold. This is related to the activation energy of enzymatic processes as expressed by Arrhenius and van't Hoff. Thus, catabolism of structural and functional cellular element is retarded for a long period—up to 3 days for some organs. The cold also suppresses microbial growth, but this can be accomplished by other means as well. The cold also allows time for the transplantation operation, and during this time it is important to be quick or to keep cooling the organ.

Textbook: Pages 455, 457 ANSWER: D.

33. Is the following statement true or false?

Organs should be preserved only for short periods of time (4 to 8 hours) because longer periods lead to too many complications, and even loss of the organ.

DISCUSSION: The logistics of organ transplantation make it very difficult to use all available cadaver organs within 4 to 8 hours. To use all the organs requires the capability to preserve them for at least 24 hours. It has been shown that most organs can be matched to a recipient within about 17 to 24 hours. For all but the heart and lung, most intra-abdominal organs tolerate preservation for 20 to 30 hours and perform as well as those preserved for 4 to 8 hours. Although undue delay should not be purposefully used, certainly, most organ transplants do not need to be done on an emergency basis. However, this is not true for hearts and lungs, which should be transplanted as quickly as possible.

Textbook: Page 455 ANSWER: False.

34. Which of the following statements about hepatic artery thrombosis following liver transplantation is/are correct?

A. Thrombosis of the hepatic artery following liver transplantation is more common in children than in adult patients.
B. Thrombosis of the hepatic artery usually occurs several weeks after transplant as a result of arteriosclerosis.
C. Thrombosis of the hepatic artery in the early days following transplantation is a serious complication leading to death unless retransplantation can be performed within 36 to 72 hours.
D. Late thrombosis of the hepatic artery may present as biliary complication or intrahepatic abscesses.
E. Thrombosis of the portal vein is more frequent than hepatic artery thrombosis following liver transplantation.

DISCUSSION: Thrombosis of the hepatic artery remains one of the most serious early complications of liver transplantation. This complication is three to five times more common in children than in adults. The major cause of this complication is related to technical error, although the hypercoagulable state may play a significant role in some situations. Early thrombosis of the hepatic artery leads to rapid liver failure with a fatal outcome unless a transplant can be performed within 36 to 72 hours. Although thrombolytic therapy through percutaneous or surgical access can be successful, most of these patients require retransplantation. Stenosis of the hepatic artery or late thrombosis of the hepatic artery can lead to multiple intrahepatic strictures of the bile duct and/or hepatic abscesses. This complication also often requires retransplantation. Portal vein thrombosis is a rarer complication. It is a devastating condition when it occurs early, but can be tolerated well if it develops after several months. Portal hypertension due to late portal vein thrombosis can often be treated successfully by a shunt procedure.

Textbook: Page 469 ANSWER: A, C, E.

35. Which of the following statements about fulminant hepatic failure (FHF) is/are correct?

A. Fulminant hepatic failure can occur in the setting of pre-existing chronic liver disease.
B. Coagulopathy and coma are important findings in patients with FHF.
C. Liver transplant should not be attempted in patients with FHF because of the high mortality rate, regardless of the treatment used.
D. The main cause of death in these patients is cerebral edema.
E. One of the most important factors in prognosis of FHF is the cause of liver disease.

DISCUSSION: FHF corresponds to the rapid loss of hepatic function in the absence of pre-existing liver disease, causing jaundice, coagulopathy, and coma. One of the major prognostic factors is the cause of the liver disease. Early admission to an intensive care unit and management by physicians experienced in liver transplantation are mandatory. The major cause of death in these patients is cerebral edema. In patients who rapidly develop coma, subdural intracerebral pressure monitoring is mandatory for optimal management as well as for identification of patients who can benefit from liver transplantation. The survival rate for patients with FHF who underwent liver transplantation is currently above 65%. This is the only cure in most patients with FHF.

Textbook: Page 462 ANSWER: B, D, E.

36. Which of the following statements about immunology in liver transplantation is/are correct?

A. Good human leukocyte antigen (HLA) matching between recipient and donor is mandatory for a good outcome for liver transplantation.
B. Hyperacute rejection is almost nonexistent following liver transplantation.
C. Acute rejection occurs in more than 50% of patients and is reversible in most patients with large doses of steroids.
D. Acute rejection is very rare later than 2 months after liver transplantation unless the patient is inadequately immunosuppressed.

E. Chronic rejection is different from acute rejection, is usually irreversible, and often requires retransplantation.

DISCUSSION: Immune-mediated reactions following liver transplantation are clearly different from those that follow other solid organ transplants. The liver is tolerated quite well, and currently donors and recipients are matched only for their ABO group. Even when the ABO barrier is not respected, survival is still over 60%. T cell–mediated acute rejection occurs in about half of the patients within 6 weeks after liver transplantation, and acute rejection is reversed by large doses of steroids in most cases. Chronic rejection, on the other hand, is a different entity that is ill-understood and corresponds to destruction of small arteries and bile ducts. Change in the immunosuppression regimen sometimes may hinder the progression of this disease, but often retransplantation is required.

Textbook: Pages 466–468 ANSWER: B, C, D, E.

37. An elevated serum amylase level following pancreas-kidney transplantation may be due to:

A. Preservation/procurement injury.
B. Rejection.
C. Reflux pancreatitis.
D. Duodenal segment leak or bladder leak.
E. Native pancreatitis.
F. Constipation.

DISCUSSION: During the immediate postoperative period, an elevated serum amylase is usually due to preservation or procurement injury to the transplanted pancreas. If UW (University of Wisconsin) solution and a good flushout technique is used in an acceptable donor, amylase is usually elevated only several hundred points and will decline in a day or two. Rejection of the pancreas can also cause elevated serum amylase and is usually accompanied by a rise in the creatinine value due to concomitant renal transplant rejection. Reflux pancreatitis is generally caused by bladder dysfunction: increased pressure transmitted back through the pancreatic ducts causes pancreatitis. It is generally relieved by bladder decompression with a Foley catheter. Naturally, leakage from the anastomosis of the pancreas transplant to the bladder causes absorption of amylase from the peritoneal cavity and an elevated serum amylase value. Constipation causes a rise in the amylase level of pancreas-kidney transplant recipients, for reasons that remain unclear. Native pancreatitis has to be borne in mind in the differential diagnosis of hyperamylasemia in transplant patients. Contributing factors may include underlying gallbladder disease, as well as side effects of steroids and Imuran.

Textbook: Pages 475–477 ANSWER: A, B, D, E, F.

38. Complications of a pancreas transplant drained into the bladder include:

A. Duodenal segment leak.
B. Recurrent urinary tract infections.
C. Recurrent hematuria.
D. Urethritis.
E. Refractory loss of bicarbonate.

DISCUSSION: All of the listed problems are potential complications of bladder drainage. The most useful diagnostic tests for a duodenal segment leak include CT cystogram and technetium-based nuclear cystogram. Cystoscopy should be performed in patients with recurrent urinary tract infections to evaluate the presence of sutures or foreign bodies acting as a nidus for infection. Severe recurrent hematuria, as well as urethritis (most commonly affecting males), may occur with bladder drainage. Finally, severe bicarbonate loss may be associated with bladder drainage, and some patients may have difficulty keeping up with the loss by oral bicarbonate replacement. All of the above situations can be effectively treated with enteric conversion

Textbook: Page 475 ANSWER: A, B, C, D, E.

39. Patient selection criteria for simultaneous pancreas-kidney transplantation should include:

A. Type I diabetes mellitus.
B. Type II diabetes mellitus.
C. Dialysis dependence.
D. Renal dysfunction with a creatinine value greater than 3.0.
E. Minimal extrarenal morbidity related to diabetes.

DISCUSSION: Simultaneous pancreas-kidney transplantation should be reserved for patients with Type I, juvenile, insulin-dependent diabetes mellitus. Although patients with Type II diabetes could potentially be helped, these older patients generally are not in good condition for simultaneous pancreas-kidney transplantation, nor are they reliably cured. In order to reliably monitor renal transplant function, the pretransplant creatinine value should be above 3, but the patient must not necessarily be on dialysis. To achieve good long-term results with pancreas-kidney transplantation it is appropriate to select patients with minimal extrarenal morbidity related to their diabetes.

Textbook: Pages 184, 473 ANSWER: A, D, E.

40. Criteria for a pancreas donor include:

A. No history of diabetes.
B. No liver donation.
C. No replaced hepatic artery vessels arising from the superior mesenteric artery (SMA).
D. No previous splenectomy.
E. No pancreatitis.

DISCUSSION: Combined liver-pancreas procurement should be routine, even if the right hepatic artery arises from the superior mesenteric artery. In this situation, since the transplanted liver is the life-saving organ, the proximal superior mesenteric artery should remain with the liver and the distal superior mesenteric artery supplying the head of the pancreas can be reconstructed on a Y-graft of iliac artery with the splenic artery. Successful pancreas transplantation can be performed using donors who have previously undergone splenectomy; however, there should be no significant pancreatitis and no history of diabetes in the donor.

Textbook: Pages 473–474 ANSWER: A, E.

41. For which of the following clinical scenarios would cardiac transplantation be an appropriate therapeutic modality?

A. A 50-year-old man with angina pectoris, three-vessel coronary artery disease, and a left ventricular ejection fraction of 25%.
B. A 75-year-old woman with irremediable heart failure secondary to critical aortic stenosis.
C. A 25-year-old male athlete with insidious onset of heart failure secondary to idiopathic dilated cardiomyopathy.
D. A 55-year-old woman who is status post two previous surgeries for coronary artery revascularization, now presenting with heart failure in the absence of angina, left ventricular ejection fraction of 15%, and insufficient target coronary arteries for a third bypass procedure.
E. A newborn infant with hypoplastic left heart syndrome and no other congenital anomalies.
F. A 30-year-old woman who develops irremediable heart failure due to postpartum cardiomyopathy after giving birth.

DISCUSSION: Scenarios *A* and *B* are not appropriate for cardiac transplantation. The patient in example *A* would be far better served by a conventional revascularization procedure such as coronary artery bypass grafting. The risk might be somewhat greater than normal because of his depressed left ventricular ejection fraction; however, cardiac transplantation is a therapy that is necessarily reserved for persons for whom no other procedure is available. That clearly is not the case in this example. In example *B*, despite the fact that this patient's disease might be benefited by cardiac transplantation, she is too old to withstand the rigors of this procedure and its attendant therapies. Examples, *C, D, E,* and *F,* all represent situations in which cardiac transplantation would be appropriate. In all these cases there is end-stage heart disease, and no other therapies are available that are likely to have any substantial benefit. Therefore, it is appropriate to consider cardiac transplantation for these patients, as a last resort.

Textbook: Page 478 ANSWER: C, D, E, F.

42. Suitable donors for heart transplantation have which of the following characteristics?

A. Normal electrocardiogram (ECG).
B. Normal echocardiogram.
C. Positive serology for HIV or hepatitis B or C.
D. Patient requiring high-dose epinephrine to maintain a systolic blood pressure of 90 mm. Hg.
E. Age over 70 years.

DISCUSSION: To be suitable for cardiac donation, individuals must have a normal ECG and a normal echocardiogram. Clearly, positive serologic tests for HIV or hepatitis B or C would render donors unsuitable for solid organ transplantation. Similarly, high-dose pressor support and age greater than 60 years, in most programs, contraindicate cardiac donation.

Textbook: Pages 478–479 ANSWER: A, B.

43. Heart-lung transplant is currently the therapy of choice for which of the following conditions?

A. Primary pulmonary hypertension with reasonably well-preserved right ventricular function.
B. Eisenmenger's syndrome due to single ventricle and truncus arteriosus.
C. Validated cardiomyopathy in a patient with cystic fibrosis and end-stage lung disease.
D. Cystic fibrosis and end-stage lung failure with normal heart function.
E. Eisenmenger's syndrome due to an atrial septal defect.
F. End-stage lung disease secondary to emphysema.

DISCUSSION: Heart-lung transplantation is now properly used only for persons with end-stage disease of the heart and lungs. Therefore, a patient with primary pulmonary hypertension and reasonably well-preserved right ventricular function is best treated with a single or bilateral lung transplant. A person with complex congenital heart disease and Eisenmenger's syndrome or one who has end-stage disease of the heart and lungs would be better treated with combined heart-lung transplantation. Patients with Eisenmenger's syndrome secondary to relatively straightforward defects (e.g., atrial septal defect, ventricular septal defect) are best treated with concomitant correction of the congenital defect and single or bilateral lung transplantation. Similarly, the patient with end-stage emphysema with normal heart function can be treated very well with single or bilateral lung transplantation, preserving the donor heart for someone who truly has heart failure.

Textbook: Pages 482–483 ANSWER: B, C.

44. Both single and bilateral lung transplantation are suitable technical alternatives for which of the following conditions?

A. Obstructive lung disease (chronic obstructive pulmonary disease, emphysema).
B. Restrictive lung disease (pulmonary fibrosis).
C. Primary pulmonary hypertension.
D. Cystic fibrosis.

DISCUSSION: Single-lung transplantation is inappropriate for cystic fibrosis or for any patient with chronic bilateral pulmonary sepsis. Leaving a septic native lung in situ in an immunocompromised patient would leave the patient at risk for local and systemic septic complications. Single-lung transplantation with contralateral pneumonectomy would be associated with a high risk of empyema in the pneumonectomy space and also disruption of the bronchial stump. Both single- and bilateral lung transplantation have been applied successfully in all of the other disease categories listed here.

Textbook: Pages 487–488 ANSWER: A, B, C.

45. Which of the following are contraindications to lung transplantation?

A. Age 65 years or older.
B. Current corticosteroid therapy.
C. History of thoracotomy.
D. Ventilator-dependent respiratory failure.

DISCUSSION: Single-lung transplantation is still offered up to age 65 years. Current low-dose corticosteroid therapy has not been demonstrated to lead to a higher risk of airway complications after lung transplantation. Advancements in operative technique have lessened the risk of surgery, so prior thoracotomy is no longer a contraindication to lung transplantation. However, patients with chronic ventilator-dependent respiratory failure who have no potential for cardiopulmonary rehabilitation currently are not accepted for evaluation for potential lung transplantation.

Textbook: Page 488 ANSWER: D.

46. Which of the following is the single most useful approach for diagnosing acute lung allograft rejection?

A. Clinical diagnosis.
B. Decline in spirometry and oxygenation.
C. Chest radiographic abnormalities.
D. Fiberoptic bronchoscopy with transbronchial lung biopsy.

DISCUSSION: Virtually all lung transplant patients experience at least one episode of acute rejection during their postoperative recovery in hospital. All of the approaches mentioned above are useful in leading to the diagnosis. Clinically, the patient experiences malaise and fever. There is also typically a slight decline in spirometry and arterial oxygenation. The chest radiograph typically shows a hilar or basal shadow; however, although these findings all suggest acute rejection, they are not specific. The one test with high specificity for detection of acute rejection is bronchoscopy with transbronchial lung biopsy.

Textbook: Pages 492–493 ANSWER: D.

47. Advantages of split-thickness skin grafts over full-thickness skin grafts include:

A. Split-thickness grafts include only part of the epidermis and none of the dermis.
B. Split-thickness grafts offer better pigment matching.
C. Split-thickness grafts offer better resistance to contraction.
D. Split-thickness grafts offer better resistance to infection.
E. Split-thickness grafts survive better on surfaces with compromised blood supply.

DISCUSSION: Split-thickness grafts include all of the epidermis but only a part of the dermis. Full-thickness skin grafts include all of both layers, so surgical closure of the donor wound is necessary whereas the portion of dermis left at the split-thickness skin donor site regenerates a skin covering. Because all layers of the skin are included in a full-thickness skin graft, pigment matching is better and less contraction occurs than with split-thickness grafts. Full-thickness grafts require a better blood supply for survival than the split-thickness grafts because the graft vessels are cut below the level of the dermal branching. Relatively fewer cut vessels are available to absorb nutrients from the wound bed to meet the relatively greater nutritional needs of the thicker graft. The poor resistance of full-thickness grafts to infection precludes their use on contaminated wounds, whereas split-thickness skin, which is more richly supplied with open blood vessels on its underside, is able to survive on compromised surfaces, including granulating wounds contaminated with bacteria.

Textbook: Pages 497–498 ANSWER: D, E.

48. The most commonly used substitutes for peripheral arteries are:

A. Dacron grafts.
B. Expanded polytetrafluoroethylene (Gore-Tex) grafts.
C. Internal, external, and/or common iliac artery autografts.
D. Bovine carotid artery xenografts.
E. Saphenous vein autografts.

DISCUSSION: The greater saphenous vein has proved to be the most satisfactory and most commonly used arterial substitute. The wall is sufficiently strong to withstand arterial pressures without becoming dilated or aneurysmal, yet is flexible and easily sutured. The diameter is sufficiently great to avoid thrombosis and nourishment is provided by the intraluminal blood flow. The smooth, natural endothelial lining is less thrombogenic than any known synthetic surface. The lining surface heals itself and may sequester white cells to fight infection, unlike Dacron grafts, which provide a haven for infecting organisms in the interstices of their synthetic fibers. Saphenous vein autografts heal even when placed into the infected bed of a previous synthetic graft.

Textbook: Pages 499–500 ANSWER: E.

49. Endocrine autografts were among the first successful transplantation procedures. The demonstration by Berkhold in 1849 that autotransplanted testes led to the acquisition of secondary sexual characteristics in castrated cocks marked the beginning of experimental endocrinology. Endocrine autografts used successfully in modern surgical practice include:

A. Adrenal medulla to the brain.
B. Thyroid to the forearm.
C. Parathyroid to the forearm.
D. Testicle to the scrotum.
E. Pancreatic islets to the liver.

DISCUSSION: The report in 1987 of open microsurgical autotransplantation of the adrenal medulla to the caudate nucleus of the brain for treatment of intractable Parkinson's disease aroused great interest in the topic. Subsequent multicenter trials showed improvement but not cure of the disease and substantial postoperative morbidity, so the technique was not recommended for widespread use. Excellent synthetic hormone replacement is available for thyroid insufficiency, so implantation of the thyroid gland in the forearm is not necessary. However, parathyroid hormone replacement is not available, and medical therapy for hypoparathyroidism is complicated. When parathyroid tissue is removed it should be autografted to prevent the deficiency symptoms of tetany, psychological disturbances, convulsions, coma and death. One-millimeter pieces may be implanted into pockets in the sternocleidomastoid muscle. When all glands are removed for diffuse parathyroid hyperplasia, implantation of fragments into the forearm muscles facilitates subsequent removal of more tissue under local anesthesia if hyperparathyroidism persists. Autotransplantation is the treatment of choice for undescended testes. The cryptorchid or ectopic testicle must be taken out of the abdomen and placed into a cooler location prior to age 6 (preferably at 1 year) for normal spermatogenesis to occur. Approximately half of the pancreatic islet transplants performed after pancreatectomy for relief of chronic pancreatitis pain have produced patients who are insulin independent. Islets for autotransplantation are difficult to isolate in sufficient quantities from the fibrotic adult pancreas. Dispersed islets injected directly into the human portal vein have occasionally produced untoward effects such as disseminated intravascular coagulation, portal hypertension, and even hepatic necrosis.

Textbook: Pages 500–501 ANSWER: C, D, E.

50. Several types of gastrointestinal autografts have been used to replace the esophagus after extirpation of carcinomas. Successful reconstructions have been achieved most frequently with:

A. Stomach.
B. Jejunum.
C. Ileum.
D. Ascending colon.
E. Descending colon.

DISCUSSION: Although all of the listed bowel segments have been used successfully for reconstruction of the esophagus following removal of carcinomas, the stomach remains the most frequently used autograft for esophageal reconstruction. Because of its excellent blood supply the procedure can be performed at little risk as a single operation and achieve satisfactory long-term relief of dysphasia in at least 90% of patients. Either the entire stomach can be drawn into the chest or a gastric tube created in an isoperistaltic or antiperistaltic manner of sufficient length to reconstruct the entire esophagus. The advantages of a mucosal lining, serosal covering, natural opening into the stomach, and excellent blood supply based on the gastroepiploic vessels make the stomach the autograft of choice in most situations.

Textbook: Pages 502–504 ANSWER: A.

NOTES

NOTES

CHAPTER 8

SURGICAL ONCOLOGY: THE BREAST (with Reconstructive and Aesthetic Breast Surgery)

1. Cytotoxic T cells (CTL) are capable of recognizing:

A. Peptide antigens associated with major histocompatibility complex (MHC) molecules.
B. Membrane-bound antigens.
C. Cytoplasmic antigens.
D. Nuclear antigens.
E. All of the above.

DISCUSSION: It was long thought that CTL recognize antigen expressed on the surface of the target cell destined to be killed, similar to the recognition of an antigen by an antibody; however, it was found that the mechanism of CTL recognition of antigens was fundamentally different from the mechanism of antibody recognition. CTL can detect antigens derived from cell surface–associated proteins, but in addition can recognize proteins that are normally in the cytoplasm or in the nucleus. In fact, the normal location of the protein can be anywhere within the cell.

To understand how a CTL can distinguish an antigen from a protein that is normally located within the cytoplasm or nucleus of the cell, investigators had to determine exactly what was being recognized by the CTL. T cells were found to recognize short linear fragments of processed or even denatured protein. It was found that proteins that were synthesized endogenously were degraded within the cytoplasm into 9– or 10–amino acid long peptides. These peptides were then transported to the endocytoplasmic reticulum and associated with newly synthesized MHC class I molecules. Certain peptides could fit within the MHC class I molecule and were then transported to the cell surface as a complex. It was this complex, consisting of a 9– to 10–amino acid peptide within a MHC class I molecule that was presented to, and recognized by, CD8+ CTL.

Textbook: Page 508 ANSWER: E.

2. Adoptive immunotherapy with lymphokine activated killer cells (LAK) and tumor infiltrate (TIL) cells are characterized by:

A. Nonspecific stimulation of effector cells.
B. Expansion *ex vivo* of large numbers of lymphocytes.
C. Infusion with interleukin 2 (IL-2).
D. Significant toxicity at high doses.
E. All of the above.

DISCUSSION: LAK cells, generated by short-term culture of peripheral blood lymphocytes in the presence of high concentrations of IL-2, lyse transformed target cells, and have minimal lytic activity for most normal tissues. Up to 10^{11} *in vitro* generated LAK cells have been administered in a single intravenous infusion to cancer patients. Therapeutic trials have also combined short courses of high-dose systemic IL-2 administration with LAK cell transfer to promote LAK function and viability, with apparently enhanced efficacy. The shortcomings of LAK and IL-2 therapy included a larger degree of toxicity (including pulmonary, renal, and hepatobiliary) with a significant proportion of patients requiring intensive care unit admissions and 2% to 5% treatment-related mortality. Despite this, response rate remained relatively low.

Another therapy using *in vitro* expanded lymphocytes derived from a TIL has been evaluated in clinical trials. In humans, TIL cell lines have been generated by mincing tumor specimens and culturing eluted lymphocytes with high concentrations of IL-2. TIL lines can be expanded to 10^8 to 10^{11} cells over 3 to 8 weeks in culture, and some lines appear to function as T cells with lytic specificity for autologous—but not allogeneic—tumor targets, whereas others function as LAK cells and lyse both autologous and allogeneic tumor targets. Adoptive transfer of 5×10^{10} TIL alone has not been associated with significant toxicity, and administration of 5×10^{10} TIL cells with concurrent systemic IL-2 has caused toxicities that are attributable to the IL-2.

Textbook: Page 510 ANSWER: E.

3. Previous clinical studies with cancer vaccines have:

A. Clearly demonstrated induction of tumor-specific immune response.
B. Repeatedly demonstrated clinical response to large tumor burden.

C. Not clearly demonstrated induction of tumor-specific immune response.
D. Not been performed to date.

DISCUSSION: Several different approaches in experimental animal studies in the 1970s formed the basis for human clinical trials of SAI against human cancers. Although several thousand patients have been injected with a variety of tumor cell preparations in this country and elsewhere during the past 25 years, the complexity of the studies has made it difficult to definitively assess the value of this approach to cancer therapy. Nonetheless, a number of clinical trials have suggested a therapeutic benefit of SAI. Most of these trials have two features in common: (1) a therapeutic effect was not seen or, if seen, has not been confirmed independently; and (2) no acceptable information was provided on the presence of tumor antigens in the vaccines and the immune response of patients to these antigens.

Textbook: Pages 511–512 ANSWER: C.

4. Which of the following statements is/are true of the epidemiology and etiology of melanoma?

A. Most patients are diagnosed after age 60 years.
B. Skin color has no association with risk of melanoma.
C. Sun exposure is the only risk factor for melanoma.
D. The per capita incidence of melanoma is highest in Australia.

DISCUSSION: The median age at diagnosis is in the late forties; so, a minority of patients are diagnosed after age 60. The risk of melanoma is closely tied to skin color: Caucasians are at highest risk, and those with a Celtic complexion at even higher risk. Australia has a large Celtic population living near the equator, and it has the highest per capita incidence of melanoma in the world. Sun exposure is believed to be an important cause of melanoma, but the data remain incomplete. Some melanomas arise in sites not exposed to the sun (e.g., mucous membranes), so sun exposure is not the only risk factor.

Textbook: Pages 515–516 ANSWER: D.

5. Which of the following variables best predicts prognosis for patients with a recent diagnosis of cutaneous melanoma and no clinical evidence of metastatic disease?

A. Breslow thickness.
B. Clark's level.
C. Ulceration.
D. Gender.
E. Celtic complexion.

DISCUSSION: The prognosis for melanoma is best predicted by the thickness, measured in millimeters (Breslow thickness). Clark's level and ulceration are also predictive, but less so. Gender is a secondary prognostic factor. Skin color may have a mild impact on outcome, but it is primarily a risk factor for developing melanoma.

Textbook: Pages 519–520 ANSWER: A.

6. A 38-year-old man presents with a melanoma on the skin of the right calf measuring 5 mm. in thickness. Several large nodes are palpable in the right inguinal region. Which of the following statements about the appropriate management of this clinical problem is false?

A. In the absence of systemic disease, the primary melanoma of the right calf should be excised with at least a 2-cm. margin.
B. Complete right inguinal node dissection should be performed if there is no evidence of systemic metastasis.
C. If further work-up reveals multiple lung metastases of melanoma, they should be excised as soon as possible.
D. Chemotherapy for melanoma is primarily palliative; so surgical therapy is preferred if there is no evidence of metastastic disease beyond the inguinal region.
E. If the nodes do not contain metastatic disease but are simply reactive, the chance of 5-year survival is 50% or less.

DISCUSSION: This patient should be evaluated with computed tomography in addition to a careful history, review of systems, and physical examination. If there is no evidence of metastatic disease beyond the inguinal region, therapy should focus on the local and regional disease. The primary lesion should be excised with a 2- to 3-cm. margin. The enlarged nodes can be evaluated by fine-needle aspiration (FNA) or node excision. If the FNA or excisional biopsy does show metastatic melanoma, then complete inguinal node dissection should be performed. Alternatively, complete node dissection can be justified simply on the basis of clinical findings. Chemotherapy does not provide any significant chance of cure, whereas a significant proportion of patients with isolated nodal metastases will live long. The depth of the primary lesion would predict chances of 5-year survival at less than 50%, even if the nodes are not metastatic. If work-up does reveal multiple pulmonary nodules, chemotherapy or experimental systemic therapies should be considered. Surgery has no role in the therapy of multiple lung metastases of melanoma.

Textbook: Pages 522–523 ANSWER: C.

7. A 42-year-old woman presents with an 8 cm. × 6 cm. × 4 cm. mass in the posterior thigh. Incisional biopsy reveals a high-grade liposarcoma. Her management should include:

A. High thigh amputation.
B. Extracompartment excision with negative margins.
C. Complete excision with negative margins.
D. Adjuvant radiation therapy.
E. Adjuvant chemotherapy.

DISCUSSION: This is a common presentation of soft tissue sarcoma. Surgery remains the principal modality for curative therapy for all soft tissue sarcomas. Provided the entire tumor is removed, less radical procedures have not been demonstrated to adversely affect local recurrence or outcome. The surgical objective is complete removal of the tumor with negative margins and maximal preservation of function. Adjuvant radiation improves local control. Adjuvant chemotherapy has not proven to be efficacious.

Textbook: Pages 530–531 ANSWER: C, D.

8. Biologic features of adult soft tissue sarcomas include the following:

A. Mutations of *p53* in metastatic liposarcoma.
B. A low (less than 1%) risk of metastasis for small, low-grade lesions.
C. Recurrent disease in at least 33% of patients.
D. Lymph node metastasis in less than 3% of patients.
E. Mutations of *p53* in Li-Fraumeni syndrome.

DISCUSSION: Inactivation of the *p53* tumor suppressor gene is involved in tumorigenesis of several sarcomas, but not specifically liposarcoma. The relevance of this gene is underscored by the frequent occurrence of soft tissue sarcomas in the Li-Fraumeni syndrome, where all families studied have *p53* germ line mutations. Low-grade lesions have a low (less than 1%) risk of subsequent metastasis, whereas high-grade lesions have a high (greater than 50%) risk of subsequent metastasis. Despite optimal multimodality treatment, at least 33% of patients develop recurrent disease (median disease-free interval 18 months). Lymph node metastasis occur in fewer than 3% of adult soft tissue sarcomas.

Textbook: Pages 528, 530–532 ANSWER: B, C, D, E.

9. Which of the following statements describes an ideal tumor marker?

A. The ideal tumor marker should be tumor specific; that is, in the normal population or patients with benign diseases, false-positive test results are rare.
B. The ideal marker must have a low false-negative rate; that means that all patients with a particular type of cancer should test positive.
C. The circulating level of an ideal tumor marker should correlate directly with the amount of viable tumor and be a measure of the response to therapy.
D. The ideal tumor marker should act as a prognostic indicator.
E. All of the above.

DISCUSSION: Each of the above is a criterion for an ideal tumor marker.

Textbook: Page 534 ANSWER: E.

10. A marker for the diagnosis of pancreatic cancer is:

A. CA 15-3.
B. CA 19-9.
C. Alphafetoprotein (AFP).
D. Carcinoembryonic antigen (CEA).
E. CYFRA 21-1.

DISCUSSION: CA 15-3 is a marker for breast cancer. AFP is a marker for hepatocellular and testicular cancer. CEA is a marker for colon cancer. CYFRA 21-1 is a marker for non–small-cell lung cancer. CA 19-9 is a marker for pancreatic cancer.

Textbook: Page 539 ANSWER: B.

11. Which of the following tumors may cause elevated CEA levels?

A. Breast cancer.
B. Colorectal cancer.
C. Gastric cancer.
D. Lung cancer.
E. All of the above.

DISCUSSION: CEA is relatively nonspecific, and each of the listed cancers can cause elevated levels of CEA.

Textbook: Pages 535–536 ANSWER: E.

12. The presence of which marker is a significant poor prognosis variable for patients with breast cancer:

A. CEA.
B. C-*erb* B-2.
C. AFP.
D. Human chorionic gonadotropin (hCG).
E. RB-1.

DISCUSSION: Some 20% to 30% of breast cancers have C-*erb* B-2 gene expression. Studies have demonstrated that it is an independent prognostic tumor marker. Tumors that express C-*erb* B-2 have a poorer prognosis.

Textbook: Page 549 ANSWER: B.

13. The most useful circulating marker for patients with hepatocellular carcinoma is:

A. CA 50.
B. Levels of vitamin B_{12}.
C. CEA.
D. AFP.
E. hCG.

DISCUSSION: Eighty percent of patients with hepatocellular carcinoma have elevated serum levels of AFP.

Textbook: Pages 536–537 ANSWER: D.

14. In patients with colorectal cancer the serum CEA level is a clinically useful measure for all reasons except:

A. Prognosis.
B. Detection of recurrence.
C. Guiding second-look operations.
D. Following treatment response.
E. Early diagnosis.

DISCUSSION: CEA levels may be used for each of the indications except early diagnosis.

Textbook: Pages 543–545 ANSWER: E.

15. Which serum markers are useful in the management of patients with testicular cancer?

A. hCG.
B. AFP.

C. CA 15-3.
D. Two of the above.
E. None of the above.

DISCUSSION: AFP and hCG are useful in managing testicular cancer. Approximately 90% of patients with testicular cancer have elevated levels of one or both of these markers.

Textbook: Pages 545–546 ANSWER: D.

16. Which tumor marker is useful for the management of patients with breast cancer?

A. CA 125.
B. Inhibin.
C. CA 19-9.
D. CA 15-3.
E. CEA.

DISCUSSION: CA 15-3 is the only useful marker for patients with breast cancer. Approximately 73% of patients with breast cancer have elevated levels.

Textbook: Page 549 ANSWER: D.

17. A new marker that has possible utility in the management of patients with non–small-cell lung cancer (NSCLC) is:

A. Calcitonin.
B. Neuron-specific enolase.
C. CYFRA 21-1.
D. Glucagon.
E. Chromogranin A.

DISCUSSION: CYFRA 21-1 is a new marker for non–small-cell lung cancer (NSCLC). Approximately 40% to 50% of patients with NSCLC will have elevated levels.

Textbook: Page 549 ANSWER: C.

18. A circulating marker that may be useful in the management of patients with any neuroendocrine tumor is:

A. Chromogranin A.
B. Neuron-specific enolase.
C. hCG.
D. Two of the above.
E. None of the above.

DISCUSSION: Although most endocrine tumors have a specific marker hormone that is the mainstay of diagnosis, both chromogranin A and neuron-specific enolase may be useful as serum markers in patients with all types of neuroendocrine tumors.

Textbook: Pages 550, 552 ANSWER: D.

19. After intraductal papilloma, unilateral bloody nipple discharge from one duct orifice is most commonly caused by which of the following pathologic conditions?

A. Paget's disease of the nipple.
B. Intraductal carcinoma.
C. Inflammatory carcinoma.
D. Subareolar mastitis.

DISCUSSION: Nipple discharge is surgically significant when it is grossly bloody and when it appears at a single duct orifice on one nipple. Bloody discharge is usually due to a benign intraductal papilloma; however, intraductal carcinoma in the large ducts under the nipple can be the cause of bloody discharge, and pathologically the lesion is frequently a large papillary tumor that has become malignant. Paget's disease of the nipple is also due to intraductal carcinoma arising in subareolar ducts, but it rarely is associated with nipple discharge. Subareolar mastitis may produce nipple discharge, but it is purulent and not bloody. Inflammatory carcinoma is not associated with nipple discharge.

Textbook: Pages 559–560 ANSWER: B.

20. Which of the following conditions is associated with increased risk of breast cancer?

A. Fibrocystic mastopathy.
B. Severe hyperplasia.
C. Atypical hyperplasia.
D. Papillomatosis.

DISCUSSION: Fibrocystic mastopathy, or fibrocystic disease, was once thought to increase the risk of breast cancer; however, later studies of the pathologic findings in fibrocystic complex found an increased cancer risk only for patients whose biopsies showed atypical hyperplasia. "Severe hyperplasia" is a pathologic term that refers to the amount of hyperplasia and is frequently seen in the biopsy specimens of young women; it is a misleading term and is not associated with a disease risk. Papillomatosis is also part of the fibrocystic complex and is a frequent finding in benign breast biopsies; it does not confer an increased risk of cancer.

Textbook: Pages 561–562 ANSWER: C.

21. Which of the following breast lesions are noninvasive malignancies?

A. Intraductal carcinoma of the comedo type.
B. Tubular carcinoma and mucinous carcinoma.
C. Infiltrating ductal carcinoma and lobular carcinoma.
D. Medullary carcinoma, including atypical medullary lesions.

DISCUSSION: Tubular, mucinous, and medullary carcinomas are histologic variants of infiltrating ductal cancer and are all invasive malignancies. Infiltrating lobular cancer is a particular histologic variant of invasive breast cancer characterized by permeation of the stroma with small cells that resemble those found in the breast lobule or acinus. Intraductal carcinoma refers to a malignancy of ductal origin that remains enclosed within duct structures. This noninvasive proliferation can undergo central necrosis, which frequently calcifies to form the microcalcifications seen on mammography. The central necrosis within enlarged and back-to-back ductal structures resembles comedoes and gives rise to the term "comedocarcinoma," now reserved for this histologic variety of intraductal carcinoma.

Textbook: Pages 561, 569–572 ANSWER: A.

22. Which of the following are the most important and clinically useful risk factors for breast cancer?

A. Fibrocystic disease, age, and gender.
B. Cysts, family history in immediate relatives, and gender.
C. Age, gender, and family history in immediate relatives.
D. Obesity, nulliparity, and alcohol use.

DISCUSSION: The most important risk factors for breast cancer are the patient's age, gender, and a family history of breast cancer in immediate relatives (sisters, mother, daughter). The age-adjusted incidence of breast cancer increases with age. Breast cancer does occur in males, but the disease is far more common in women. Family history is important when breast cancer occurs within the immediate family; history of breast cancer in more distant relatives (grandmothers, cousins, aunts) is less important. In addition, age factors into the risk associated with family history. An affected young primary relative is far more significant as a risk factor than an older relative with breast cancer. The other important risk factor not listed here is a history of breast cancer, either within the conserved ipsilateral breast or in the contralateral breast. Again, age plays an important modifying role; as the age at which breast cancer was first diagnosed increases, the risk of a subsequent second cancer decreases. Although patients with fibrocystic disease are at increased risk for breast cancer, risk concentrates in those patients with fibrocystic disease who show atypical epithelial hyperplasia within breast ducts. Obesity, nulliparity, and alcohol all appear to increase risk slightly and are important to the epidemiologic study of breast cancer; however, the effect of these factors is not sufficient to warrant their use in common clinical practice.

Textbook: Pages 561–562 ANSWER: C.

23. Which of the following pathologic findings is the strongest contraindication to breast preservation (lumpectomy with breast radiation) as primary treatment for a newly diagnosed breast cancer?

A. Grade 3, poorly differentiated, infiltrating ductal carcinoma.
B. Extensive intraductal cancer around the invasive lesion.
C. Tumor size greater than 3 cm.
D. Positive surgical margin for invasive cancer.

DISCUSSION: The only firm contraindication to wide excision and radiation (breast preservation, lumpectomy) as the primary surgical treatment for a newly discovered breast cancer is the inability to achieve an uninvolved surgical margin after excision of the tumor. A positive surgical margin requires, at least, reoperation with an attempt at re-excision of the cancer. If the margin of removal is positive after attempts at re-excision, this is a strong reason to recommend mastectomy in preference to breast conservation. Tumor size is a relative contraindication when the cancer is so large in relation to the breast that excision to a clean surgical margin seems unreasonable. Other histologic findings, such as tumor grade or vascular invasion, are not strong reasons to recommend mastectomy if the patient would prefer breast conservation.

Textbook: Pages 575–576 ANSWER: D.

24. Axillary lymph node dissection is routinely used for all of the following conditions except:

A. 2-cm. pure comedo-type intraductal carcinoma.
B. 1-cm. infiltrating lobular carcinoma.
C. 8-mm. infiltrating ductal carcinoma.
D. A pure medullary cancer in the upper inner quadrant.

DISCUSSION: Intraductal carcinoma is carcinoma *in situ* and does not metastasize to regional or distant sites. Lymph node dissection is not routinely required for a pure *in situ* cancer of the breast. In contrast, all of the other cancers listed above (infiltrating lobular, infiltrating ductal, and medullary carcinoma) are invasive malignancies that are capable of nodal and distant metastasis. Lymph node dissection is commonly recommended for these invasive malignancies. Intraductal lesions that have grown larger than 5 cm. are more apt to have become focally invasive. Since this invasive component might be missed histologically, many surgeons advocate selective use of axillary node dissection for large intraductal lesions, particularly high-grade tumors such as the comedo variant. However, a purely intraductal 2-cm. cancer would most likely be treated without performing node dissection.

Textbook: Pages 559–560 ANSWER: A.

25. Failure to perform radiation after wide excision of an invasive cancer risks which of the following outcomes?

A. Recurrence of cancer in the ipsilateral breast.
B. Shorter survival time.
C. Regional nodal recurrence.
D. Greater chance of breast cancer mortality.

DISCUSSION: Retrospective reviews and prospective surgical trials agree that omission of breast radiation after wide excision leads to a higher rate of ipsilateral breast recurrence. However, survival and the risk of distant disease are not altered in patients treated by excision alone, within the follow-up time of the studies and given their inherent power to detect differences in outcome. Regional node metastasis is not affected by the choice of mastectomy versus wide excision and radiation.

Textbook: Pages 577–578 ANSWER: A.

26. Which of the following treatments should never be recommended to a patient with purely intraductal carcinoma?

A. Modified radical mastectomy.
B. Lumpectomy to clear surgical margins, followed by observation.
C. Incisional biopsy with an involved margin, followed by radiation.
D. Excisional biopsy to clear margins, followed by radiation.

DISCUSSION: The treatment approach to intraductal carcinoma depends on the extent of the disease, its multifocality, and the involvement of the surgical margin. For extensive disease, modified radical mastectomy is appropriate, particularly if there is a great likelihood of occult invasive disease, making axillary dissection logical. For small foci of disease excised to clear surgical margins, observation is an acceptable recommendation to a well-informed patient. Several noncontrolled reviews and the National Surgical Adjuvant Breast and Bowel Project (NSABP) trial for intraductal disease would indicate a greater chance of ipsilateral breast recurrence for lumpectomy only; however, the magnitude of the risk is small, and survival is excellent and unaffected. The only mode of treatment that cannot be recommended for routine management is leaving residual disease in the breast and treating only with radiation.

Textbook: Pages 569–570, 576–580 ANSWER: C.

27. The proper treatment for lobular carcinoma *in situ* (LCIS) includes which of the following components?

A. Close follow-up.
B. Radiation after excision.
C. Mirror-image biopsy of the opposite breast.
D. Mastectomy and regional node dissection.

DISCUSSION: LCIS is best thought of as a precursor lesion that confers increased risk for eventual cancer. The magnitude of this risk appears to be in the range of seven- to ninefold over baseline risk. The chance of breast cancer is equal in both breasts, not just in the biopsied breast, and the type of cancer is not confined to a lobular histology. After a diagnosis of LCIS, patients are at increased risk for invasive and noninvasive ductal carcinoma in both breasts. Therefore, mirror-image biopsy as practiced in the past has little to offer. Since LCIS is purely noninvasive, nodal dissection is not required if mastectomy is chosen. There are no data on the use of breast radiation therapy for LCIS. Most surgical oncologists recommend close follow-up for patients who have LCIS only; the alternative surgical treatment that makes most sense is bilateral simple mastectomies, with or without reconstruction.

Textbook: Pages 570, 583–584 ANSWER: A.

28. Which of the following statements most accurately reflects the findings of large overview analyses of clinical trials in which adjuvant chemotherapy for early-stage breast cancer was compared to a control group treated only with surgery?

A. The benefit of adjuvant therapy is confined to young patients.
B. Adjuvant therapy benefits all patients and is independent of age or node status.
C. Adjuvant therapy does not work in estrogen-positive patients.
D. The magnitude of benefit is very large.

DISCUSSION: An overview analysis (meta-analysis) examined nearly all randomized clinical trials in which chemotherapy after surgery was compared to surgery alone for treatment of early-stage breast cancer. This examination of the world's published literature revealed that the magnitude of benefit (the reduction in the odds of recurrence) from chemotherapy was relatively small and in the range of a 20% reduction in the chance of recurrence or death; however, this benefit extended to patients of all ages (young and older) and to both node-positive and node-negative patients. The value of adjuvant chemotherapy does not depend on the hormone receptor content of the cancer. It is useful to remember that a constant reduction in the odds of recurrence results in a higher absolute benefit as the prognosis worsens. If the chance of recurrence is 50% (for node-positive groups) the absolute reduction will be in the range of 10% or 15%. In contrast, if the recurrence rate is 10%, the absolute difference between treated and control groups will be less than 5%. This means that many patients need to be exposed to the risks and side effects of chemotherapy to benefit a very small number. This kind of thinking is currently used to decide who should receive adjuvant chemotherapy after primary treatment (mastectomy or lumpectomy).

Textbook: Pages 586–587 ANSWER: B.

29. Which of the following statements are true about reconstruction of the breast following mastectomy?

A. A permanent prosthesis or tissue expander may be inserted at the time of the ablative surgery.
B. If the patient requires adjuvant chemotherapy or radiation therapy, reconstruction of the breast is delayed until completion of the treatment.
C. Extensive postmastectomy defects require the use of a flap.

DISCUSSION: Reconstruction can be initiated at the time of the ablative surgery, using a 6-cm. slightly curved incision at the level of the sixth rib through the serratus muscle. A pocket is created beneath the serratus and pectoralis major muscles, extending medially to the perforating internal mammary vessels and inferiorly beneath the fascial insertion of the rectus abdominis muscle. A tissue expander prosthesis is inserted into the pocket. If the patient requires adjuvant chemotherapy or radiation therapy, reconstruction of the breast is delayed until treatment is completed and an adequate recovery period has passed. If the quantity or quality of the chest skin or the pectoralis major muscle is insufficient, tissue must be brought in from adjacent areas. A latissimus dorsi musculocutaneous flap may be transferred on its blood supply via the thoracodorsal artery and vein. Extensive postmastectomy defects necessitate the use of the larger rectus abdominis musculocutaneous flap, which is based on the superior epigastric vessels. A "free" microvascular rectus abdominis or other myocutaneous flaps may be used. The thoracodorsal or anterior serratus vessels can usually be anastomosed to the inferior epigastric vessels of the rectus abdominis flap.

Textbook: Pages 595–597 ANSWER: A, B, C.

30. Which of the following statements are true about the management of mammary hyperplasia?

A. Reduction mammaplasty can be performed only on women younger than 40 years.
B. Removal of breast tissue to reduce size of the breast is usually predicated on the use of a nipple, areola, and dermal pedicle flap.
C. If removal of 2000 gm. of breast tissue is needed, breast amputation with immediate free nipple-areola grafting is performed.

DISCUSSION: Reduction mammaplasty can be performed at any age. Because of the increased weight of the breast considerable shoulder and back pain, accompanied by excoriation of the skin in the inframammary area and the shoulders, can occur. Older women frequently seek relief from these problems, which can be resolved by a reduction mammaplasty. The reduction in breast volume is usually accomplished by moving the nipple and areola on a dermal pedicle flap. The flap can be based inferiorly, medially, superiorly, laterally, vertically, or horizontally. It is possible to remove up to 3000 gm. of breast tissue utilizing a pyramidal-based breast flap with an inferior dermal nipple-areola pedicle since the blood supply to the tissues is preserved by this technique. Breast reduction involving removal of more than 3000 gm. requires a breast amputation technique with immediate free nipple grafting.

Textbook: Page 594 ANSWER: B, C.

NOTES

NOTES

NOTES

CHAPTER 9

ENDOCRINE DISORDERS

1. When progressive enlargement of a multinodular goiter causes symptomatic tracheal compression, the preferred management in otherwise good-risk patients is:

A. Iodine treatment.
B. Thyroid hormone treatment.
C. Surgical resection of the abnormal thyroid.
D. Radioactive iodine treatment.

DISCUSSION: When a multinodular goiter enlarges enough to cause symptoms of tracheal compression, surgical treatment is usually required if the patient is considered a reasonable operative risk. Medical treatment may be effective in preventing the initial growth of the goiter but is unlikely to cause enough regression to relieve symptoms. Radioactive iodine can occasionally be used to cause some regression in patients who are poor anesthesia risks, but this is a temporizing treatment rather than a definitive one.
Textbook: Page 628 ANSWER: C.

2. The most precise diagnostic screening procedure for differentiating benign thyroid nodules from malignant ones is:

A. Thyroid ultrasonography.
B. Thyroid scintiscan.
C. Fine-needle-aspiration biopsy (FNAB).
D. Thyroid hormone suppression.

DISCUSSION: Analysis of multiple series in which patients with thyroid nodules have undergone FNAB has demonstrated a false-negative rate of 2.4% and a false-positive rate of 3.3%. Sensitivity for this method is 92%; specificity 74%. This surpasses the other methods for accurate selection of patients who require surgical resection.
Textbook: Page 632 ANSWER: C.

3. The preferred operation for initial management of a thyroid nodule that is considered suspicious for malignancy by FNAB is:

A. Excision.
B. Partial lobectomy.
C. Total lobectomy and isthmusectomy.
D. Total thyroidectomy.

DISCUSSION: There is a consensus that the initial minimum operation for a nodule suspected to be malignant is total lobectomy and isthmusectomy. Partial lobectomy or excision of the nodule is associated with a higher risk of local recurrence if the nodule proves to be malignant. Reoperation on the side of a partial lobectomy can be technically difficult and associated with a higher risk of recurrent nerve injury. Ordinarily, total thyroidectomy is not performed until a conclusive diagnosis of malignancy is established.
Textbook: Pages 634–635 ANSWER: C.

4. Advantages of total thyroidectomy for management of papillary carcinomas of the thyroid larger than 1.5 cm. include:

A. Possibility of using radioactive iodine postoperatively to identify and treat metastases.
B. The ability to use thyroglobulin levels as a marker for recurrence.
C. Lower overall recurrence rate.
D. Lower risk of hypoparathyroidism.

DISCUSSION: Following total thyroidectomy iodine 131 can be used more efficiently because of the absence of normal thyroid tissue, which has greater affinity for iodine than papillary carcinoma tissue. When all normal thyroid tissue is removed, serum thyroglobulin, which is produced by normal and malignant thyroid tissue, becomes a more effective marker for recurrence. The overall recurrence rate is lower for patients undergoing total thyroidectomy, but the risk of hypoparathyroidism is higher for patients who have total thyroidectomy instead of unilateral lobectomy.
Textbook: Pages 634–635 ANSWER: A, B, C.

5. Which of the following statements about follicular carcinoma is/are true?

A. It presents at a later age than papillary carcinoma.
B. It disseminates via hematogenous routes.
C. It is the most common type of well-differentiated thyroid carcinoma.
D. Extensive angioinvasion portends a poor prognosis.
E. Follicular carcinomas are frequently multicentric.

DISCUSSION: Follicular carcinoma is more common in older patients (peak incidence in the fifth decade). The tumor has a marked propensity for vascular invasion and spreads hematogenously to bone, lung, liver, and central nervous system sites. Local nodal metastases are less common than in papillary carcinoma. Extensive angioinvasion indicates a less favorable prognosis. Papillary carcinoma is the most common type of well-differentiated thyroid carcinomas. Follicular carcinomas are rarely multicentric.

Textbook: Page 635 ANSWER: A, B, D.

6. A familial form of medullary thyroid carcinoma (MTC) should be suspected whenever:

A. The tumor is multifocal.
B. The tumor is bilateral (foci of tumor are present in both thyroid lobes).
C. Pathologic examination of the resected thyroid gland reveals the presence of C-cell hyperplasia in areas of the gland adjacent to foci of MTC.
D. All of the above.

DISCUSSION: Sporadic MTC is unilateral in at least 80% of cases. However, in patients with MTC occurring as a component of the multiple endocrine neoplasia (MEN) type 2A or type 2B syndromes, the tumor is virtually always multifocal and bilateral. Typically, in this setting the MTC appears as multiple whitish-tan tumor nodules in the middle and upper thirds of each thyroid lobe.

A diffuse premalignant proliferation of the C cells of the thyroid is thought to precede the development of MTC in patients with familial MTC. This proliferation, known as *C-cell hyperplasia* (CCH), consists of parafollicular clusters of increased numbers of C cells. The finding of CCH in areas of the thyroid adjacent to gross foci of MTC is strong evidence for familial MTC.

Textbook: Pages 639–642 ANSWER: D.

7. All of the following are components of the MEN type 2B syndrome except:

A. Multiple neuromas on the lips, tongue, and oral mucosa.
B. Hyperparathyroidism.
C. MTC.
D. Pheochromocytoma.

DISCUSSION: MTC and pheochromocytoma occur in both MEN 2A and MEN 2B syndromes. Patients with MEN 2A may also develop hyperplasia of the parathyroid glands. Although some investigators have reported equivocal histologic abnormalities in the parathyroid glands of patients with MEN 2B, hyperparathyroidism is not a component of this syndrome.

In contrast to patients with MEN 2A, those with MEN 2B have a characteristic phenotype, including a tall, thin "marfanoid" habitus. Patients with MEN 2B also develop multiple neuromas on the lips, tongue, and oral mucosa, creating the appearance of thick lips.

Textbook: Pages 640–641 ANSWER: B.

8. MEN 2A and MEN 2B syndromes are associated with germline mutations in:

A. The p53 tumor suppressor gene.
B. The H-*ras* gene.
C. The N-*myc* gene.
D. The *RET* proto-oncogene.

DISCUSSION: Germline mutations in the *RET* proto-oncogene, a receptor tyrosine kinase that maps to chromosome 10, are associated with MEN 2A and MEN 2B syndromes. Homozygous loss of the tumor suppressor gene p53 is associated with the Li-Fraumeni syndrome, and mutations of p53 are present in a variety of human neoplasms. Point mutations in the H-*ras* gene are associated with carcinoma of the colon, lung, and pancreas. Amplification of the N-*myc* gene, when present in neuroblastoma, suggests a poorer prognosis.

Textbook: Page 640 ANSWER: D.

9. Which of the following are true concerning islet cell neoplasms of the pancreas in patients with MEN type 1?

A. Islet cell neoplasms in patients with MEN 1 are characteristically multicentric.
B. The most common islet cell neoplasm in patients with MEN 1 is gastrinoma.
C. Islet cell neoplasms in patients with MEN 1 may be malignant.
D. All of the above.

DISCUSSION: The pathologic change in the pancreas of patients with MEN 1 is typically multicentric. Diffuse hyperplasia of islet cells and microadenoma formation are often identified in areas of the gland distant from grossly evident tumor. Tumors are commonly multifocal. Islet cell neoplasms of the pancreas occur in 30% to 80% of patients with MEN 1. The most common islet cell neoplasm in these patients is gastrinoma. Gastrinomas associated with MEN 1 probably account for 20% to 50% of all cases of the Zollinger-Ellison syndrome. The second most common islet cell tumor is insulinoma. Other pancreatic islet cell neoplasms, such as glucagonoma, somatostatinoma, or vasoactive intestinal polypeptide neoplasm (VIPoma), are rarely associated with MEN 1. Approximately 10% of insulinomas and approximately 15% or more of gastrinomas in patients with MEN 1 are malignant.

Textbook: Pages 638–639 ANSWER: D.

10. Which of the following statements about the differential diagnosis of hypercalcemia is/are correct.

A. Malignant tumors typically cause hypercalcemia by ectopic production of parathyroid hormone (PTH).
B. The diagnosis of primary hyperparathyroidism is supported by these serum levels: calcium, 10.8 mg. per dl.; chloride, 104 mmol. per liter; bicarbonate 21 mmol. per liter; phosphorus, 2.4 mg. per dl.; elevated parathyroid hormone.
C. Familial hypocalciuric hypercalcemia is

distinguished from primary hyperparathyroidism by parathyroid imaging.

D. Although serum albumin binds calcium, the measured total calcium value is usually unaffected in patients with severe hypoproteinemia.

E. Thiazide diuretics are a good treatment for hypercalcemia and can be given to patients with apparent hypercalcemia of malignancy.

DISCUSSION: Malignant tumors rarely secrete PTH itself; they can secrete PTHrP or cytokine activators of osteoclast activity. The diagnosis of primary hyperparathyroidism is supported by hypercalcemia with mild hyperchloremic metabolic acidosis and a chloride-phosphate ratio greater than 33 or a modified chloride (mmol. per liter/mg. per dl.) phosphate ratio greater than 500. Familial hypocalciuric hypercalcemia is distinguished from primary hyperparathyroidism by a low urine calcium. Serum calcium changes approximately 0.8 mg. per dl. for every 1 gm. per dl. change in serum albumin. Thiazide diuretics can cause hypercalcemia and should not be given to patients who are hypercalcemic.

Textbook: Pages 654, 655, 657 ANSWER: B.

11. Indications for operation in a patient with previously asymptomatic hyperparathyroidism include:

A. Age older than 60.
B. Nephrolithiasis.
C. A substantial decline in renal function.
D. A substantial decline in bone mass.
E. Depression and fatigue.

DISCUSSION: Age younger than 50 is considered an indication for operation.

Textbook: Pages 657–658 ANSWER: B, C, D, E

12. The parathyroid glands:

A. Develop from the second and third pharyngeal pouches, along with the palatine tonsil and the thymus.
B. Migrate caudally in the neck in normal development but can be found anywhere from the pharyngeal mucosa to the deep mediastinum.
C. Secrete PTH and calcitonin to manage calcium homeostasis.
D. Usually number four, but frequently number only two or three.
E. Contain enzymes that catalyze the conversion of 25(OH) vitamin D_3 to $1,25(OH)_2$ vitamin D_3.

DISCUSSION: The parathyroid glands develop from the third and fourth pharyngeal pouches, along with the thymus and the thyroid ultimobronchial body; there are four glands in the vast majority of persons. Calcitonin is secreted by the C cells of the thyroid. Vitamin D_3 hydroxylation occurs in the kidney.

Textbook: Pages 647–649 ANSWER: B.

13. Hyperparathyroidism can affect which of the following organs and body systems?

A. Gastrointestinal tract.
B. Kidneys.
C. Skeleton.
D. Neuromuscular system.
E. Cardiovascular system.

DISCUSSION: Gastrointestinal involvement includes pancreatitis and peptic ulcer disease. The kidneys can be affected by nephrocalcinosis or nephrolithiasis. The bones can be severely affected by bone resorption. Neuromuscular complaints can include weakness and fatigue. Hypertension is present in as many as 70% of people with hyperparathyroidism and may be related to the renal disease.

Textbook: Pages 651–653 ANSWER: A through E.

14. Secondary hyperparathyroidism:

A. Is a metabolic disease in which the primary abnormality is decreased glomerular filtration rate.
B. Is best treated initially by subtotal parathyroidectomy.
C. Is caused by increased production of $1,25(OH)_2$ vitamin D_3, causing increasing intestinal calcium absorption and hypercalcemia.
D. Can have severe effects on bones exacerbated by aluminum contained in phosphate binders and dialysate water.
E. Is best treated initially by total parathyroidectomy with autotransplantation.

DISCUSSION: Secondary hyperparathyroidism is caused by renal disease, including decreased glomerular filtration rate and decreased $1,25(OH)_2$ vitamin D_3 production. It is best treated by medical management restricting dietary phosphate, administering vitamin D and calcium with phosphate-binding gels, and limiting aluminum exposure, which can exacerbate bone disease.

Textbook: Page 656 ANSWER: A, D.

15. Hypoparathyroidism:

A. Is most commonly encountered as a postviral syndrome.
B. Can be associated with marked hypocalcemia after parathyroidectomy in patients with bone disease.
C. Can cause anxiety, depression, or confusion.
D. Can cause physical signs such as Chvostek's and Trousseau's signs.
E. Is treatable acutely with intravenous calcium salts and chronically with oral calcium and vitamin D.

DISCUSSION: Hypoparathyroidism is most commonly encountered after thyroid surgery. It can be temporarily severe after parathyroidectomy in patients with bone disease ("postoperative bone hunger"). The signs and symptoms can include anxiety, depression, confusion, Chvostek's sign, and Trousseau's sign, as

well as circumoral or extremity tingling, tetany with carpopedal spasms, or seizures. Treatment is as noted.
Textbook: Pages 662–663 ANSWER: B, C, D, E.

16. True statements about pituitary anatomy and physiology include:

A. The pituitary has dual embryonic origin: the anterior pituitary arises from embryonic ectoderm; the posterior pituitary, from the diencephalon.
B. The hypophyseal portal system integrates function of the anterior and posterior pituitary.
C. Adrenocorticotropin (ACTH), formed by posttranslational processing of the precursor POMC, is normally controlled by hypothalamic CRF but may be released by immune-related mechanisms.
D. Growth hormone (GH) directly stimulates longitudinal growth of the skeleton and growth of muscles.
E. Cell types of the anterior pituitary are classified by their position in the anterior pituitary and by their staining characteristics with histologic dyes.

DISCUSSION: The anterior pituitary arises from Rathke's pouch (embryonic ectoderm), and it includes the pars distalis, pars intermedia, and pars tuberalis. The posterior pituitary arises from the diencephalon and includes the neural stalk, infundibulum, and posterior lobe. The hypophyseal portal system drains from the hypothalamus and integrates function of the hypothalamus and anterior pituitary by carrying hypothalamus-derived releasing factors to target cells in the anterior pituitary. ACTH may be released during stress in response to interleukin-1, -2, and -6. Somatotrophic actions of GH are indirect and are mediated by the insulinlike growth factors formerly known as somatomedins. Current classification of anterior pituitary cells is based on immunochemical identification of their secretory products (i.e., corticotropes produce ACTH, lactotropes produce prolactin, and thyrotropes produce thyroid-stimulating hormone [TSH]).
Textbook: Pages 665–668 ANSWER: A, C.

17. Antidiuretic hormone (ADH):

A. Is related to oxytocin, and both are released from the posterior pituitary in conjunction with neurophysins.
B. Is released into the circulation by the posterior pituitary in response to a rise in plasma osmolality above 285 mOsm. or a decrease in circulating blood volume.
C. May be stimulated by catecholamines and inhibited by phenytoin, alcohol, and lithium.
D. In excess, may produce a syndrome of euvolemic hyponatremia with inappropriately concentrated urine that is responsive to free water restriction.
E. Deficiency causes prolonged polyuria and polydipsia and may be diagnosed by a combination of high plasma osmolality and low urine osmolality following water deprivation.

DISCUSSION: ADH and oxytocin are nine–amino acid peptides derived from a common ancestral peptide, vasotocin. ADH is released from the posterior pituitary with neurophysin II in response to a rise in plasma osmolality greater than 285 mOsm/kg. H_2O. by a 5% or greater decrease in blood volume, and by catecholamines. The syndrome of inappropriate ADH release (SIADH) produces euvolemic hyponatremia and is responsive to free water restriction. Diabetes insipidus (DI) reflects a deficiency of ADH and causes prolonged polyuria and polydipsia. Diabetes insipidus is diagnosed by a combination of high plasma osmolality and low urine osmolality following water deprivation. Exogenously administered ADH differentiates central (ADH-responsive) DI from nephrogenic (ADH-unresponsive) DI.
Textbook: Pages 668, 670–671 ANSWER: A, B, C, D, E.

18. Signs and symptoms of acute pituitary apoplexy include:

A. Severe headache.
B. Meningismus.
C. Vision loss.
D. Shock.
E. May be relieved by emergent transsphenoidal decompression of the sella turcica.

DISCUSSION: Acute pituitary apoplexy follows sudden hemorrhage into a pre-existing pituitary tumor or following closed head trauma. Symptoms, including headache, meningismus, and vision loss, are attributable to the intracerebral blood. Pituitary insufficiency, as well as the accompanying secondary adrenal insufficiency, may cause hypotension and shock. Other manifestations may include DI and myxedema. Acute pituitary apoplexy is a neurosurgical emergency that requires transsphenoidal decompression of the sella turcica.
Textbook: Page 674 ANSWER: A, B, C, D.

19. Prolactinomas of the pituitary:

A. Most often produce dysfunctional uterine bleeding in women.
B. Most commonly produce infertility in men.
C. When asymptomatic, are best treated surgically early in the microadenoma stage.
D. May enlarge during pregnancy, requiring treatment with bromocriptine or surgery.
E. Commonly occur in patients with MEN 2.

DISCUSSION: Pituitary prolactinomas are the most common pituitary tumor and cause amenorrhea, galactorrhea, or both in women. Men usually have macroprolactinomas and experience symptoms of a space-occupying lesion of the sella (i.e., headache). A minority of men experience impotence and infertility. Asymptomatic prolactinomas remain stable over time and require observation only. Symptomatic prolactinomas require treatment, usually with bromocriptine.

Prolactinomas may enlarge during pregnancy and can produce symptoms requiring treatment with either bromocriptine or surgery. Prolactiomas are seen in as many as 40% of patients with MEN 1.

Textbook: Pages 672–673 ANSWER: D.

20. Hypercortisolism:

A. Is most often ACTH-dependent, owing to an ACTH-producing pituitary adenoma.
B. Is best diagnosed by measurement of cortisol from a serum sample collected at 8 A.M.
C. Is attributable to an adrenal source if the basal serum ACTH level is above 10 pg. per ml., if the hypercortisolism is suppressed by high-dose dexamethasone, and if an adrenal tumor is visualized radiographically.
D. May be caused by small cell carcinoma of the lung, carcinoid tumors, tumors of the endocrine pancreas, pheochromocytoma, or medullary thyroid carcinoma (MTC).
E. In children is most often caused by adrenocortical neoplasia.

DISCUSSION: Cushing's syndrome is most often (80% to 90%) ACTH-dependent and is most often due to an ACTH-secreting pituitary adenoma (Cushing's disease). Some 10% to 20% of ACTH-dependent Cushing's syndrome is caused by ectopic production of ACTH from small cell carcinoma of the lung, carcinoid tumors, tumors of the endocrine pancreas, pheochromocytoma, and MTC. ACTH-independent Cushing's syndrome secondary to primary adrenal pathology occurs in 10% to 20% of cases in adults and is the most common form in children. Measurement of cortisol in two to three consecutive 24-hour collections of urine is the best screening test for Cushing's syndrome: plasma levels of cortisol show marked variability, and a single random level is not helpful in establishing the diagnosis. ACTH-independent Cushing's syndrome suppresses the pituitary and is diagnosed if the basal serum ACTH level is suppressed below 5 pg. per ml., if the hypercortisolism is not suppressed by high-dose dexamethasone, or if the metyrapone stimulation test is negative. The dexamethasone suppression and metyrapone tests do not, however, distinguish an adrenal from an ectopic ACTH cause of Cushing's since both suppress the pituitary. Radiographic evidence of an adrenal tumor must be supported by biochemical testing to confirm that the adrenal is the primary cause of Cushing's syndrome.

Textbook: Pages 678–682 ANSWER: A, D, E.

21. Primary aldosteronism:

A. Produces a syndrome of diastolic hypertension, hypokalemia, and edema.
B. Is suggested by findings of serum potassium less than 3.5 mEq. per liter, urinary potassium excretion greater than 30 mEq. per day, upright plasma renin below 3 ng. per ml., and a plasma aldosterone concentration–plasma renin activity ratio greater than 20:1.
C. Is most often due to an aldosterone-producing adrenal adenoma, which may be distinguished from idiopathic adrenal hyperplasia by its sensitivity to diurnal changes in ACTH and insensitivity to changes in posture.
D. May be diagnosed in hypertensive patients by demonstration of an adrenal mass larger than 1 cm. on computed tomography alone.
E. Is best treated surgically if it is due to either aldosteronoma or idiopathic adrenal hyperplasia.

DISCUSSION: Primary aldosteronism is a syndrome of diastolic hypertension and hypokalemia; edema typically is absent. The diagnosis relies on demonstration of hypokalemia with inappropriate kaliuresis and inappropriately elevated plasma aldosterone with suppression of plasma renin following sodium loading. Primary aldosteronism most often is due to an adrenal adenoma, which must be distinguished from idiopathic adrenal hyperplasia since resection of the adenoma is nearly always curative, whereas adrenal resection for idiopathic adrenal hyperplasia is curative less than 20% of the time. CT evidence of adrenal tumor alone is inadequate to diagnose aldosteronism, even in a hypertensive patient.

Textbook: Pages 682–684 ANSWER: B, C.

22. Adrenocortical carcinoma:

A. May be suspected in a patient with rapidly progressive Cushing's syndrome and virilizing features or in asymptomatic patients with adrenal tumors larger than 6 cm on CT.
B. Most often is diagnosed early in its course when disease is confined to the adrenal gland.
C. Is differentiated from benign adrenocortical adenoma by tumor necrosis, hemorrhage, and cellular features of large hyperchromatic nuclei and more than 20 mitoses per high-power field.
D. Should be resected only if disease is localized to the adrenal gland; otherwise treatment with mitotane is indicated.
E. Carries a poor prognosis: overall 5-year survival less than 25%.

DISCUSSION: Patients with adrenocortical carcinoma often present with rapidly progressive syndromes of combined adrenocortical hormone excess. However, approximately half do not have syndromes of hormone excess but present with abdominal pain, increased abdominal girth, weight loss, and anorexia. Furthermore, incidentally discovered adrenal masses larger than 6 cm. harbor carcinoma in as many as 92% of cases. Adrenocortical carcinoma is differentiated from adenoma by pathologic demonstration of either local invasion or distant metastases. Most patients with adrenocortical carcinoma present with locally advanced (stage III) or metastatic (stage IV) disease. Prognosis for these patients is poor: 5-year survival is less than 25% in most series. Patients with adrenocortical carcinoma should undergo primary surgical resection or palliative surgical debulking of locally advanced, metastatic, or even recurrent disease since response of these tumors to medical therapy, including mitotane, is poor.

Textbook: Page 687 ANSWER: A, E.

23. Addisonian crisis, or acute adrenocortical insufficiency:

A. Occurs only in patients with known adrenal insufficiency or in those receiving long-term supraphysiologic doses of exogenous steroids.
B. Can mimic an acute abdomen with fever, nausea and vomiting, abdominal pain, and hypotension.
C. May cause electrolyte abnormalities, including hypernatremia, hypokalemia, hypoglycemia, and hypercalcemia, as well as eosinophilia on peripheral blood smear.
D. Should be diagnosed with the rapid ACTH stimulation test before steroid replacement is instituted.
E. May be effectively treated with intravenous "stress-dose" glucocorticoid and mineralocorticoid replacement.

DISCUSSION: Addisonian crisis, or acute adrenal insufficiency, may be seen following even mild illness in patients with suppression of the hypothalamic-pituitary-adrenal axis. This suppression can be produced by as little as 1 week of supraphysiologic stress dose steroids in the year before the stressful event. Addisonian crisis is a medical emergency that requires prompt treatment based on clinical suspicion. Clinical findings include fever, nausea and vomiting, abdominal pain, and hypotension. Laboratory analysis may reveal electrolyte abnormalities, including hyponatremia, hyperkalemia, hypoglycemia, and hypercalcemia, as well as eosinophilia on peripheral blood smear. The rapid ACTH test is diagnostic, but it should not delay treatment with intravenous fluid resuscitation, glucose replacement, and high-dose dexamethasone. Dexamethasone, not hydrocortisone, should be given initially, since it does not interfere with subsequent determination of plasma cortisol. Stress dose steroids are inadequate once adrenal crisis has occurred, and exogenous mineralocorticoids are given when the patient resumes oral intake.

Textbook: Pages 687–689 ANSWER: B.

24. Preparation for surgical removal of a pheochromocytoma includes:

A. Beta-adrenergic blockade followed by alpha-adrenergic blockade.
B. Hydration.
C. Alpha-adrenergic blockade, with or without beta-adrenergic blockade.
D. Preoperative Swan-Ganz monitoring in all patients.
E. Planning removal through an anterior, posterior, or laparoscopic approach based upon tumor localization with CT, magnetic resonance imaging (MRI), and/or ^{131}I-MIBG.

DISCUSSION: Principles of preoperative management for pheochromocytoma include preoperative alpha-adrenergic blockade using phenoxybenzamine or phentolamine. Beta-adrenergic blockade with propranolol is then used selectively in patients who develop tachycardia, have a history of cardiac arrhythmia, or have primarily epinephrine-secreting tumors. Beta-adrenergic blockade should be undertaken only after successful alpha blockade is established. Patients with pheochromocytoma frequently exhibit intravascular volume depletion, and careful hydration is mandatory. Central venous pressure monitoring alone is helpful to guide hydration; more intensive monitoring with a Swan-Ganz catheter is indicated for patients with pre-existing heart disease. Formerly, the anterior approach was preferred for adrenalectomy as it facilitated complete abdominal exploration and search for extra-adrenal pheochromocytoma. Accurate preoperative localization with CT, MRI, and ^{131}I-MIBG has allowed selective use of the posterior, or even the laparoscopic, approach for adrenalectomy.

Textbook: Pages 692–693 ANSWER: B, C, E.

25. Indications for surgical adrenalectomy include:

A. An adrenal mass larger than 6 cm.
B. Hypertensive patients with aldosteronism that is ACTH insensitive and posture sensitive and who also have multiple adrenal nodules on CT.
C. Cushing's syndrome secondary to adrenal neoplasms or to persistent ectopic ACTH syndrome when the primary tumor is inoperable.
D. Pheochromocytoma in adults and children.
E. Congenital adrenal hyperplasia secondary to 21-hydroxylase deficiency.

DISCUSSION: Adrenalectomy is indicated for the management of adrenal masses larger than 6 cm. on CT since tumors of this size harbor carcinoma in more than 90% of cases. Surgical adrenalectomy is also the treatment of choice for primary adrenal causes of Cushing's syndrome. Surgical adrenalectomy may be considered as an alternative to medical adrenalectomy with metyrapone, aminoglutethimide, or mitotane in patients with ectopic ACTH syndrome when treatment of the primary tumor is unsuccessful. Patients with aldosteronism that is ACTH sensitive and posture insensitive likely have an adrenal adenoma that is curable by adrenalectomy. Aldosteronism that is ACTH insensitive and posture sensitive is likely caused by idiopathic adrenal hyperplasia, which is best managed medically with spironolactone, triamterene, amiloride, or nifedipine. Adrenalectomy following preoperative alpha-adrenergic blockade, with or without beta-adrenergic blockade, and hydration is the treatment of choice of all pheochromocytomas. Adrenalectomy is not indicated in the management of any of the congenital adrenal hyperplasias.

Textbook: Pages 682, 685, 687, 692–683 ANSWER: A, C, D.

26. Incidental adrenal masses:

A. May be seen in as many as 10% of abdominal CT studies.
B. Most commonly represent pheochromocytoma; adrenocortical adenoma, adrenocortical carcinoma, and metastases from other primary cancers occur less frequently.
C. May represent adrenocortical carcinoma if greater than 6 cm. in diameter.
D. Should be routinely evaluated by measurement of 24-hour urine levels of catecholamines and their metabolites, cortisol, and aldosterone plus fine-needle aspiration.
E. Should be resected if biochemically active, if greater than 6 cm., or if they grow over six months' follow-up.

DISCUSSION: The incidental adrenal mass is seen in as many as 1.3% of abdominal CT scans performed for other reasons. Adrenocortical adenomas are most common, followed by adrenocortical carcinoma, metastases from other primary cancers, and pheochromocytoma. Biochemical evaluation must weigh the prevalence of adrenal neoplasms against the consequences of a missed life-threatening diagnosis, as in pheochromocytoma. All adrenal masses should be evaluated for pheochromocytoma with measurement of 24-hour urine catecholamines and their metabolites. Aldosterone and cortisol measurement are indicated if clinical features suggest aldosteronism or Cushing's syndrome. Fine-needle aspiration of adrenal masses is indicated for clearly cystic lesions or if metastasis is suspected based on the presence of another known primary. Fine-needle aspiration is not routinely indicated in the evaluation of adrenal lesions and is contraindicated until pheochromocytoma is definitively excluded. Adrenal lesions should be resected if they are functional, are larger than 6 cm., or have enlarged during follow-up.

Textbook: Pages 695–696 ANSWER: C, E.

27. Which of the following statements is true about the synthesis of thyroid hormone and its physiology?

A. The iodine utilized in hormone synthesis is derived principally from dietary sources.
B. The role of thyroid-stimulating hormone (TSH) in thyroid physiology is limited to regulation of the release of thyroid hormone in plasma.
C. Enough thyroxine (T_4) is stored in the normal thyroid to provide a euthyroid state for 3 weeks despite absence of iodine intake.
D. The regulation of thyroid function involves pituitary, but not hypothalamic, input.

DISCUSSION: Iodine is necessary for the synthesis of thyroid hormone, and approximately 200 to 500 mg is ingested daily. Most of it is absorbed from the small intestine and is cleared from the plasma by secretion of thyroid hormone. TSH is required for the normal production and secretion of thyroid hormone. It is generally accepted that TSH also has a major role in thyroid growth. The thyroid gland has a storage reserve of approximately 3 weeks. The principal regulatory mechanisms of the thyroid gland are the hypothalamic-pituitary-thyroid control system and the intrathyroidal regulatory systems. TRH is produced by the superoptic and paraventricular nuclei within the hypothalamus and passes down their axones. Following secretion into the hypophyseal portal blood systems TRH passes to the pituitary and induces stimulation of TSH secretion.

Textbook: Pages 599–601 ANSWER: A, C.

28. Correct statements about thyroid function tests include which of the following?

A. Contraceptive pills and pregnancy increase the amount of thyroxin-binding globulin (TBG), and, consequently, the total T_4 level.
B. Anticonvulsive medications and chronic debilitating illnesses decrease the amount of TBG and, consequently, the total T_4 level.
C. Intravenous pyleography can lower the rate of active iodine uptake by the thyroid.
D. A triiodothyronine (T_3) suppression test that demonstrates nonsuppressibility of thyroid function is compatible with the diagnosis of Graves' disease, toxic adenoma, or functioning carcinoma.
E. An increased serum cholesterol level in a hypothyroid patient indicates a thyroid cause.

DISCUSSION: Hormone binding proteins are the principal intravascular factors influencing total hormone concentration. Various factors may cause changes in the concentration of TBG. Contraceptive pills and pregnancy increase the amount of TBG, while anticonvulsive medications and chronic debilitating disease may decrease the amount of TBG. Administration of excess amounts of iodine may lower the rate of active iodine uptake in the thyroid gland. The thyroid suppression test is based on the principle that administration of thyroid hormone does not suppress the patient's thyroid function when normal homeostatic mechanisms are disrupted. Thyroid function is nonsuppressible in hyperthyroidism or in the presence of thyroid hormone–secreting tumors. Serum cholesterol, deep tendon reflex time, and cardiovascular functions can be measured to reflect hypothyroidism and hyperthyroidism but do not give an indication of the etiology of hypothyroidism.

Textbook: Pages 603–606 ANSWER: A, B, C, D.

29. Hyperthyroidism can be caused by all of the following except:

A. Graves' disease.
B. Plummer's disease.
C. Struma ovarii.
D. Hashimoto's disease.
E. Medullary carcinoma of the thyroid.

DISCUSSION: Common types of hyperthyroidism include diffuse toxic goiter (Graves' disease, named after the Dublin physician Robert Graves who described it in 1835 but known since its original descrip-

tion by Parry in 1786 and described by von Basedow in 1840) and toxic adenoma or toxic multinodular goiter (Plummer's disease). Uncommon causes include thyrotoxicosis factitia, functioning metastatic thyroid carcinoma, trophoblastic tumors that secrete human chorionic gonadotropin (having thyroid-stimulating properties), inappropriate secretion of thyrotropin by pituitary tumors, struma ovarii, iodide-induced hyperfunction, and thyroiditis.
Textbook: Page 611. ANSWER: E.

30. Which of the following is true about the use of radioiodine to treat hyperthyroidism?

A. If hyperthyroidism is secondary to radioiodine use, it will occur within 2 years of treatment.
B. There is a markedly increased risk of future thyroid cancer following radioiodine therapy.
C. The risk of leukemia following radioiodine therapy is approximately 10%.
D. Mutation abnormalities occur in 15% of fetuses in utero following internal treatment of the mother with radioiodine during pregnancy.
E. Radioiodine may pass through the placenta and lactating breast to produce hypothyroidism in a fetus or infant.

DISCUSSION: Hypothyroidism secondary to radioiodine therapy increases in frequency with time to 85% after 5 years. There has been no demonstration of an increase in malignancies following radioiodine therapy. Radioactive iodine can cross the placenta and lactating breast to produce hypothyroidism in a fetus or a nursing infant and is, therefore, contraindicated.
Textbook: Pages 612–613. ANSWER: E.

31. Arrange the following complications of thyroid surgery (bilateral subtotal thyroidectomy) in decreasing order of incidence in patients with Graves' disease.

A. Laryngeal nerve paralysis.
B. Hypoparathyroidism.
C. Hypothyroidism.
D. Recurrent hyperthyroidism.

DISCUSSION: The incidence of recurrent disease is inversely related to the incidence of hypothyroidism and is 1% to 5%. Within 1 to 2 years, hypothyroidism may develop in 5% to 50% of patients (with a slight additional increase in subsequent years). The associated morbidity—related primarily to damage to the recurrent laryngeal nerves and parathyroid glands—is estimated to be 0.5% to 3.0%.
Textbook: Page 613–620. ANSWER: C, D, A, B

32. The most common cause of goitrous hypothyroidism in adults is:

A. Graves' disease.
B. Riedel's thyroiditis.
C. Hashimoto's disease.
D. de Quervain's thyroiditis.

DISCUSSION: Hashimoto's disease was first described in Japan by Hakaru Hashimoto in 1912 and is the best-known of the immunologic thyroid diseases. It is the most common cause of goitrous hypothyroidism in adults and of sporadic goiter in children. The incidence is 0.3 to 1.5 cases per 1000 population per year and it is 10 to 15 times more common in women than in men, with the highest incidence in the group aged 30 to 50 years.
Textbook: Page 623. ANSWER: C.

33. Therapy for Hashimoto's disease includes:

A. Radioiodine.
B. Antithyroid medications.
C. Subtotal thyroidectomy.
D. None of the above.

DISCUSSION: There is no specific treatment for Hashimoto's disease. Patients are usually followed medically, and replacement therapy with T_4 is begun in patients with hypothyroidism that is symptomatic or associated with a goiter that is causing pressure symptoms. Early initiation of thyroid hormone therapy has been recommended by many to prevent further thyroid enlargement and reduce the risk of myxedema, especially in postpartum patients. Surgical reduction of goiter should be performed if severe pressure symptoms that have not responded to corticosteroid therapy are present. This usually consists of subtotal thyroidectomy. Biopsy to rule out malignancy in nodules suspicious for thyroid carcinoma (usually papillary) or lymphoma is indicated. If carcinoma is suspected, lobectomy should be performed, and if frozen section demonstrates carcinoma, subtotal or total thyroidectomy should be performed.
Textbook: Page 624. ANSWER: D.

NOTES

NOTES

CHAPTER 10

GASTROINTESTINAL SYSTEM

1. Which of the following statements about the anatomic course of the esophagus is correct?

A. The cervical esophagus passes behind and to the right of the trachea.
B. The thoracic esophagus enters the posterior mediastinum anterior to the aortic arch.
C. The thoracic esophagus passes behind the right mainstem bronchus and the pericardium.
D. The esophagus enters the diaphragmatic hiatus at the level of T8.
E. The esophagus deviates anteriorly and to the left as it enters the abdomen.

DISCUSSION: Knowledge of the normal course of the esophagus is important in operative and endoscopic procedures. The cervical esophagus lies just anterior to the prevertebral fascia and courses through the neck posterior to the trachea and to the *left* of the midline. The cervical esophagus is therefore more readily approached surgically through a left neck incision. The thoracic esophagus enters the posterior mediastinum *posterior* to the aortic arch. Therefore, when operating on the upper esophagus, a right thoracotomy is preferred, since the aortic arch overlies the esophagus in the left chest. The esophagus descends in the posterior mediastinum behind the left mainstem bronchus and pericardium. It is the proximity of the esophagus and left mainstem bronchus that is responsible for the development of malignant tracheoesophageal fistulas between these two structures. The esophagus enters the diaphragmatic hiatus, which is located at the level of T11. As it enters the abdomen, the esophagus deviates *anteriorly* and to the *left.* Therefore, when performing rigid esophagoscopy as the distal esophagus is entered, the patient's head must be turned to the right and the esophagoscope elevated anteriorly to avoid perforation.

Textbook: Page 703 ANSWER: E.

2. Which of the following statements about esophageal anatomy is correct?

A. The esophagus has a poor blood supply, which is segmental in distribution and accounts for the high incidence of anastomotic leakage.
B. The esophageal serosa consists of a thin layer of fibroareolar tissue.
C. The esophagus has two distinct muscle layers, an outer, longitudinal one and an inner, circular one, which are striated in the upper third and smooth in the distal two thirds.
D. Injury to the recurrent laryngeal nerve results in vocal cord dysfunction but does not affect swallowing.
E. The lymphatic drainage of the esophagus is relatively sparse, localized primarily to adjacent paraesophageal lymph nodes.

DISCUSSION: Poor technique, not poor blood supply, explains most esophageal anastomotic leaks. While the major blood supply of the esophagus is from four to six segmental aortic esophageal arteries, there are extensive submucosal collaterals from the inferior thyroid, intercostal, bronchial, inferior phrenic, and left gastric arteries. The esophagus lacks serosa and instead is surrounded by mediastinal connective tissue (adventitia). There are two muscle layers in the esophagus, an outer longitudinal and an inner circular one. Both layers of the upper third of the esophagus consist of striated muscle, while in the lower two thirds they are (nonstriated) smooth muscle. The recurrent laryngeal branches of the vagus nerves provide both parasympathetic innervation to the cervical esophagus and innervation to the upper esophageal sphincter (UES). Injury to the recurrent laryngeal nerve therefore results in improved UES function with secondary aspiration on swallowing as well as vocal cord dysfunction and hoarseness. The esophagus has extensive lymphatic drainage, with lymphatic capillaries coursing longitudinally in the esophageal wall and communicating with paraesophageal, paratracheal and subcarinal, other mediastinal, perigastric, and internal jugular lymph nodes. This accounts for the biologically aggressive nature of esophageal carcinoma, which tends to metastasize early in its course.

Textbook: Pages 703–706 ANSWER: C.

3. Which of the following statements about the lower esophageal sphincter (LES) mechanism, or high-pressure zone (HPZ), is true?

A. The LES is a circular smooth muscle ring that is 3 to 5 cm. long.
B. In assessing esophageal manometric data, mean HPZ pressure less than 6 mm. Hg or overall length less than 2 cm. is more likely to be associated with incompetence of the LES and gastroesophageal reflux.
C. Esophageal manometry and the acid perfusion

(Bernstein) test reliably identify the patient with an incompetent LES mechanism.
D. Distal HPZ relaxation occurs within 5 to 8 seconds of initiating a swallow.
E. Twenty-four–hour distal esophageal pH monitoring is achieved with an intraesophageal pH electrode positioned at the esophagogastric junction.

DISCUSSION: The LES is not an anatomic muscular sphincter like the anus or pylorus, but rather, is *a functional sphincter* that serves as a barrier against abnormal regurgitation of gastric contents into the esophagus and is more appropriately termed the *distal esophageal HPZ.* While, in general, *no HPZ value absolutely indicates either competence or incompetence of the LES mechanism,* patients with a mean HPZ pressure less than 6 mm. Hg or a sphincter length less than 2 cm. are likely to have an incompetent LES and gastroesophageal reflux. Esophageal manometry defines the amplitude and length of the distal HPZ and the character of esophageal peristalsis. It does *not* determine whether or not the LES is competent. The Bernstein test identifies the patient with an acid-sensitive esophagus but does *not* indicate whether or not the patient has gastroesophageal reflux or esophagitis. Reflex distal HPZ relaxation occurs within 1.5 to 2.5 seconds after a swallow is initiated and lasts 4 to 6 seconds. Twenty-four–hour distal esophageal pH monitoring is achieved by means of an intraesophageal pH electrode positioned 5 cm. proximal to the HPZ, as determined by prior manometric evaluation.
Textbook: Pages 708–711 ANSWER: B.

4. Which of the following statements about esophageal motility is/are true?

A. The act of swallowing initiates UES relaxation, which persists until the bolus of food passes the LES.
B. The primary peristaltic wave normally propels the swallowed bolus through the esophagus in 4 to 8 seconds.
C. Normally, a progressive peristaltic contraction (primary wave) follows 50% of all swallows, the remainder being secondary or tertiary contractions.
D. Secondary peristalsis is initiated when the entire swallowed bolus of food fails to empty from the esophagus into the stomach.
E. Tertiary esophageal contractions are high-amplitude progressive peristaltic contractions that produce the "corkscrew" appearance of esophageal spasm on barium esophagography.

DISCUSSION: Swallowing initiates UES relaxation, which lasts only 0.5 to 1.0 second, considerably less than the 4 to 8 seconds required for a swallowed bolus to pass through the esophagus and into the stomach. A progressive peristaltic contraction normally follows 97% of all swallows. If the swallowed bolus does not empty completely into the stomach, distention of the esophagus initiates secondary peristalsis, which is progressive and sequential and persists until the retained intraesophageal contents have passed into the stomach. Tertiary contractions are simultaneous, *nonprogressive,* incoordinated contractions of the esophageal smooth muscle that produce the contraction rings responsible for the corkscrew esophagus of diffuse esophageal spasm on barium esophagography.
Textbook: Pages 707–708 ANSWER: B, D.

5. Which of the following statements about UES dysfunction are correct?

A. This condition is diagnosed by the characteristic manometric findings of UES spasm.
B. Typical symptoms include cervical dysphagia, expectoration of saliva, and hoarseness.
C. The classic finding on barium esophagogram is a posterior cricopharyngeal bar.
D. Medical or surgical therapy of gastroesophageal reflux may be curative.
E. A cervical esophagomyotomy for UES dysfunction should be limited to 2 to 3 cm. in length so that normal muscle is not damaged.

DISCUSSION: The unique anatomic characteristics of the UES and the limitations of existing equipment in recording the rapid sequence of events associated with swallowing make standard manometric definition of UES motor abnormalities extremely difficult. Characteristic consistent abnormalities of UES function in patients with cricopharyngeal dysfunction have not been well documented. UES dysfunction results in cervical dysphagia, expectoration of saliva that is no longer swallowed freely, and, often, intermittent hoarseness due to alteration of the larynx and vocal cords by the pull of the abnormal cricopharyngeal sphincter. Barium esophagography in the patient with UES dysfunction frequently shows a posterior cricopharyngeal "bar," representing the prominent impression of the sphincter on the esophageal lumen. Patients with gastroesophageal reflux may present with cervical dysphagia due to secondary UES dysfunction. Successful medical or surgical treatment of the reflux may eliminate the cervical complaints. Since the UES is normally 3 to 5 cm. long, when a cervical esophagomyotomy is required for treatment of cricopharyngeal dysfunction, a generous myotomy, 7 to 10 cm. long, is carried out to ensure complete division of all incoordinated UES muscle fibers.
Textbook: Pages 712–714 ANSWER: B, C, D.

6. Which of the following statements about achalasia is/are correct?

A. In most cases in North America the cause is a parasitic infestation by *Trypanosoma cruzi.*
B. Chest pain and regurgitation are the usual symptoms.
C. Distal-third esophageal adenocarcinomas may occur in as many as 20% of patients within 10 years of diagnosis.
D. Manometry demonstrates failure of LES relaxation on swallowing and absent or weak

simultaneous contractions in the esophageal body after swallowing.
E. Endoscopic botulinum toxin injection of the LES, pneumatic dilatation, and esophagomyotomy provide highly effective curative therapy for achalasia.

DISCUSSION: While in South America achalasia is the result of Chagas' disease caused by parasitic infestation by the leishmanial forms of *T. cruzi,* in Europe and North America the cause of achalasia is unknown. The common presenting symptoms of achalasia are dysphagia, regurgitation, and weight loss. Chest pain is an infrequent symptom in achalasia and is more characteristic of esophageal spasm. Achalasia is a premalignant esophageal lesion: the retention esophagitis leads to metaplasia and *squamous cell carcinoma,* which occurs after 15 to 25 years in the middle third of the thoracic esophagus in 10% of patients. The classic manometric findings of achalasia are failure of relaxation of the LES on swallowing and absent or weak simultaneous contractions in the esophageal body after swallowing. Achalasia is currently incurable, and, though the recently described endoscopic botulinum toxin injection of the lower esophageal sphincter, pneumatic dilatation, and esophagomyotomy effectively relieve dysphagia in the majority of patients, all of these treatments are strictly palliative. The motility disturbance persists throughout life.

Textbook: Pages 715–718 ANSWER: D.

7. Which of the following statements about diffuse esophageal spasm is/are true?

A. Chest pain due to esophageal spasm is readily differentiated from angina pectoris of cardiac origin.
B. Bouts of esophageal obstruction and regurgitation of food are characteristic.
C. Associated psychiatric disorders are common.
D. During manometric assessment, unless the patient is having pain there may be no detectable multiphasic, high-amplitude, simultaneous esophageal contractions.
E. The treatment of choice is a long esophagomyotomy from the aortic arch to the esophagogastric junction.

DISCUSSION: The chest pain of diffuse esophageal spasm is often indistinguishable from that of angina pectoris of cardiac origin. Many patients undergo cardiac catheterization to rule out coronary artery disease. Patients may experience slow emptying of the esophagus, but obstructive symptoms and regurgitation of food are unusual. Psychiatric disorders (depression, psychosomatic complaints, anxiety) have been documented in more than 80% of patients with esophageal contraction abnormalities. The classic manometric criteria of diffuse esophageal spasm are simultaneous, multiphasic, repetitive, high-amplitude contractions occurring after a swallow and spontaneously. These changes may not be detected if manometry is performed when the patient is having no pain. As the cause of esophageal spasm is unknown, treatment is far from ideal. Conservative management—avoidance of "trigger" foods and drinks, psychiatric counseling, treatment of reflux, esophageal dilatations, use of histamine H_2 blockers, anti-spasmodics, and smooth muscle relaxants—should always be attempted first. Esophagomyotomy provides no lasting relief of esophageal spasm for as many as 50% of patients and should be used only in a minority of these patients.

Textbook: Pages 721–723 ANSWER: C, D.

8. Which of the following statements about epiphrenic diverticula of the esophagus is/are correct?

A. They are traction diverticula that arise close to the tracheobronchial tree.
B. They characteristically arise proximal to an esophageal reflux stricture.
C. The degree of dysphagia correlates with the size of the pouch.
D. They are best approached surgically through a right thoracotomy.
E. The operation of choice is a stapled diverticulectomy, long esophagomyotomy, and partial fundoplication.

DISCUSSION: Epiphrenic diverticula are pulsion diverticula that arise in the distal 10 cm. of the esophagus. The cause is elevated intraesophageal pressure, which forces mucosa and submucosa to herniate through the muscle layers. Though this may occur with an esophageal reflux stricture or tumor, primary disordered esophageal motility is the most common cause. Many patients are asymptomatic when their epiphrenic diverticula are diagnosed by barium esophagography, symptoms being related more to the degree of disordered motility than to the size of the pouch. Distal esophageal diverticulum is best approached through a left thoracotomy. When surgery is indicated, the preferred approach is transthoracic diverticulectomy using a surgical stapler, a long esophagomyotomy to relieve the elevated intraesophageal pressure, and a nonobstructing partial (e.g., Belsey's) fundoplication.

Textbook: Page 731 ANSWER: E.

9. Which of the following statements about Schatzki's ring is correct?

A. The ring represents a panmural fibrotic stricture resulting from gastroesophageal reflux.
B. Dysphagia occurs when the ring diameter is 13 mm. or less.
C. The ring occurs within 1 to 2 cm. of the squamocolumnar epithelial junction.
D. Schatzki's ring indicates reflux esophagitis.
E. Schatzki's ring signifies the need for an antireflux operation.

DISCUSSION: Schatzki's ring is seen radiographically as an annular weblike constriction at the esophagogastric junction in a patient with a sliding hiatalhernia.

It represents prominence of the esophagogastric junction with slight submucosal fibrosis but *not* true panmural fibrotic reflux stricture. Intermittent dysphagia may occur when the ring size is 20 mm. or less, but dysphagia is almost invariable when the ring measures 13 mm. or less. Schatzki's ring occurs *precisely* at the squamocolumnar epithelial junction. It is indicative of the presence of a hiatal hernia but not of gastroesophageal reflux or esophagitis. An asymptomatic Schatzki's ring requires no therapy per se. Patients with refractory severe reflux symptoms after dilation therapy are candidates for antireflux surgery.

Textbook: Pages 732–733 ANSWER: B.

10. Choose the distance in centimeters from the upper incisor teeth at which the following radiographically identified esophageal lesions would be encountered endoscopically:

A. 10 cm.
B. 15 cm.
C. 25 cm.
D. 30 cm.
E. 40 cm.

1. Zenker's diverticulum
2. Traction diverticulum
3. Tumor 10 cm. proximal to the esophagogastric junction

DISCUSSION: A barium esophagogram should be obtained routinely before performing elective esophagoscopy. The location of an esophageal lesion seen on the barium swallow study can be related to adjacent anatomic landmarks. This allows the endoscopist to anticipate the level (as measured from the upper incisor teeth) where he should expect to see the abnormality at esophagoscopy. For example, the upper esophageal (cricopharyngeal) sphincter is generally seen at the level of the C7–T1 vertebrae radiographically and at 15 cm. endoscopically. This is the level at which the mouth of a Zenker's diverticulum is seen. The tracheal bifurcation occurs at the level of the T4 or 25 cm. from the upper incisors endoscopically; a traction (parabronchial) diverticulum at the level of the carina on a barium esophagogram will be seen at approximately 25 cm. The esophagogastric junction occurs at approximately the level of T11, 40 cm. from the upper incisors; a tumor 10 cm. proximal to the esophagogastric junction stricture is seen endoscopically at 30 cm.

Textbook: Pages 703–704, 729, 730, 736 ANSWER: 1. B.
2. C.
3. D.

11. Which of the following statements about pathology encountered at esophagoscopy is/are correct?

A. Reflux esophagitis should be graded as *mild, moderate,* or *severe,* to promote consistency among different observers.
B. An esophageal reflux stricture with a 2-mm. lumen is not dilatable and is best treated with resection.
C. A newly diagnosed radiographic distal esophageal stricture warrants dilation and antireflux medical therapy.
D. In patients with Barrett's mucosa, the squamocolumnar epithelial junction occurs 3 cm. or more proximal to the anatomic esophagogastric junction.
E. After fasting at least 12 hours, a patient with megaesophagus of achalasia can safely undergo flexible fiberoptic esophagoscopy.

DISCUSSION: The traditional subjective grading of reflux esophagitis as *mild, moderate,* or *severe* has inherent wide variations in meaning among observers. Consistent use of standardized grading systems for endoscopic reflux esophagitis (e.g., that of Belsey or Savary) provides a more objective description of the changes seen and allows more meaningful evaluation of patients at different times and by different observers. The size of the lumen does not predict whether or not a reflux stricture is dilatable. Even a tight 2-mm. lumen can be traversed with a guidewire over which Savary dilators can be used to achieve an acceptable lumen size. Every newly diagnosed esophageal stricture warrants esophagoscopy with brushings and biopsies of the stricture (to exclude carcinoma) and an assessment of its "dilatability." Antireflux medical therapy is not justified until carcinoma has been ruled out. Because the squamocolumnar epithelial junction may normally be found within 2 to 3 cm. of the anatomic esophagogastric junction, the diagnosis of Barrett's mucosa requires identification of the columnar epithelium at least 3 mm. proximal to the junction of the tubular esophagus and the stomach. In advanced achalasia with megaesophagus, the dilated esophagus may have a capacity of 1 to 2 liters, and simply fasting overnight does not ensure that the esophagus is empty of food and drink consumed the day before. Life-threatening massive regurgitation and aspiration may occur as the endoscope is being introduced unless an effort is made to evacuate the esophagus first by means of a nasogastric tube.

Textbook: Pages 738–742 ANSWER: D.

12. Which of the following statements about the diagnosis and treatment of esophageal leiomyomas is/are correct?

A. The majority are diagnosed after they cause dysphagia and chest pain.
B. Biopsy is indicated at the time of esophagoscopy, to rule out carcinoma.
C. Full-thickness elliptical excision of the esophageal wall is the preferred surgical approach.
D. Endoscopic ultrasonography is a reliable means of following leiomyomas conservatively.
E. Recurrence of resected leiomyomas is minimized by wide local excision.

DISCUSSION: Most esophageal leiomyomas are asymptomatic when discovered incidentally on a barium esophagogram or upper gastrointestinal tract series. When suspected on the basis of its radiographic appearance, biopsy of the mass should *not* be performed at the time of esophagoscopy, so that subsequent extramucosal resection will not be complicated by scarring at the biopsy site. The preferred surgical approach is submucosal enucleation of the mass, *not* full-thickness excision. Leiomyomas have a characteristic hypoechogenic homogeneous appearance on esophageal ultrasonography that allows a noninvasive diagnosis and means of surveillance. Submucosal enucleation of leiomyomas, without wide local excision, provides excellent long-term results with virtually no local recurrence rate.

Textbook: Pages 744–745 ANSWER: D.

13. Which of the following statements regarding the pathology of esophageal carcinoma is/are correct?

A. Worldwide, adenocarcinoma is the most common esophageal malignancy.
B. Squamous cell carcinoma is most common in the distal esophagus, whereas adenocarcinoma predominates in the middle third.
C. Patients with Barrett's metaplasia are 40 times more likely than the general population to develop adenocarcinoma.
D. Metastases from esophageal carcinoma are characteristically localized to regional mediastinal lymph nodes adjacent to the tumor.
E. Achalasia, radiation esophagitis, caustic esophageal stricture, Barrett's mucosa, and Plummer-Vinson syndrome are all premalignant esophageal lesions that predispose to the development of squamous cell carcinoma.

DISCUSSION: Histologically, 95% of esophageal cancers worldwide are squamous cell carcinomas, but the incidence of adenocarcinoma is increasing dramatically in the United States and Europe. Squamous cell carcinoma predominates in the upper and middle thirds of the esophagus, whereas adenocarcinoma is the most frequent distal esophageal cancer. A columnar lined lower esophagus (Barrett's metaplasia) is associated with an incidence of adenocarcinoma approximately 40 times greater than that of the general population. Esophageal cancer is a biologically aggressive tumor that characteristically metastasizes widely to regional and distant lymph nodes as well as to liver and lungs. Recognized premalignant esophageal lesions include achalasia, radiation esophagitis, caustic stricture, Plummer-Vinson syndrome, leukoplakia, esophageal diverticula, and Barrett's metaplasia. All but Barrett's metaplasia are associated with the development of squamous cell carcinoma.

Textbook: Pages 747–748 ANSWER: C.

14. Which of the following statements about the surgical treatment of esophageal carcinoma is/are correct?

A. The finding of severe dysphagia in association with Barrett's mucosa is an indication for an antireflux operation to prevent subsequent development of carcinoma.
B. Long-term survival is improved by radical *en bloc* resection of the esophagus with its contained tumor, adjacent mediastinal tissues, and regional lymph nodes.
C. The morbidity and mortality rates for cervical esophagogastric anastomotic leak are substantially less than those associated with intrathoracic esophagogastric anastomotic leak.
D. The leading complications of transthoracic esophagectomy and intrathoracic esophagogastric anastomosis are bleeding and wound infection.
E. Transhiatal esophagectomy without thoracotomy achieves better long-term survival than transthoracic esophagectomy.

DISCUSSION: Severe dysplasia in Barrett's mucosa is indicative of carcinoma *in situ* and is an indication for *resectional* therapy, not an antireflux operation. In the majority of patients, local tumor invasion or distant metastases preclude cure when esophageal carcinoma is diagnosed, and attempts to improve survival with a more radical local operation performed in the face of systemic disease have been disappointingly futile. A cervical esophagogastric anastomotic leak causes a relatively minor cervical salivary fistula that heals in 7 to 10 days in 95% of patients. In contrast, an intrathoracic esophagogastric anastomotic leak results in mediastinitis, which is fatal in 50%. The leading complications of transthoracic esophagectomy and an intrathoracic esophagogastric anastomosis are respiratory insufficiency (from combined thoracic and abdominal incisions) and anastomotic leak resulting in mediastinitis and sepsis. Both complications are minimized by transhiatal esophagectomy without thoracotomy plus cervical esophagogastric anastomosis. No single operative approach to the treatment of esophageal cancer has proved superior to others in terms of long-term survival. The biologic behavior of the tumor (its stage and aggressiveness)—not the number of lymph nodes resected with the tumor—determines survival.

Textbook: Pages 748, 750, 752–755 ANSWER: C.

15. The best management for a 48-hour-old distal esophageal perforation is:

A. Antibiotics and drainage.
B. Division of the esophagus and exclusion of the perforation.
C. Primary repair with buttressing.
D. Resection with cervical esophagostomy, gastrostomy, and jejunostomy.
E. T-tube fistula and drainage.

DISCUSSION: When the esophagus is repaired primarily and covered by well-vascularized autologous tissue, the rates of fistula and death are significantly less than those observed for patients who receive simple repair without any protection. Primary repair with buttressing is the first choice for treatment. Resection is reserved for esophageal perforations with extensive damage to the esophageal wall or with advanced mediastinal infection and sepsis. Exclusion of the perforated esophagus and T-tube drainage of a perforation are alternative approaches that cannot be considered for primary treatment. Antibiotics and drainage as the sole treatment is reserved for a very small, selected population of patients with well-contained esophageal perforation.

Textbook: Pages 762–765 ANSWER: C.

16. A 50-year-old patient develops sudden left lower chest pain and epigastric pain after vomiting. The patient shows diaphoresis, breath sounds are decreased on the left, and there is abdominal guarding. The most appropriate diagnostic test is:

A. Aortography.
B. Esophagoscopy.
C. Electrocardiogram.
D. Film of the chest.
E. White blood count.

DISCUSSION: The history of pain after vomiting efforts suggests esophageal rupture. Pain is often described as excruciating and frequently masquerades as a dissecting aneurysm, perforated ulcer, or myocardial infarction. Decreased breath sounds suggest the possibility of hydropneumothorax. The diagnostic procedure is a chest film. More than 90% of patients with an esophageal perforation show abnormalities suggestive of perforation. The findings are influenced by the interval between perforation and the examination, by the site of the perforation, and by the integrity of the mediastinal pleura. Esophagoscopy is not indicated.

Textbook: Pages 760–762 ANSWER: D.

17. The following statements about the influence of diet and lifestyle on lower esophageal sphincter (LES) function are true *except one.* Identify the incorrect statement.

A. A high-protein diet increases LES pressure.
B. A fat meal results in sustained decrease in LES pressure.
C. Chocolate ingestion causes a decrease in LES pressure.
D. Peppermint produces a transient decrease in LES values.
E. Cigarette smoking produces no significant changes in LES pressures.

DISCUSSION: There is a dramatic decrease in LES pressure following the ingestion of fat. Chocolate has the same effect on LES resting pressures. Peppermint was shown to produce transient decreases in LES pressures of 20 to 30 seconds, which occur approximately 10 minutes after ingestion. The ingestion of carbohydrates produces no significant change in sphincter pressures, but a high-protein meal increases LES pressure. Cigarette smoking has also been shown to produce significant decreases in LES pressure that persist throughout the duration of active smoking.

Textbook: Pages 773–774 ANSWER: E.

18. When a stricture is present in association with gastroesophageal reflux, each of the following is an acceptable repair for reflux control except one. Identify the poorest repair.

A. Intrathoracic total fundoplication.
B. Lengthening gastroplasty with total fundoplication.
C. Total fundoplication.
D. Lengthening gastroplasty with partial fundoplication.
E. Partial fundoplication.

DISCUSSION: When a stricture is present, periesophagitis and shortening limit the chances of obtaining a sufficient length of intra-abdominal esophagus. Even extensive mobilization of the esophagus to the aortic arch and freeing of the esophagogastric junction does not afford a comfortable 4 to 5 cm. of esophagus under the diaphragm. A tension-free repair is not possible in such circumstances. Partial fundoplication at this stage of the disease is followed by a 45% failure rate. Excellent results have been reported using a total fundoplication following dilatation of the stricture, and intrathoracic fundoplication provided good results. The lengthening gastroplasty with a partial fundoplication or with total fundoplication shows satisfactory control of reflux in a majority of patients.

Textbook: Pages 780–782 ANSWER: E.

19. When assessing gastroesophageal reflux disease by manometry each of the following statements is correct except one. Identify the incorrect one.

A. Absent or extremely low LES pressures have predictive value in identifying more severe reflux.
B. Peristaltic dysfunction increases with increasing severity of esophagitis.
C. With established reflux disease the UES is hypertensive.
D. Esophageal functional changes are worst in patients with a circumferential columnar-lined esophagus.
E. Absence of peristalsis may be associated with more severe forms of reflux disease.

DISCUSSION: In reflux disease when LES pressure is below 10 mm. Hg, manometry is too imprecise to identify a potential for significant reflux. If the pressure is less than 6 mm. Hg, this shows a reasonable high specificity as compared with abnormal reflux on pH testing. When LES pressure is extremely low or nonexistent, this identifies a more severe degree of reflux and a poorer prognosis for long-term medical therapy. In the esophageal body, active reflux esophagitis causes altered function. Failed peristalsis increases, and the contractions become weaker. Patients with a columnar-lined esophagus have the worst functional abnormalities. Although distention or acid perfusion in the proximal esophagus can produce a significant increase in UES resting pressure, there is at present no solid evidence relating UES resting pressures to active reflux disease.

Textbook: Page 773 ANSWER: C.

20. The presence of a nonmalignant mid- or upper esophageal stricture always indicates the presence of:

A. Alkaline reflux esophagitis.
B. Barrett's esophagus.
C. Idiopathic reflux disease.
D. Mediastinal fibrosis.
E. Scleroderma.

DISCUSSION: A stricture at or above the aortic arch is almost certainly situated above an esophagus lined at its lower end with columnar epithelium. Barrett's esophagus is suggested radiographically when local esophagitis, ulcer, or stricture is at the limits of a normal-looking segment of esophagus under the stricture but above a herniated stomach. The columnar-lined esophagus is not always associated with a high stricture; however Messiaen and Halpert documented strictures in 80% of their Barrett's patients. These high strictures, when seen with alkaline reflux esophagitis, with idiopathic reflux disease, or in association with scleroderma, always suggest the presence of a columnar-lined esophagus. Mediastinal fibrosis is a rare condition that can cause multilevel strictures on the esophagus.

Textbook: Page 777 ANSWER: B.

21. Which of the following is most reliable for confirming the occurrence of a significant esophageal caustic injury?

A. History of the event.
B. Physical examination of the patient.
C. Barium esophagraphy.
D. Endoscopy.

DISCUSSION: In the absence of physical or radiographic evidence of upper airway obstruction or esophagogastric perforation, the presence of a significant caustic injury can be defined reliably only by direct visualization at the time of endoscopy. Although the history may shed light on the possibility of a burn and its severity, all too often the event goes unwitnessed or the type and amount of ingested substance are not known with certainty. The identification of oropharyngeal burns clearly indicates the need for endoscopy, but as many as 70% of patients with such lesions escape associated esophageal injury. Conversely, 10% to 30% of patients with no external evidence of burns have subsequently been confirmed by esophagoscopy to have sustained damage. In the absence of an identifiable perforation, a barium esophagogram can rarely be considered unequivocally diagnostic of acute injury, though such an injury may be suggested when the esophagus appears atonic and dilated, rigid and persistently narrowed, or excessively irritable. Because of the importance of early confirmation of the presence or absence of a significant esophageal burn as a guide to formulating appropriate treatment, esophagoscopy should be performed expeditiously as soon as sufficient time has elapsed to allow gastric emptying and stabilization of the patient, preferably within the first 12 to 48 hours after ingestion.

Textbook: Page 785 ANSWER: D.

22. Indications for surgical reconstruction of the esophagus include which of the following?

A. Continuing requirement for frequent dilation of an extensive esophageal stricture for a minimum of 2 years.
B. Failure or refusal of the patient to comply with a treatment regimen of regular dilation.
C. Development of a fistula between the esophagus and tracheobronchial tree.
D. Iatrogenic perforation of the esophagus during attempted dilation.

DISCUSSION: Development of a tracheobronchial fistula almost always necessitates some form of esophageal reconstruction because of the extensive damage usually associated with it. Failure of the patient to cooperate effectively condemns to failure any attempt at restoring esophageal patency by bougienage, because sporadic attempts at dilation do not allow progressive lumen enlargement but, rather, invite additional injury because of the necessity for repeated instrumentation of a recurrent, tight stricture. The need for repeated dilation of extensive or multiple strictures over a period exceeding 6 months should prompt surgical reconstruction of the esophagus, especially in young children, for whom the psychological and physical hazards are intensified by prolonged treatment. In such circumstances, a 2-year period of attempted bougienage is excessive. Although iatrogenic perforation often signals the need for esophageal reconstruction, this misadventure should not be considered an absolute indication but should be assessed in relation to (1) the extent and complexity of the stricture, (2) the potential for eventually achieving successful bougienage, and (3) the severity of complications caused by the secondary injury.

Textbook: Pages 787–788 ANSWER: B, C, D.

23. Which of the following statements about desmoid tumors are correct?

A. These abdominal wall tumors are benign fibrous tumors that arise from the musculoaponeurotic abdominal wall.
B. They are histologically benign but frequently are locally invasive.
C. They usually present as a rapidly growing subcutaneous mass.
D. They have a high propensity toward metastasis.

DISCUSSION: Desmoid tumors of the abdominal wall are benign fibrous tumors that arise from the musculoaponeurotic abdominal wall. Histologically benign but frequently locally invasive, they are prone to recurrence following local excision. They present as firm, subcutaneous masses that grow slowly. They should be widely excised to prevent local recurrence. They do not have a propensity toward metastasis.

Textbook: Page 815 ANSWER: A, B.

24. The following statements about retroperitoneal fibrosis are correct.

A. Retroperitoneal fibrosis is relatively rare, and

about two thirds of all cases are considered idiopathic.

B. Presentation may vary from mild back pain to uremia or sepsis.

C. The characteristic findings are hydronephrosis and hydroureter proximal to the site of extrinsic compression of the ureters.

D. The ureters are generally deviated laterally.

DISCUSSION: Retroperitoneal fibrosis is a rare and unusual disease that has some similarities to hypersensitivity reactions and to autoimmune diseases. The cause is unknown, and two thirds of all cases are considered idiopathic in that no specific cause can be proved. A correlation between ingestion of methysergide and the disease has been reported. The most important clinical aspect of retroperitoneal fibrosis is that the fibrotic process frequently entraps and constricts the ureters, thus causing obstructive uropathy. Patient's signs and symptoms depend on the presence or absence of urinary tract infection. The characteristic findings are hydronephrosis and hydroureters proximal to the site of extrinsic compression of the ureters. The disease is usually bilateral and results in deviation of the ureters toward the midline.

Textbook: Pages 821–822 ANSWER: A, B, C.

25. During a routine laparoscopic cholecystectomy (LC) the anesthesiologist reports a declining end-tidal CO_2. Intra-abdominal pressure is 1.5 mm. Hg. Breath sounds are equal. Heart rate is 110; systolic blood pressure, 75 mm. Hg; oxygen saturation, 88; and a heart murmur is noted. Which of the following is the most likely cause?

A. Anesthetic overdose.
B. Hemorrhage.
C. Tension pneumothorax.
D. Carbon dioxide embolus.
E. Vasovagal reaction.
F. Vena caval compression.

DISCUSSION: See next question.

26. Treatment of the above situation should include which of the following?

A. Type and cross-match and give rapid blood transfusion.
B. Evacuate the pneumoperitoneum.
C. Place patient in head-down, left lateral decubitus position.
D. Place patient in Trendelenburg position.
E. Place patient in reverse Trendelenburg position.
F. Stick a needle into the right chest.
G. Place an emergent central venous line.

DISCUSSION: Hemodynamic compromise following insufflation of CO_2 pneumoperitoneum is a rare but potentially lethal event. The differential diagnosis should include CO_2 embolism, vena caval compression, tension pneumothorax, hemorrhage, arrhythmias, and anesthesia-related causes. In addition to CPR, if necessary, and supportive measures, treatment should consist of immediate evacuation of the pneumoperitoneum and treatment aimed at specific causes. A sudden decrease in oxygen saturation with a drop in end-tidal CO_2, and the presence of a new continuous murmur, with or without hemodynamic compromise, should alert one to the possibility of a CO_2 embolus. Treatment should include immediate evacuation of the pneumoperitoneum and placement of the patient in Trendelenburg position, left side down, to direct the air bubble into the right atrium so that absorbtion may occur away from the right ventricular outflow. Aspiration via a central venous catheter may be diagnostic as well as therapeutic.

Textbook: Pages 799–800 ANSWER: 1, D. 2, B, C, G.

27. Pulmonary function following LC as compared with open cholecystectomy is characterized by which of the following findings?

A. No changes in oxygen saturation.
B. A relatively smaller decrease in FEV_1 on the first postoperative day, returning to preoperative levels after the tenth postoperative day.
C. An increase in the rate of atelectasis due to the reduction in lung volume caused by the pneumoperitoneum.
D. No effect on pulmonary complications.
E. A relatively smaller decrease in lung volume.

DISCUSSION: Numerous studies have demonstrated that LC as compared with open cholecystectomy results in a significantly reduced compromise in pulmonary function and narcotic requirement, leading to fewer postoperative pulmonary complications. Patients undergoing LC have a significant reduction in postoperative pulmonary impairment (30% to 38%) in all areas studied including FVC, FEV_1, $FEF_{25-75\%}$, FEF_{max}, MVV, TLC, and oxygen saturation. Pulmonary function returns to baseline levels 4 to 10 days sooner after LC. Pulmonary complications, including atelectasis and hypoxia and pneumonia are less frequent after LC. There is a significant reduction in postoperative pain medication requirement in patients undergoing LC, which may partially account for the observed benefits in pulmonary function.

Textbook: Page 798 ANSWER: E.

28. Laparoscopic access for abdominal surgery, as compared with laparotomy, results in which of the following?

A. A greater increase in the catecholamine response as compared to open procedures, owing to the stress of the pneumoperitoneum.
B. A more pronounced suppression of immune function due to impairment of T-cell function as determined by skin antigen testing.
C. A reduction in the rate of postoperative ileus.
D. A threefold increase in the rate of deep venous thrombosis because of pneumoperitoneum-induced venous stasis.
E. An increase in wound infection rates related to laparoscopic methods of specimen removal.

DISCUSSION: Compared to laparotomy, laparoscopic surgery has a positive effect on many organ systems other than the pulmonary system. The stress response to surgical injury as measured by the neuroendocrine response is attenuated. Immune function is better preserved, as determined by response to skin antigens, levels of immune cytokines (IL-6), and tumor growth in mice. Reduced cardiac complications after laparoscopic surgery suggest reduced cardiac impairment. Clinical and laboratory evidence demonstrates reduced impairment of postoperative gastrointestinal motility. Although pneumoperitoneum may increase venous stasis, a reduction in the postoperative hypercoagulable state may negate a potential increase in venous thrombosis after laparoscopic procedures. The incidence of postoperative venous thrombosis after laparoscopic procedures is currently unknown. Postoperative adhesion formation and wound-related complications are less common after laparoscopic surgery.
Textbook: Pages 795–800 ANSWER: C.

29. Regarding complications of laparoscopic surgery, which of the following are true?

A. The overall morbidity of LC is greater than that of open cholecystectomy.
B. Only trocar sites greater than 12 mm. require fascial closure to prevent abdominal wall hernia.
C. Visceral injuries related to trocar insertion can be completely avoided by using an "open" Hassan technique.
D. Spilled gallstones should be retrieved because they may result in development of an intra-abdominal abscess.
E. Prior abdominal surgery, and the presence of acute inflammation, are absolute contraindications to laparoscopic surgery.

DISCUSSION: The reduction in overall morbidity is the primary benefit of LC. Reports of hernia formation from unclosed trocar sites as small as 10 mm. support the recommendation that fascial incisions 10 mm. or greater should be closed. Visceral injuries have been reported using the open technique (e.g., bowel laceration); however, they tend to be less severe and are more likely to be recognized at the time of occurrence. Prior abdominal surgery and acute inflammation were once thought to be contraindications to laparoscopic surgery. Many reports have demonstrated that patients with these pre-existing conditions may safely undergo LC.
Textbook: Pages 801, 804 ANSWER: D.

30. Which of the following statements concerning the abdominal wall layers are correct?

A. Scarpa's fascia affords little strength in wound closure.
B. The internal abdominal oblique muscles have fibers that continue into the scrotum as cremasteric muscles.
C. The transversalis fascia is the most important layer of the abdominal wall in preventing hernias.
D. The lymphatics of the abdominal wall drain into the ipsilateral axillary lymph nodes above the umbilicus and into the ipsilateral superficial inguinal lymph nodes below the umbilicus.

DISCUSSION: The integrity of the abdominal wall is maintained principally by the transversalis fascia. Scarpia's fascia affords little strength in wound closure, but its approximation contributes considerably to the creation of an aesthetically acceptable scar. The cremasteric muscles of the spermatic cord are a continuation of muscle fibers from the internal abdominal oblique musculature. The lymphatic supply of the abdominal wall follows a simple pattern. These superficial lymphatics run parallel to the superficial veins, which above the umbilicus drain into the ipsilateral axillary vein and below it into the ipsilateral femoral vein.
Textbook: Pages 809–813 ANSWER: A, B, C, D.

31. Which of the following congenital abnormalities are correctly defined?

A. *Omphalocele* represents a defect in the abdominal wall lateral to the umbilical cord.
B. The *herniated viscera* associated with omphaloceles are usually covered with a membranous sac.
C. An *umbilical polyp* is a small excrescence of omphalomesenteric duct mucosa that is retained in the umbilicus.
D. *Meckel's diverticulum* results when the intestinal end of the omphalomesenteric duct persists and represents a true diverticulum.

DISCUSSION: Omphalocele may be seen in newborns and represents a defect in the closure of the umbilical ring. The herniated viscera are usually covered with a sac. Gastroschisis, a defect of the abdominal wall lateral to the umbilical cord, is caused by failure of closure of the body wall. The intestines protrude through the defect, and no sac is present to cover the herniated intestine. In the fetus, the omphalomesenteric duct may present as abnormalities related to the abdominal wall when the duct fails to obliterate. Meckel's diverticulum is the result of the failure of obliteration of the intestinal end of the omphalomesenteric duct. This is a true diverticulum with all layers of the intestinal wall represented. An umbilical polyp is a small excrescence of omphalomesenteric duct mucosa retained in the umbilicus. Such polyps resemble umbilical granulomas except that they do not disappear after silver nitrate cauterization. Appropriate treatment is excision of the mucosal remnant.
Textbook: Pages 813–814 ANSWER: B, C, D.

32. Which of the following statements concerning intraperitoneal fluid collections are correct?

A. Ascites occurs when either the peritoneal fluid secretion rate increases or the absorption rate decreases.
B. Accumulation of lymph within the peritoneal cavity usually results from trauma as tumor

involving the intra-abdominal lymphatic structures.

C. Choleperitoneum (intraperitoneal bile) generally occurs following biliary surgery, but spontaneous perforation of the bile duct has been reported.

D. The most common cause of hemoperitoneum is trauma to the liver or spleen.

DISCUSSION: Normally, there is a balance between fluid secretion and absorption in the peritoneal cavity. Ascites occurs when either the secretion rate increases or the absorption rate decreases disproportionately. Accumulation of lymph in the peritoneal cavity usually results from trauma or tumor involving lymphatic structures. Proposed treatment regimens range from salt restriction and diuretics to surgical ligation and peritoneovenous shunting. Uninfected bile is a mild irritant to the peritoneal cavity and causes increased production of peritoneal fluid, resulting in bile ascities or choleperitoneum. Most cases of choleperitoneum follow biliary tract surgery, but cases of spontaneous bile duct perforation have been reported in infants and some adults. The most common cause of hemoperitoneum is trauma to the liver or spleen. Less common causes include ruptured ectopic pregnancy, ruptured aortic aneurysms, and other intra-abdominal injuries.

Textbook: Pages 816–817 ANSWER: A, B, C, D.

33. The following statement about peritonitis are all true except:

A. Peritonitis is defined as inflammation of the peritoneum.

B. Most surgical peritonitis is secondary to bacterial contamination.

C. Primary peritonitis has no documented source of contamination and is more common in adults than in children and in men than in women.

D. Tuberculous peritonitis can present with or without ascites.

DISCUSSION: Peritonitis is inflammation of the peritoneum and can be septic or aseptic, bacterial or viral, primary or secondary, acute or chronic. Most surgical peritonitis is secondary to bacterial contamination from the gastrointestinal tract. Primary peritonitis refers to inflammation of the peritoneal cavity without a documented source of contamination. It is more common in children than in adults and in women than in men. The female predominance is felt to be explained by entry of organism into the peritoneal cavity through the fallopian tubes. The clinical manifestations of tuberculous peritonitis are of two types. The moist form consists of fever, ascites, abdominal pain, and weakness. The dry form presents in a similar manner but without ascites.

Textbook: Pages 817–818 ANSWER: C.

34. True or false?

A. Mesenteric cysts are most often due to congenital lymphatic spaces that gradually fill with lymph.

B. Mesenteric cysts usually present as abdominal masses accompanied by pain, nausea, or vomiting.

C. Mesenteric cysts are best treated by marsupialization.

D. Omental cysts are frequently asymptomatic unless they undergo torsion.

DISCUSSION: Mesenteric cysts are most often due to congenital lymphatic spaces that gradually enlarge as they fill with lymph. They generally present as abdominal masses accompanied by pain, nausea, and vomiting. They usually can be diagnosed by physical examination and have characteristic lateral mobility. They are best treated by surgical excision, and intestinal resection may be necessary for complete removal. Omental cysts are frequently asymptomatic but may present with vague discomfort or as a mobile abdominal mass that can cause torsion of the omentum. Torsion generally presents with signs and symptoms compatible with acute cholecystitis, appendicitis, or a twisted ovarian cyst. Treatment entails local resection.

Textbook: Pages 819–820 ANSWER: A, True; B, true; C, false; D, true.

35. Which of the following statements about acute salpingitis are true?

A. The disease rarely occurs after menopause.

B. Gonococcal infection is most common.

C. There is minimal cervical tenderness to palpation.

D. Vaginal discharge occurs rarely.

Textbook: Pages 843–844 ANSWER: A, B.

36. Acute appendicitis is most commonly associated with which of the following signs?

A. Temperature above 104° F.

B. Frequent loose stools.

C. Anorexia, abdominal pain, and right lower quadrant tenderness.

D. White blood cell count greater than 20,000 per cu. mm.

Textbook: Pages 838–839 ANSWER: C.

37. The best type of x-ray to locate free abdominal air is:

A. A posteroanterior view of the chest.

B. A flat and upright view of the abdomen.

C. Computed tomograph (CT) of the abdomen.

D. A lateral decubitus x-ray, right side up.

Textbook: Page 829 ANSWER: D.

38. The most helpful diagnostic radiographic procedure in small bowel obstruction is:

A. CT of the abdomen.

B. Contrast study of the intestine.

C. Supine and erect x-rays of the abdomen.

D. Ultrasonography of the abdomen.

Textbook: Pages 829–830 ANSWER: C.

39. The most commonly used imaging method for diagnosis of acute cholecystitis is:

A. CT of the abdomen.
B. Ultrasonography of the gallbladder.
C. Oral cholecystogram.
D. Radionuclide (HIDA) scan of the gallbladder.

Textbook: Page 831 ANSWER: B.

40. Acute salpingitis occurs most often:

A. After menopause.
B. In patients with unilateral lower abdominal pain.
C. During the menstrual cycle.
D. In patients with cervical tenderness and vaginal discharge.

Textbook: Pages 843–844 ANSWER: D.

41. Meckel's diverticulitis most often occurs in the:

A. Proximal jejunum.
B. Distal jejunum.
C. Proximal ileum.
D. Distal ileum.

Textbook: Pages 843–844 ANSWER: D.

42. First-line therapy for routine peptic duodenal ulcer disease includes:

A. Vagotomy and antrectomy.
B. Upper endoscopy and biopsy to rule out tumor.
C. Evaluation for *Helicobacter pylori.*
D. Serum gastrin determination.
E. Cream or milk-based "Sippy" diet.

DISCUSSION: Vagotomy and antrectomy is the definitive surgical therapy for peptic ulcer disease but should be applied only for complications of the disease or after refractory disease has been documented. Biopsy of routine peptic duodenal ulcer is not indicated to rule out malignancy except in special circumstances, such as an endoscopic appearance typical of malignancy. *H. pylori* is found in a large percentage of peptic ulcer patients, and treatment alters the rate of recurrence if therapy is directed toward reduction of *H. pylori* in addition to acid. Measurement of serum gastrin is recommended for patients with resistant or persistent peptic ulcer disease for patients undergoing surgery for peptic ulcer disease. The Sippy diet has not been recommended clinically for years. Formerly it was recommended as a bland diet that would not exacerbate peptic ulcer disease. It is now known that these diets are heavily calcium-laden and probably exacerbate peptic ulcer disease.

Textbook: Pages 853–854 ANSWER: C.

43. Appropriate management of severe vomiting associated with gastric outlet obstruction from peptic ulcer disease includes all of the following except:

A. Nasogastric suction.
B. Intravenous hydration.
C. Nutritional assessment; upper endoscopy to rule out malignancy.
D. Intravenous H_2 antagonist.
E. Oral antacid therapy.

DISCUSSION: All patients should undergo nasogastric suction, rehydration, and control of acid secretion. This control of acid secretion requires an H_2 antagonist since oral antacids are often inadequate to neutralize the large volume of acid often present in the obstructed stomach. Patients with a long history of obstruction are often nutritionally compromised and need careful nutritional assessment before operative planning.

Textbook: Page 858 ANSWER: E.

44. All of the following are complications of peptic ulcer surgery except:

A. Duodenal stump blowout.
B. Dumping.
C. Diarrhea.
D. Delayed gastric emptying.
E. Steatorrhea.

DISCUSSION: Duodenal stump blowout occurs after Billroth II operations, where back-pressure in the duodenal stump results in breakdown of this stump closure, leading to abdominal sepsis. Dumping syndrome and postvagotomy diarrhea are complications of peptic ulcer surgery. They represent two different syndromes, both of which are predominately related to the vagotomy portion of the operation. Delayed gastric emptying occurs frequently after peptic ulcer surgery, for a variety of reasons, but it is most common after elective peptic ulcer surgery for gastric outlet obstruction. Steatorrhea is not necessarily related to peptic ulcer surgery but is a complication of pancreatic insufficiency.

Textbook: Pages 861–865 ANSWER: E.

45. The presentation of Zollinger-Ellison syndrome includes all of the following except:

A. Hyperparathyroidism in patients with multiple endocrine neoplasia type 1 (MEN 1) syndrome.
B. Diarrhea.
C. Migratory rash.
D. Jejunal ulcers.
E. Duodenal ulcers.

DISCUSSION: Zollinger-Ellison syndrome occurs in two settings: sporadically and in association with MEN 1 syndrome. MEN 1 syndrome includes parathyroid adenomas, and the initial presentation is often related to this parathyroid disease. Diarrhea is a common presentation for Zollinger-Ellison syndrome, since hyperacidity can result in diarrhea due to the volume of acid secreted or from a steatorrhea-type diarrhea when the high levels of acids inactivate the pancreatic enzymes. Migratory rash is commonly associated with glucagonoma but not with Zollinger-Ellison syndrome. Both jejunal and duodenal ulcers can be found with Zollinger-Ellison syndrome.

Textbook: Pages 866–867 ANSWER: C.

46. All are true about the dumping syndrome except:

A. Symptoms can be controlled with a somatostatin analog.
B. Diarrhea is always part of the dumping syndrome.
C. Flushing and tachycardia are common features of the syndrome.
D. Separating solids and liquids in the patient's oral intake alleviates some of the symptoms of the syndrome.
E. Early postoperative dumping after vagotomy often resolves spontaneously.

DISCUSSION: The somatostatin analog octreotide has been used to control the dumping syndrome and is currently the only known medical therapy for this disease. Other therapies include dietary measures such as six small meals a day and separation of solids and liquids. Pcstvagotomy diarrhea is a secondary complication of vagotomy and is not strictly associated with the dumping syndrome itself. The vast majority of patients with dumping syndrome experience spontaneous resolution of their symptoms without intervention in the postoperative period.

Textbook: Pages 863–864 ANSWER: B.

47. In patients with bleeding duodenal ulcers, the endoscopic finding associated with the highest incidence of rebleeding is:

A. Visible vessel.
B. Cherry-red spot.
C. Clean ulcer bed.
D. Duodenitis.
E. Shallow, 3-mm. ulcer.

DISCUSSION: A visible vessel in an ulcer bed is associated with a 50% chance of rebleeding and, other than an actively bleeding vessel, is the worst endoscopic prognostic indicator for rebleeding. Cherry-red spot, adherent clot, and clean small ulcers all are associated with a lower incidence of rebleeding.

Textbook: Page 859 ANSWER: A.

48. All of the following are contraindications for highly selective vagotomy except:

A. Intractable duodenal ulcer disease.
B. Peptic ulcer disease causing gastric outlet obstruction.
C. Fundic peptic ulceration.
D. Cigarette chain smoking.
E. Perforated peptic ulcer disease with more than 24 hours' soilage.

DISCUSSION: Intractable peptic ulcer symptoms are a classic indication for highly selective vagotomy. Patients with gastric outlet obstruction often do poorly with highly selective vagotomy and develop recurrent ulceration. Highly selective vagotomy is not indicated for gastric ulceration. Heavy chain smokers often get recurrent peptic ulceration after highly selective vagotomy; therefore, vagotomy and antrectomy is indicated for them. Patients who experience long periods of perforation before exploratory laparotomy should receive either patch plus vagotomy or pyloroplasty or patch of the ulcer alone. Extensive operations, such as highly selective vagotomy, are usually not indicated in this acute setting.

Textbook: Pages 859–861 ANSWER: A.

49. All the following are true of omeprazole except:

A. It is the only drug available that has the potential to achieve pharmacologically induced achlorhydria.
B. It works by blocking the hydrogen-potassium ATPase in the parietal cell.
C. It is parietal cell specific.
D. It has a short half-life (about 90 minutes) when taken orally.
E. It has been associated with gastric neoplasm in a rat model.

DISCUSSION: Omeprazole and drugs in this category are the only drugs that can produce achlorhydria. All other antiacid drugs reduce acid secretion without producing achlorhydria. Omeprazole inhibits acid at the final common pathway by blocking the hydrogen-potassium ATPase in parietal cells. It is gastric parietal cell specific and has a very long half-life, allowing once daily dosing when given orally. When it was given to rats in pharmacologic doses the gastric mucosa formed carcinoid-type tumors. This problem has not been identified in humans.

Textbook: Pages 779, 854–857 ANSWER: D.

50. All of the following statements about gastrin-releasing peptide (GRP) are true except:

A. In species other than man and dog GRP is commonly referred to as *bombesin.*
B. GRP serves as a neurotransmitter.
C. GRP inhibits pancreatic secretion when given intravenously.
D. GRP stimulates gastric acid secretion when given intravenously.
E. GRP is released in response to cholinergic stimulation of the parietal cells to stimulate release of gastrin.

DISCUSSION: Gastrin-releasing peptide and bombesin are homologous peptides of different amino acid lengths. GRP functions as a neurotransmitter at the cholinergic nerve ending on the parietal cell and releases gastrin after cholinergic stimulation. It functions to increase gastric acid secretion and also pharmacologically increases pancreatic secretion.

Textbook: Page 849 ANSWER: C.

51. Cholecystokinin (CCK) is believed to function in all of the following processes except:

A. It physiologically delays gastric emptying.
B. It appears to have a role in satiety regulation.
C. It contracts the gallbladder.

D. It stimulates pancreatic secretion.
E. It is important in the control of the anal sphincter.

DISCUSSION: CCK has a physiologic role in the regulation of gastric emptying, eating behavior, gallbladder contraction, and pancreatic secretion. There is experimental evidence that it may serve as a neurotransmitter in the function of the lower esophageal sphincter. It probably also has a role in augmenting the release of insulin after a meal. It has no known role in the function of the anal sphincter.

Textbook: Page 852 ANSWER: E.

52. All of the following measures have been recommended for control of acid secretion in patients with Zollinger-Ellison syndrome except:

A. Antrectomy.
B. Highly selective vagotomy.
C. Total gastrectomy.
D. Vagotomy and pyloroplasty.
E. Medical therapy with Prilosec (omeprazole).

DISCUSSION: Patients with MEN 1 syndrome or sporadic-metastatic Zollinger-Ellison syndrome should be palliated with omeprazole to control their acid secretion. Patients who undergo exploration may have a variety of operations to control their ulcer diathesis, including total gastrectomy or various vagotomy-type operations. Antrectomy alone is not indicated, since the gastrin that is contributing to the production of acid is not coming from the antrum but coming from the tumor.

Textbook: Pages 866–867 ANSWER: A.

53. All of the following contribute to peptic ulcer disease except:

A. Cigarette smoking.
B. Nonsteroidal anti-inflammatory drugs.
C. *Helicobacter pylori.*
D. Gastrinoma.
E. Spicy foods.

DISCUSSION: Cigarettes and nonsteroidal anti-inflammatory drugs are common contributors to peptic ulceration. *H. pylori* is found in most patients with peptic ulceration, and eradication of this bacterium decreases the recurrence rate for peptic ulcer disease. Gastrinoma results in much acid secretion and commonly presents with peptic ulcer disease. Dietary factors such as spicy foods have little or no effect on postprandial acid secretion and do not contribute to peptic ulceration.

Textbook: Pages 853–854 ANSWER: E.

54. Which of the following statements about gastric polyps is/are true?

A. Like their colonic counterparts, gastric epithelial polyps are common tumors.
B. They are analogous to colorectal polyps in natural history.
C. Endoscopy can uniformly predict the histology of a polyp based on location and appearance.
D. In a given patient, multiple polyps are generally of a single histologic type.
E. Gastric adenomatous polyps greater than 2 cm. in diameter should be excised because of the risk of malignant transformation.

DISCUSSION: As early as 1895 Hauser reported an association between familial adenomatous polyposis of the colon and multiple gastric polyps. This early association may have given rise not only to the confusing nomenclature of gastric polyps but also to the mistaken notion that they are analogous to colorectal polyps in microscopic appearance and natural history. Unlike colonic polyps, gastric epithelial polyps are very uncommon tumors (prevalence 0.4% to 0.8%). Their histologic appearance cannot be predicted on the basis of location in the stomach, although the endoscopic literature is beginning to define predictive algorithms based on location and ultrasound. Multiple polyps are almost always of a single histologic type. Gastric adenomatous polyps have long been associated with adenocarcinoma. This association is directly related to the size of the polyps. Up to 24% of polyps 2 cm. or greater in diameter are associated with adenocarcinoma. In contrast, only 4% of polyps with a diameter less than 2 cm. are associated with carcinoma. The risk, if any, of carcinoma in patients with hyperplastic polyps appears to be associated with the atrophic gastritis that frequently accompanies them rather than with the polyps themselves.

Textbook: Pages 870–871 ANSWER: D, E.

55. Which of the following statements about gastric leiomyomas is/are true?

A. They are the most common type of gastric tumor of the stomach at autopsy.
B. The leiomyoblastoma cell type reflects malignant transformation of gastric leiomyomas.
C. A conservative surgical approach is indicated for their resection since regional lymphadenectomy has not been proved reliable even when they turn out to be malignant.
D. Severe hemorrhage may occur from deep ulcerations overlying the intramural tumor.

DISCUSSION: Approximately 40% of benign tumors of the stomach are leiomyomas derived from the smooth muscle of the stomach or its associated blood vessels. Because it is rare for gastric leiomyomas smaller than 3 cm. in diameter to be symptomatic, considerably fewer than 2% of gastric neoplasms resected surgically are of smooth muscle origin. Gastric leiomyomas may be smooth or lobulated, but in time a central ulceration occurs in the mucosal bulge of the tumor in approximately half of submucosal leiomyomas. Ulceration may be present in smaller tumors but absent in very large tumors. Overlying central mucosal ulceration, which may penetrate deeply into the tumor, results in hematemesis, melena, or anemia and draws attention to the tumor. Bleeding from the tumor may be massive and/or intermittent.

Gastric leiomyomas are not encapsulated, even though on section they appear to be well-circumscribed. Microscopically, the tumor cells at the margin may intermingle with cells of the surrounding gastric wall. Along with the presence of occasional large cells with hyperchromatic nuclei, this has led to confusion in distinguishing benign tumors from malignant ones. Stout described a reasonably distinct variety of gastric smooth muscle tumor that he called *leiomyoblastoma* (bizarre smooth muscle tumor). They were characterized histologically by polyhedral smooth muscle cells with central nuclei and abundant cytoplasm rather than elongated cells. A clear zone that surrounds the central nucleus may be an artifact of fixation. Leiomyoblastoma may be benign or malignant. Carney has described a syndrome characterized by the triad of multiple malignant leiomyoblastoma, pulmonary chondroma, and functioning extra-adrenal paraganglioma.

The principle of surgical treatment of smooth muscle tumors is local excision with a 2- to 3-cm. margin of surrounding gastric wall. In view of the difficulty in distinguishing between the benign and malignant variants, enucleation is not an appropriate method of treatment. Regional lymphadenectomy is not of proven value, even if malignancy is strongly suspected and is not consistent with the known property of these tumors to spread by the hematogenous route.

Textbook: Pages 870–871 ANSWER: A, C, D.

56. The *sine qua non* of the histologic diagnosis of a gastric pseudolymphoma is:

A. Extragastric extension of the gastric lesion.
B. Nodal involvement beyond the immediate stomach.
C. A germinal center in the gastric lesion.
D. Extension into esophagus and duodenum.
E. Unresponsive to conservative gastric resection.

DISCUSSION: Pseudolymphoma represents approximately 10% of all gastric lymphomas. These are benign conditions involving mostly the mucosa without evidence of nodal disease and without extragastric extension. The *sine qua non* for the diagnosis is a germinal center within the gastric lesion. These are premalignant lesions but can be cured completely with conservative resection.

Textbook: Page 876 ANSWER: C.

57. All of the following statements about surgical management of gastric lymphomas are true except:

A. Stage I gastric lymphomas (small lesions confined to the stomach wall) can be cured completely with surgical therapy alone.
B. Extensive gastric lymphomas that initially are treated with radiation and/or chemotherapy occasionally perforate during treatment and require secondary resection.
C. Patients explored with a presumptive diagnosis of gastric lymphoma should undergo an attempt at curative resection when this is safe and feasible.
D. Without a preoperative diagnosis resection for gastric mass should not be attempted unless lymphoma can be excluded.
E. Appropriate staging for primary gastric lymphoma includes bone marrow biopsy.

DISCUSSION: Operation alone is adequate treatment for very early-stage lymphoma, although chemotherapy is commonly added. For more advanced disease, particularly stages III and IV, preoperative radiation chemotherapy is often indicated, even though some of these patients suffer perforation during therapy and require emergent resection. Patients who undergo exploration for gastric mass without a preoperative diagnosis can safely be resected with potential for cure even if the diagnosis includes gastric lymphoma.

Textbook: Pages 876–877 ANSWER: D.

58. Which of the following risk factors have been shown to increase significantly the incidence of gastrointestinal bleeding from stress gastritis in intensive care unit (ICU) patients?

A. Glucocorticoid administration.
B. Respiratory failure.
C. Coagulopathy.
D. Organ transplantation.
E. Jaundice.

DISCUSSION: Prophylactic measures such as H_2-receptor antagonists and antacid titration effectively reduce the incidence of gastrointestinal bleeding; however, prophylaxis against stress gastritis is expensive and may have adverse effects. Therefore, it should be used selectively in patients with high risk factors. In a prospective multicenter study in which 10 potential risk factors were evaluated for stress gastritis bleeding in ICU patients, respiratory failure and coagulopathy are two independent risk factors for clinically significant bleeding. Therefore, a strong recommendation for prophylaxis of stress gastritis can be made for ICU patients who have either respiratory failure or coagulopathy.

Textbook: Pages 879–880 ANSWER: B, C.

59. Which of the following measures are effective in preventing stress gastritis bleeding in critically ill patients?

A. Improving systemic circulation by correcting any shocklike state resulting from blood loss or sepsis.
B. Correcting systemic acid-base abnormality.
C. Maintaining adequate nutrition.
D. Reducing intragastric acidity by either antacid titration or H_2 antagonists.

DISCUSSION: Despite the lack of documentation, a strong impression exists among clinicians and clinical investigators that the incidence and prevalence of stress gastritis have decreased significantly during the past decade, perhaps owing to improved general care

for critically ill patients. The improvement in general care of these critically ill patients includes vigorous efforts to correct any shocklike state secondary to blood loss or sepsis, better ventilatory support, and maintenance of adequate nutrition. These prophylactic measures enhance the ability of the gastric mucosa to protect itself against acid injury. In addition, several prospective, randomized studies have shown that antacid titration and/or H_2-receptor antagonists are effective in preventing gastrointestinal bleeding in these patients.
Textbook: Pages 879–880 ANSWER: A, B, C, D.

60. The most common site of adenocarcinoma of the small intestine is the:

A. Duodenum.
B. Jejunum.
C. Ileum.

Textbook: Page 884 ANSWER: A.

61. The most common benign tumor of the small intestine is:

A. Adenoma.
B. Hemangioma.
C. Leiomyoma.

Textbook: Page 883 ANSWER: C.

62. Vigorous bleeding from a small bowel lesion is most likely caused by:

A. Adenocarcinoma.
B. Arteriovenous malformation.
C. Leiomyoma.

Textbook: Page 885 ANSWER: C.

63. Which of the following have been used successfully to treat patients with vascular compression of the duodenum?

A. Subtotal gastrectomy and Roux-en-Y gastrojejunostomy.
B. Total parenteral nutrition.
C. Division of the ligament of Treitz and duodenal mobilization.
D. Percutaneous endoscopic gastrostomy.
E. Duodenojejunostomy.

DISCUSSION: Vascular compression of the duodenum is best treated initially with supportive care. Of paramount importance is supplying adequate nutrition, since most patients have significant weight loss with this syndrome. This can best be done with a nasojejunal feeding tube placed past the ligament of Treitz (and the obstructed area). Gastrostomy alone does not provide unobstructed enteral access. Parenteral nutrition may be used successfully when enteral access cannot be established. When operative therapy is needed, duodenojejunostomy has been the most common and successful operation and is the treatment of choice for adults. In the pediatric population, division of the ligament of Treitz and duodenal mobilization has also proved successful. Gastrojejunostomy has been used, but with a lower overall success rate. Distal gastrectomy usually worsens duodenal obstruction by preventing duodenogastric reflux.
Textbook: Pages 890–892 ANSWER: B, C, E.

64. Which of the following statements about the anatomic basis for the syndrome of vascular compression of the duodenum are true?

A. The duodenum is obstructed in its distal third as it crosses over the lumbar vertebral column.
B. Structures crossing beneath the superior mesenteric artery include the duodenum, the uncinate process of the pancreas, and the left renal vein.
C. Hyperextension of the back allows the angle of origin of the superior mesenteric artery to widen, lessening the obstruction of the duodenum.
D. Patients are at significant risk for vascular compression of the duodenum if the angle between the takeoff of the superior mesenteric artery and the aorta is less than 45 degrees.
E. Arteriographic studies show a typical area of extrinsic compression and narrowing of the arterial lumen due to duodenal pressure.

DISCUSSION: The superior mesenteric artery originates behind the neck of the pancreas at the level of the first lumbar vertebra. It arises from the aorta at an acute angle, usually about 37 degrees in normal patients, through which passes the left renal vein, the uncinate process of the pancreas, and the distal third of the duodenum. The duodenum crosses the lumbar spine from right to left and passes upward. It is at this point of passage of the duodenum upward and over the spine that the obstruction occurs. Arteriographic studies show that the aortomesenteric angle in patients with the syndrome is only about 8 degrees. There is no narrowing of the superior mesenteric artery or disturbance of arterial flow, but the area of duodenal obstruction corresponds to the compression of the bowel by the artery. The duodenal compression may often be relieved by assuming the knee-chest, the left lateral, or even the prone position. Increasing lumbar lordosis, as with hyperextension of the back, exacerbates the problem.
Textbook: Pages 888–889 ANSWER: A, B.

65. Numerous epidemiologic associations have been made between (1) environmental and dietary factors and (2) the incidence of gastric cancer, including all except:

A. Dietary nitrites.
B. Dietary salt.
C. *Helicobacter pylori* infection.
D. Dietary ascorbic acid.

DISCUSSION: Numerous epidemiologic studies support the role of certain foods in the development of gastric cancer. Salt, which can act as a gastric irritant, and nitrates and nitrites, which can be converted to the active carcinogens *N*-nitrosamines, are implicated in the development of gastric cancer. *H. pylori* infection is associated with atrophic gastritis, a known precursor to gastric cancer. Important studies of large populations indicate that the majority of patients with gastric cancer are *H. pylori* positive. The bacteria produce toxins such as ammonia and acetaldehyde, which could lead to chronic inflammation and epithelial damage. Dietary ascorbic acid has been associated with overall improvements in diet and is not associated with the development of gastric cancer.

Textbook: Page 893 ANSWER: D.

66. All of the following benign conditions are associated with increased rates of gastric cancer except:

A. Pernicious anemia.
B. Multiple endocrine neoplasia type I (MEN 1).
C. Adenomatous polyps.
D. Chronic atrophic gastritis.

DISCUSSION: Adenomatous polyps are unusual but carry the distinct potential for malignancy. They occur most often between the fifth and seventh decades of life. The adenocarcinoma sequence in gastric polyps is thought to be analogous to that of colonic polyps. An adenomatous polyp is a marker for increased risk of carcinoma in the remaining stomach. Both pernicious anemia and chronic atrophic gastritis are associated with gastric cancer. Many of these patients develop chronic achlorhydria, a condition also associated with an increased risk of cancer. Neither multiple MEN 1 nor MEN 2, is associated with gastric cancer.

Textbook: Pages 893–895 ANSWER: B.

67. Which of the following statements concerning the pathology of gastric cancer is true?

A. Distal gastric cancers are becoming more common.
B. Intestinal-type gastric tumors resemble colon carcinomas and have a better prognosis than diffuse type.
C. Early gastric cancers are confined to the mucosa and are lymph node negative.
D. Broders' histologic grading system correlates well with survival: patients with grade IV tumors have 5-year survival rates around 65%.

DISCUSSION: Distal gastric cancers are decreasing in incidence in several populations. Lesions of the gastroesophageal junction and cardia have increased in incidence over the past two decades. Early gastric cancers are confined to the mucosa and submucosa of the stomach. Six to 10% of these early lesions are lymph-node positive. The survival rates from early gastric cancer is related to node positivity, just as in advanced gastric cancer. Broders' histologic grades do correlate well with survival. Grade I and IV tumors are associated with a 65% and 11% 5-year survival, respectively. The Lauren classification system is divided into intestinal and diffuse-type tumors. The intestinal-type tumor is more analogous to colon carcinoma and has a better prognosis than the diffuse type.

Textbook: Pages 895–897 ANSWER: B.

68. An 80% distal gastrectomy is performed for a 6-cm. antral cancer with extension to the muscularis propria and three positive lymph nodes less than 3 cm. from the tumor. The stage of this tumor was:

A. Stage I.
B. Stage II.
C. Stage III A.
D. Stage III B.

DISCUSSION: The American Joint Committee on Cancer Staging system depends on primary tumor, lymph node involvement, and distant metastasis. The tumor described is a T2N1M0 tumor, which categorizes it as stage II.

Textbook: Pages 898–899 ANSWER: B.

69. Which of the following statements about the surgical treatment of gastric cancer is false?

A. Patients with tumors of the middle and proximal thirds should undergo total gastrectomy.
B. Adenocarcinoma of the cardia-gastroesophageal junction may require reconstruction in the abdomen, chest, or neck.
C. Palliative resection yields better results than palliative bypass.
D. Japanese patients who undergo gastric resection are, on average, 10 years younger and much leaner than their Western counterparts.

DISCUSSION: Depending on the size and extent of the tumor, cancers of the gastroesophageal junction may extend proximally into the esophagus for a varying distance. Reconstruction may be required in the abdomen, chest, or neck, depending on extension and whether the operation is to be palliative or curative. Palliative resection yields better results than palliative bypass, which is unreliable for relieving obstruction. Japanese patients typically are younger and thinner than their Western counterparts. In addition, they have a higher prevalence (up to 50%) of early gastric cancer. Depending on the size and particular location of the tumor, patients with small middle-third tumors or small lesions of the cardia may undergo subtotal proximal gastrectomy and reconstruction with a gastric tube. If 6-cm. margins can be obtained on either side of the lesion, total gastrectomy is unnecessary and may be associated with a higher risk of morbidity.

Textbook: Pages 898, 901–905 ANSWER: A.

70. The lamina propria between the intestinal epithelium and the muscularis mucosae contains:

A. Blood and lymph vessels.
B. Undifferentiated epithelial cells.
C. Nerve fibers.
D. Enterochromaffin cells.
E. Macrophages.
F. Connective tissue.

DISCUSSION: The mucosa of the small intestine encompasses the epithelium, the lamina propria, and the muscularis mucosae. The lamina propria between the epithelium and the muscularis mucosae contains blood and lymph vessels, nerve fibers, smooth muscle fibers, fibroblasts, macrophages, plasma cells, lymphocytes, eosinophils, and mast cells, as well as connective tissue elements.

Textbook: Page 910 ANSWER: A, C, E, F.

71. The intestinal epithelial cells, 22 to 26 μm. tall, exhibit a striated luminal border (brush border). The brush border microvilli:

A. Produce the brush border appearance.
B. Contain amylase.
C. Contain dissacharidases.
D. Increase absorptive area.
E. Play an important role in digestion.
F. Contain trypsinogen.

DISCUSSION: The columnar epithelial cells are responsible for absorption. These cells exhibit a striated luminal border or brush border. The microvilli account for the appearance of the brush border. The microvilli greatly increase the absorption surface of the epithelial cell. The brush border contains disaccharidase in high concentrations. In addition to increasing surface area the microvilli perform an important digestive function.

Textbook: Pages 910–911 ANSWER: A, C, D, E.

72. Which of the following statements about carbohydrate digestion are true?

A. Amylopectin has 1-4 straight chains and 1-6 side chains.
B. Amylase has 1-4 straight chains and 1-6 side chains.
C. Amylase breaks 1-4 glucose linkages.
D. Amylase breaks 1-6 side chains.
E. An adult may ingest about 350 gm. of carbohydrate daily.
F. Dietary starch contains two glucose polymers, amylopectin and amylase.

DISCUSSION: Amylopectin, the most abundant constituent of starch, is a 1-4–linked straight chain of glucose molecules. In addition, amylopectin possesses a 1-6 branching side chain at approximately every 25 glucose units along the straight chain. Amylase has only 1-4 linkages of glucose molecules. Pancreatic and salivary amylase break the interior 1-4 glucose linkages.

Textbook: Page 912 ANSWER: A, C, E, F.

73. Which of these statements about the digestion of fat are true?

A. Micellar solution provides an optimal environment for the action of pancreatic lipase.
B. Decreasing the pH below 5.5 increases the effectiveness of pancreatic lipase in hydrolyzing fat.
C. Co-lipase blocks triglyceride hydrolysis.
D. Lipase catalyzes the hydrolysis of dietary triglyceride into 2-monoglyceride and fatty acids.
E. Fatty acids and 2-monoglyceride are held in micellar solutions.
F. Fatty acid and 2-monoglyceride enter the intestinal cell by active transport.

DISCUSSION: Micellar solution provides an optimal environment for the action of pancreatic lipase. Pro-colipase is converted to co-lipase by trypsin. Co-lipase binds to triglyceride, then lipase complexes with colipase, and triglyceride hydrolysis access. Pancreatic lipase hydrolyzes triglyceride into 2-monoglyceride and fatty acids. The 2-monoglyceride and fatty acid enter the micellae. An alkaline pH allows lipase to function optimally. Micellar fatty acids and 2-monoglyceride pass into the epithelial cell by diffusion.

Textbook: Pages 912–913 ANSWER: A, D, E.

74. Complete mechanical small bowel obstruction can cause dehydration by:

A. Interfering with oral intake of water.
B. Inducing vomiting.
C. Decreasing intestinal absorption of water.
D. Causing secretion of water into the intestinal lumen.
E. Causing edema of the intestinal wall.

DISCUSSION: One of the most important events during simple mechanical small bowel obstruction, loss of water and electrolytes from the body, is caused mainly by intestinal distention. Distention may produce reflex vomiting. Distention causes intestinal secretion. Distention causes decreased absorption.

Textbook: Page 917 ANSWER: A, B, C, D, E.

75. History and physical examination permit the diagnosis of intestinal obstruction in most cases. Which of the following are important for the clinical diagnosis of small bowel obstruction?

A. Crampy abdominal pain.
B. Fever.
C. Vomiting.
D. Abdominal distention.
E. Leukocyte count above 12,000.
F. Abdominal tenderness.

DISCUSSION: History and physical examination permit the diagnosis of intestinal obstruction. Any patient having crampy abdominal pain, vomiting, obstipation, abdominal distention, abdominal tenderness, and peristaltic rushes should be managed for intestinal obstruction until the diagnosis can confidently be excluded.

Textbook: Pages 917–918 ANSWER: A, B, C, D, F.

76. Patients with established, complete, simple, distal small bowel obstruction usually have the following findings on plain and upright abdominal radiographs:

A. Distended small bowel identifiable by the valvulae conniventes.

B. Multiple air-fluid levels.
C. Modest amount of gas in the pelvis.
D. Peripheral, rather than central, distribution of gas.
E. Prominent haustral markings.
F. Free air.

DISCUSSION: Abdominal x-ray examination of patients with intestinal obstruction usually reveals abnormally large quantities of gas in the bowel. One can usually identify distended small intestine or colon. Gas in the small bowel outlines the valvulae conniventes, which usually occupy the entire transverse diameter of the bowel image. Colonic haustral markings occupy only a portion of the transverse diameter of the bowel.

Typically, the small bowel pattern occupies the more central portion of the abdomen, whereas the colon shadow is on the periphery of the abdominal files or in the pelvis. Patients with mechanical small intestinal obstruction usually have minimal colonic gas, if any.

Textbook: Pages 918–919 ANSWER: A, B.

77. Which answers are true? In contrast to ulcerative colitis, Crohn's disease of the colon:

A. Is not associated with increased risk of colon cancer.
B. Seldom presents with daily hematochezia.
C. Is usually segmental rather than continuous.
D. Has a lower incidence of perianal fistulas.
E. Never develops toxic megacolon.

DISCUSSION: Crohn's disease of the colon is a patchy, segmental, chronic, transmural inflammatory process that penetrates the bowel wall to form fistulas but seldom causes rectal bleeding. In contrast, ulcerative colitis is a mucosal ulcerating process that extends continuously from the rectum to the more proximal colon and frequently bleeds. Both diseases can develop toxic megacolon, and both predispose the patient to increased risk of malignancy of the large intestine over the long term.

Textbook: Pages 925–926, 928 ANSWER: B, C.

78. Which answers are true? Options to consider when operating for Crohn's disease of the large intestine include:

A. Colectomy and ileorectostomy.
B. Colectomy, closure of the rectal stump, and ileostomy.
C. Colectomy and continent ileostomy (Kock pouch).
D. Proctocolectomy and ileostomy.
E. Proctocolectomy and ileal pouch–anal canal anastomosis.

DISCUSSION: Patients with colonic Crohn's disease who have minimal or mild rectal involvement can be treated by colectomy and ileorectostomy or by colectomy, closure of the rectal stump, and ileostomy. When severe rectal involvement is also present, proctocolectomy with permanent ileostomy is required. The Kock pouch (continent ileostomy) and the ileal pouch–anal canal operation are not performed for Crohn's disease because of the risk of recurrence of Crohn's disease in the ileal pouch in the postoperative period.

Textbook: Page 930 ANSWER: A, B, D.

79. Crohn's disease:

A. Is caused by *Mycobacterium paratuberculosis.*
B. Is more common in Asians than in Jews.
C. Tends to occur in families.
D. Is less frequent in temperate climates than in tropical ones.
E. Is improved by smoking.

DISCUSSION: The cause of Crohn's disease is unknown. No specific microorganism has been identified as a pathogen, and no clear-cut environmental factor, such as smoking, has been implicated, even though many patients with Crohn's disease are heavy smokers. The disease does tend to occur in families. It is more common among Jews than Asians and among people who live in temperate climates than those in tropical ones.

Textbook: Pages 923–924 ANSWER: C.

80. Recurrence after operation for Crohn's disease:

A. Occurs after operations for ileal Crohn's but not colonic Crohn's.
B. Is usually found just proximal to an enteric anastomosis.
C. Rarely requires reoperation.
D. Occurs in 1% of patients at risk per year during the first 10 years after the operation.
E. Is prevented by maintenance therapy with corticosteroids.

DISCUSSION: Recurrence after operation for Crohn's disease often occurs just proximal to an enteric anastomosis or stoma and occurs at a rate of about 6% per year over the first 10 years after operation. Recurrence follows operations for both ileal and colonic Crohn's and is not prevented by medical therapy using corticosteroids. Reoperation is required for 30% to 50% of subjects at risk.

Textbook: Page 932 ANSWER: B.

81. Excision rather than bypass is preferred for surgical treatment of small intestinal Crohn's because:

A. Excision is safer.
B. Bypass does not relieve symptoms.
C. Excision cures the patient of Crohn's disease but bypass does not.
D. Fewer early complications appear with excision.
E. The risk of small intestine cancer is reduced.

DISCUSSION: Bypass of segments of small bowel affected with Crohn's disease is a safe operation with few complications, and one that usually relieves

symptoms promptly. It leaves diseased bowel behind, however, which can flare in the future and can develop carcinoma. Excision, though it does not cure the Crohn's disease, removes the areas of severe involvement and so eliminates the risk of developing cancers in these segments.

Textbook: Pages 928–929 ANSWER: E.

82. Which statements about anorectal Crohn's disease are true?

A. It may be the only overt manifestation of Crohn's disease.
B. It accompanies large intestine Crohn's more often than small-intestine Crohn's.
C. It subsides when associated small intestinal Crohn's is excised.
D. It should not be treated operatively.
E. It may subside in response to metronidazole, 250 mg. q.i.d.

DISCUSSION: Anorectal Crohn's disease may be the sole gross manifestation of Crohn's disease. It more often accompanies large-intestinal Crohn's than small-intestinal Crohn's. When present with small-intestinal Crohn's, resection of the small-intestinal disease does not affect the course of the anorectal disease. The anorectal disease may subside with metronidazole therapy alone, but local conservative therapy, such as draining abscesses or unroofing anal fistulas, may also relieve symptoms and promote healing.

Textbook: Page 930 ANSWER: A, B, E.

83. The most common indication for operation in Crohn's disease of the colon is:

A. Obstruction.
B. Chronic debility.
C. Bleeding.
D. Perforation.
E. Carcinoma.

DISCUSSION: Crohn's disease of the colon usually leads to operation because of chronic debility and inanition unresponsive to medical therapy. Obstruction, perforation, and bleeding are uncommon complications of colonic Crohn's. While for persons with Crohn's colitis the risk of carcinoma of the colon is four to six times that of a healthy control population, the presence of cancer in the colon is an unusual cause for operation for Crohn's colitis. In fact, most patients with Crohn's have their colons excised before sufficient time has elapsed for cancers to appear. Cancers usually do not appear until 10 years or more after the onset of disease.

Textbook: Pages 927–928 ANSWER: B.

84. Which of the following measures of obesity correlates best with mortality?

A. The 1983 Metropolitan Life Insurance Company tables for ideal body weight.
B. Hydroimmersion measurements of body fat composition.
C. Body mass index (BMI).
D. Skinfold thickness.
E. Waist to hip ratios (WHR).

DISCUSSION: The measurement of obesity is still an inexact science. The Metropolitan Life Insurance tables, although widely used, do not distinguish between lean muscle mass and fat. Accordingly, the BMI (weight in kg./height in meters)^2, was developed to place greater emphasis on "fatness." The measure correlates linearly with mortality tables. Hydroimmersion data are still too sparse to relate to outcome tables. Skinfold thickness and waist-hip ratios have not been shown to have the accuracy or relevance of the BMI.

Textbook: Pages 933–934. ANSWER: C.

85. The most effective therapy for morbid obesity, in terms of weight control, is:

A. Intensive dieting with behavior modification.
B. A multidrug protocol with fenfluramine, phenylpropanolamine, and mazindol.
C. A gastric bypass with a 40-ml. pouch, a 10- to 20-cm. Roux-en-Y gastroenterostomy.
D. A gastric bypass with a 15-ml. pouch, a 40- to 60-cm. Roux-en-Y gastroenterostomy.
E. Daily exercise with strong emphasis on utilizing all four limbs.

DISCUSSION: Although the various nonsurgical measures listed in the question have proved effective for obese persons, they work only rarely for those who are morbidly obese. None have proved as effective as gastric bypass with a 15-ml. pouch and a 40- to 60-cm. Roux-en-Y gastroenterostomy.

Textbook: Pages 936–937, 940–941 ANSWER: D.

86. Which of the following statements about intestinal bypass is/are correct?

A. The operation produced weight loss similar to that of the gastric bypass.
B. The operation produced severe metabolic disturbances, including hypocalcemia, increased bile salts and glycine synthesis.
C. Bacterial overgrowth in the bypassed segment led to liver failure.
D. The operation demonstrated that an adult human could survive with 40 to 50 cm. of small intestine.

DISCUSSION: Unfortunately, all of the answers are true. Even though the intestinal bypass proved initially to be an effective procedure to induce weight loss, the side effects proved to be so severe that almost all of the operations had to be reversed or revised to gastric bypass to avert death from liver failure or severe illnesses due to malnutrition.

Textbook: Pages 937–938 ANSWER: A, B, C, D.

87. Which of the following is/are contraindications to gastric bypass surgery?

A. Diabetes mellitus.
B. Hypertension.
C. Pickwickian syndrome.

D. Failure to agree to long-term follow-up.
E. Sleep apnea.

DISCUSSION: The gastric bypass represents the best known therapy for diabetes mellitus, hypertension, the Pickwickian syndrome, and sleep apnea. In fact, no other therapy provides such complete control of hyperglycemia and hyperinsulinemia, reversal of hypertension, and total correction of the Pickwickian syndrome and most cases of sleep apnea. The only contraindication to bariatric surgery listed is failure to agree to long-term follow-up. The gastric bypass represents controlled malnutrition and, therefore, vitamin therapy is especially important. If patients are not followed closely, vitamin deficiencies, especially of B_6 and B_{12}, can develop with serious consequences including a Korsakoff-Wernicke syndrome.
Textbook: Page 943 ANSWER: D.

88. A 34-year-old morbidly obese diabetic woman underwent a gastric bypass about 12 hours ago. The operation was technically difficult but finally went well. You are called because she now has a temperature of 99.2° F, pulse of 134, and some pain in her incision and her back. She looks well; the incision is clean; and her examination is otherwise negative. A bolus of 500 ml. of dextrose/lactated Ringer's did not change her vital signs, except that her pulse rose to 140 without an increase in urine output. Your next step should be:

A. Another bolus of crystalloids.
B. Posterioanterior and lateral chest films.
C. Obtain white cell count, differential count, and electrolyte values.
D. Call the operating room and warn them that you need to re-explore for a leak.
E. Increase her pain medication.

DISCUSSION: Morbidly obese patients are malnourished and brittle and have little resistance. Serious life-threatening infections may soil the peritoneal cavity without producing any sign except a persistently high pulse rate. The usual tests listed in *A, B,* and *C,* should be done, but the most likely explanation for a continued high pulse is soiling in the area of the surgery due to either a leak or contamination and development of sepsis. Because of the unreliability of clinical evaluation, the indications for re-exploration are very liberal, and this approach has saved a number of lives. The risk of such an exploration is small, whereas failure to contain the infection with lavage and drainage may be followed by a surprisingly rapid death.
Textbook: Page 944 ANSWER: D.

89. All of the following statements about the embryology of Meckel's diverticulum are true except:

A. Meckel's diverticulum usually arises from the ileum within 90 cm. of the ileocecal valve.
B. Meckel's diverticulum results from the failure of the vitelline duct to obliterate.
C. The incidence of Meckel's diverticulum in the general population is 5%.
D. Meckel's diverticulum is a true diverticulum possessing all layers of the intestinal wall.
E. Gastric mucosa is the most common ectopic tissue found within a Meckel's diverticulum.

DISCUSSION: Meckel's diverticulum is a true diverticulum containing all layers of the intestinal wall, usually arising from the antimesenteric border of the ileum 45–90 cm. proximal to the ileocecal valve. It is a vestige of the omphalomesenteric or vitelline duct, which usually undergoes complete obliteration during the seventh week of gestation. Autopsy studies have estimated the incidence of Meckel's diverticulum to be 1% to 2% with men being more commonly affected than women by a ratio of 2:1. Gastric mucosa is present in 50% of all Meckel's diverticula, but in over 75% of symptomatic individuals.
Textbook: Pages 946–948 ANSWER: C.

90. Meckel's diverticulum most commonly presents as:

A. Gastrointestinal bleeding.
B. Obstruction.
C. Diverticulitis.
D. Intermittent abdominal pain.

DISCUSSION: It is estimated that only 4% of patients who possess a Meckel's diverticulum will become symptomatic during their lifetimes. The most common clinical presentation is incidental identification during abdominal exploration. Symptomatic presentations are secondary to hemorrhage, small bowel obstruction, diverticulitis, perforation, associated umbilical abnormalities, and tumors. Over half of patients presenting with symptoms are under the age of 2. The most common clinical problem associated with Meckel's diverticulum is gastrointestinal bleeding presenting as bright red blood per rectum. The usual source of the bleeding is a chronic acid-induced ileal ulcer in the ileum adjacent to a Meckel's diverticulum that contains gastric mucosa. Another common symptom associated with a Meckel's diverticulum is intestinal obstruction. The cause of this obstruction may be volvulus of the small bowel around a diverticulum associated with a fibrotic band attached to the abdominal wall, intussusception, or rarely, incarceration of the diverticulum in an inguinal hernia (Littre's hernia). Volvulus is usually an acute event and if allowed to progress, may result in strangulation of the involved bowel. In intussusception, a broad-based diverticulum invaginates and then is carried forward by peristalsis.
Textbook: Pages 948–949 ANSWER: A.

91. Which of the following statements about the surgical treatment of carcinoid tumors are true?

A. Carcinoid tumors should be treated by resection, regardless of the presence of metastases.

B. Appendiceal tumors larger than 1.5 cm. should be treated by ileocolectomy.
C. Local excision with margins is adequate for a rectal carcinoid of any size.
D. Carcinoid tumors are associated with a large percentage of other synchronous or metachronous neoplasms.

DISCUSSION: Carcinoid tumors should be treated by resection, regardless of the presence of metastases, because growth of the primary neoplasm is slow and local complications, such as obstruction and intussusception, are frequent. At clinical discovery a large percentage (as many as 70%) of small-intestinal carcinoids are metastatic to lymph nodes and/or liver. All tumors should be managed by wide *en bloc* resection, regardless of the size of the primary lesion or the presence of distant metastases. Lesions in the distal ileum require ileocolectomy. Appendiceal tumors larger than 1.5 cm. should be treated by ileocolectomy. The incidence of metastases depends on the size and location of the primary tumor. Appendiceal carcinoid tumors smaller than 1.5 cm. are rarely malignant and may be treated safely by routine appendectomy. This is not true of larger tumors. Like carcinoid tumors elsewhere in the gastrointestinal tract, the malignancy potential of rectal carcinoid tumors is directly proportional to their size. Tumors smaller than 1 cm. have little or no malignant potential and may be treated by endoscopic excision. Tumors measuring 1 to 2 cm. should be excised operatively with margins, but when they are larger than 2 cm. rectal carcinoid tumors may require anterior resection. In patients with ileal carcinoid tumors, the evidence of a second tumor has been reported as high as 40%. Thus, the search for synchronous metachronous and metastatic neoplasms should be undertaken.

Textbook: Page 952 ANSWER: A, B, D.

92. Which of the following statements about carcinoid syndrome are true?

A. Carcinoid syndrome occurs only when hepatic metastases are present.
B. Serotonin is thought to be responsible for the diarrhea, cardiac lesions, and flushing in patients with carcinoid syndrome.
C. Foregut carcinoid tumors cause atypical carcinoid syndrome; hindgut tumors are rarely, if ever, associated with the syndrome.
D. The long-acting somatostatin analog provides the best symptomatic treatment for carcinoid syndrome.

DISCUSSION: Carcinoid syndrome occurs when venous drainage from the tumor gains access to the systemic circulation, escaping hepatic degradation. Although hepatic metastases are most often responsible, retroperitoneal metastases and bronchial, ovarian, and testicular carcinoid tumors can also cause the carcinoid syndrome. Serotonin is thought to be largely responsible for both the diarrhea and the fibrosing cardiac lesions associated with the carcinoid syndrome. The vasomotor changes, however, are mediated by kinins and such vasoactive peptides as substance P, neuropeptide K, neurokinin A, and neurotensin. Other substances, such as histamine, vasoactive intestinal peptide (VIP), and prostaglandins, may also contribute to systemic manifestations in the carcinoid syndrome. Foregut carcinoid tumors, of which stomach and bronchial tumors are the most common, can cause atypical carcinoid syndrome. It is thought that these tumors are deficient in the enzyme dopa-decarboxylase and have impaired conversion of 5-hydroxytryptophan (5-HTP) into 5-hydroxytryptamine (5-HT), leading to secretion of 5-HTP into the vascular compartment. Some of the 5-HTP is converted into 5-HT and 5-hydroxyindoleacetic acid (5-HIAA) in extrarenal sites, and some is decarboxylated in the kidney and excreted into the urine as 5-HT; but some of the 5-HTP is excreted directly into the urine. Thus, in patients with foregut tumors, the urine contains relatively little 5-HIAA (but more than normal) but large amounts of 5-HTP and 5-HT, in contrast to patients with midgut carcinoid tumors in which large amounts of 5-HIAA are secreted into the urine but relatively little 5-HTP. Carcinoid tumors of the hindgut contain no argentaffin or argyrophil cells, they have no secretory products, and therefore they are not associated with the carcinoid syndrome. The long-acting somatostatin analog provides the best symptomatic therapy, because somatostatin inhibits both release and action of humoral mediators of the carcinoid syndrome. By contrast, serotonin antagonists are of little value and the efficacy of interferon therapy has yet to be established.

Textbook: Page 953 ANSWER: C, D.

93. Metabolic complications of subtotal gastrectomy with Billroth I or Billroth II reconstruction include:

A. Hypothyroidism.
B. Anemia.
C. Reactive hypoglycemia.
D. Dumping syndrome.
E. Metabolic bone disease.

DISCUSSION: Anemia develops in as many as 30% of patients within 15 years of surgery. The cause is multifactorial and includes malabsorption of iron, folate, and vitamin B_{12}. A metabolic bone disease occurs in as many as 33% of patients, is similar to osteomalacia, and is probably a result of malabsorption of calcium and vitamin D. Reactive hypoglycemia occurs with rapid gastric emptying, resulting in increased glucose absorption immediately after a meal. Initially there is hyperglycemia, leading to hyperinsulinemia and subsequent rapid glucose clearance and symptomatic hypoglycemia. Dumping syndrome varies from very mild symptoms to significantly disabling ones. The severe syndrome occurs in fewer than 5% of patients. Small, frequent, dry meals of low osmolality reduces symptoms, and somatostatin analog has been of some clinical use.

Textbook: Page 957 ANSWER: B, C, D, E.

94. Simple screening tests for malabsorption include:

A. Microscopic examination.
B. D-xylose absorption.
C. A 72-hour stool collection for fats.
D. Small bowel x-ray series.

DISCUSSION: The 72-hour stool collection is quite sensitive and detects even mild malabsorption. As it requires careful stool collection timed by carmen red markers and documented dietary fat intake, it is not useful for screening. Microscopic examination of the stool can detect muscle fibers if protein malabsorption is present and with Sudan II staining can estimate fat content. D-Xylose absorption from oral ingestion of 5 gm., detected by a blood sample after 1 hour, is a simple and quite accurate test to identify carbohydrate malabsorption. Small bowel x-ray series, using barium contrast, can give very useful information on mucosal abnormalities, enteric fistulas, mechanical obstructions, and very importantly, intestinal motility and transit time.

Textbook: Page 955 ANSWER: A, B, D.

95. Extensive resection of the small bowel, leaving only 2 or 3 feet beyond the ligament of Treitz anastomosed to the transverse colon, can lead to the following metabolic complications:

A. Gastric hyperacidity and hypersecretion.
B. Hyperoxaluria.
C. Hypermetabolic response.
D. Fat-soluble vitamin deficiency.

DISCUSSION: Once the stress of the surgical procedure is over, there is no further hypermetabolic response, nor does there appear to be any reduced energy expenditure from loss of the metabolically active small bowel. Energy needs are unaltered. Gastric secretion and hyperacidity are directly related to the extent of small bowel resection and is due in part to increased concentrations of gastrin in the serum. H_2 blockers are effective in reducing acidity and volume of gastric secretions. Hyperoxaluria develops owing to binding of calcium to fat in the diet with steatorrhea, leaving less to bind with dietary oxalate. The soluble oxalate is absorbed by the colon and excreted in the urine. If oxalate is excessive, oxalate kidney stones can form. With fat malabsorption due to bile salt depletion and rapid intestinal transit, absorption of the fat-soluble vitamins A, E, K, and D is reduced. Even with oral supplementation, deficiencies can develop.

Textbook: Pages 958–959 ANSWER: A, B, D.

96. Which of the following physical factors of irradiation is/are related to the potential for radiation injury?

A. The dimension of the radiation portals.
B. The number of portals.
C. The number of fractions.
D. The total amount of irradiation.
E. All of the above.

DISCUSSION: These physical factors are interactive. Less energy is delivered through a small portal than through a large one. Multiple portals permit concentration of the radiation in the area to be treated and spare skin and viscera from damage. There is less risk of injury from irradiation of a given intensity if more fractions are applied.

Textbook: Pages 961–962 ANSWER: E.

97. For which of the following consequences of radiation injury of the intestine is urgent laparotomy required?

A. Small bowel obstruction.
B. Colonic perforation.
C. Rectovaginal fistula.
D. Malabsorption and diarrhea.
E. Rectal stenosis.

DISCUSSION: Patients who have symptoms of vascular compromise or evidence of perforation require urgent laparotomy. Patients with small bowel obstruction may require a laparotomy if a complete obstruction persists, but gastrointestinal decompression and hydration are first steps. Patients with radiation-induced rectovaginal fistula may require temporary or even permanent colostomy, but the first steps are evaluation and control of sepsis. Malabsorption and diarrhea can generally be controlled pharmacologically. Rectal stenosis can usually be managed without laparotomy.

Textbook: Page 963 ANSWER: B.

98. Which of the following most often initiates the development of acute appendicitis?

A. A viral infection.
B. Acute gastroenteritis.
C. Obstruction of the appendiceal lumen.
D. A primary clostridial infection.

DISCUSSION: The majority of patients with acute appendicitis have an obstructed lumen that is due to either hyperplasia of the lymph follicles in the wall of the appendix or a fecalith. The obstruction creates a site where the bacteria in the lumen multiply rapidly, producing exotoxins and endotoxins that then ulcerate the mucosa, allowing pathogenic organisms to enter the wall of the appendix. An inflammatory process follows that can extend to the serosa, and penetration through the serosal layer causes generalized peritonitis.

Textbook: Page 965 ANSWER: C.

99. The diagnosis of acute appendicitis is most difficult to establish in:

A. Persons aged 60 and older.
B. Women aged 18 to 35.
C. Infants younger than 1 year.
D. Pregnant women.

DISCUSSION: It is very difficult to establish a firm diagnosis of acute appendicitis in an infant of 1 year or younger since the patient cannot provide a history or be helpful during the physical examination. It is rare to make a definitive diagnosis preoperatively in such infants, and in such cases the appendix is usually perforated at the time of operation. While appendicitis is somewhat more difficult to diagnose in the elderly because of the reduced response to inflammation; nevertheless, it is usually possible to make the diagnosis. With pregnant women it is wise to remember that the enlarging uterus in the last trimester dislocates the appendix higher in the abdomen and that the signs and symptoms follow this anatomic shift accordingly.

Textbook: Page 966 ANSWER: C.

100. Once a diagnosis of acute appendicitis has been made and appendectomy decided upon, which of the following is/are true?

A. Prophylactic antibiotics should be administered.
B. Prophylactic antibitics are not necessary unless there is evidence of perforation.
C. If the appendix is not ruptured and not gangrenous, antibiotics may be discontinued after 24 hours.
D. Multiple antibiotics are in all cases preferable to a single agent.

DISCUSSION: It is generally held that patients with a diagnosis of acute appendicitis should receive antibiotics such as cefoxitin or cefotetan. Administration can be discontinued after 24 hours if the appendix is not gangrenous or ruptured. Multiple antibiotics are unnecessary in straightforward cases.

Textbook: Pages 966–969 ANSWER: A, C.

101. Which of the following statements about surgical anatomy of the colon and rectum is/are correct?

A. The cecum has the largest inner diameter of all segments of the colon (13 to 15 cm.).
B. The rectosigmoid junction is situated at approximately 15 to 18 cm. from the anus.
C. The rectum is entirely an intraperitoneal organ.
D. The ileocolic, right colic, and middle colic arteries are branches from the inferior mesenteric artery.
E. The arterial arcade created by communicating vessels at 1 to 2 cm. from the mesenteric is called the *artery of Drummond.*

DISCUSSION: The cecum has, indeed, the largest inner diameter of all segments of the colon; however it usually measures between 7 and 9 cm. In patients with a distal obstruction and a continent ileocecal valve the cecum dilates. A diameter of 13 cm. or more is considered at high risk of perforation, and therefore surgery is often needed. The rectosigmoid junction is situated approximately 15 to 18 cm. from the anus, which places lesions in the sigmoid colon within reach of a rigid sigmoidoscope. The rectum is covered by peritoneum only in the anterior and superior aspect. The remainder of the rectum, or most of it, is extraperitoneal. The ileocolic, right colic, and middle colic arteries are branches from the superior mesenteric artery and supply blood to the ascending colon and the right half of the transverse colon. The artery of Drummond is an arcade that runs 1 to 2 cm. from the mesenteric border of the entire colon and provides communication between the superior mesenteric and inferior mesenteric arteries.

Textbook: Pages 971–972 ANSWER: B, E.

102. Which of the following statements about surgical procedures on the colon and rectum is/are correct?

A. Successful healing of colonic anastomoses depends on the adequacy of the blood supply.
B. In excising part of the colon containing cancer, the lymphatics should be avoided by dividing the mesentery close to the wall of the colon.
C. Despite complete removal of the colon and rectum, transanal fecal flow can be preserved by means of an ileal pouch–anal anastomosis.
D. When a colostomy is created it cannot be reversed.
E. Colostomy can be life saving in patients with colonic perforation or obstruction.

DISCUSSION: Healing of colonic anastomoses depends on the adequacy of blood supply, which in turn depends on the tension on the anastomosis. Oncologic principles for surgery of colon cancer dictate that the mesentery be divided as close as possible to the origin of the blood vessels, to include the lymphatic vessels and nodes draining that area. In patients at risk for colon cancer, such as those with ulcerative colitis or familial polyposis, the construction of an ileal pouch–anal anastomosis allows for transanal fecal flow despite complete excision of the colon and rectum. Colostomies can often be life saving, especially in patients with colon perforation or obstruction, and are usually reversed unless the patient requires abdominoperineal resection of the rectum for cancer.

Textbook: Pages 972–974 ANSWER: A, C, E.

103. Which of the following statements about colon physiology is/are correct?

A. Colonic recycling of urea is accomplished by the splitting of urea by bacterial ureases.
B. Fermentation by colonic bacteria may rescue malabsorbed carbohydrates.
C. The preferred fuel of the colonic epithelium is glucose.
D. Absorption by the colonic mucosa is a passive process.
E. Insoluble fibers create bulk in the stool.

DISCUSSION: One of the functions of the colon is to recycle nutrients used in the digestive process, such as bile salts, water, and electrolytes. Urea reaching the colon via either the ileal effluent or the mucosal circulation is split by bacterial ureases. The reabsorbed ammonia is returned to the liver, where it is used for amino acid and protein synthesis. Fermentation is the anaerobic process by which bacteria can degrade carbohydrates and proteins. The normal substrate for colonic fermentation is dietary fiber, which resists degradation by alpha-amylases in the small intestine. Starch polysaccharides are normally degraded by amylases and absorbed in the small intestine; however, when starch polysaccharides are not adequately degraded and absorbed, they can also be fermented and the caloric value recovered as short-chain fatty acids. *n*-Butyrate, one of the short-chain fatty acids produced by bacterial fermentation, is the preferred fuel of the colonic epithelium. The colonic epithelium utilizes *n*-butyrate as a fuel for the absorption of sodium and water. Insoluble fibers retain water and are poorly fermented by bacteria, thus producing fecal bulk.

Textbook: Pages 975–976 ANSWER: A, B, E.

104. Which of the following statements about colonic motility is/are true?

A. Mass contractions involve only the rectum.
B. "Antiperistaltic" contractions occur in the descending colon.
C. The rectum can accommodate stool by receptive relaxation.
D. Stool in the colon is propelled by tonic contractions.
E. Defecation involves both sensory and motor pathways.

DISCUSSION: Various patterns of motility are present in the colon. In the ascending colon "antiperistalsis" waves generate retrograde flow of colonic contents back to the cecum. In the descending colon contents are propelled caudad by tonic contractions, separating them into a series of globular masses. A third type of contraction, called *mass peristalsis,* occurs at varying intervals through the entire colon's length. Finally, the rectum will undergo receptive relaxation to accommodate stool until defecation takes place. Normal defecation involves the perception and discrimination of stool and gas in the rectum, deferment of stool elimination until a socially acceptable time, expulsion of stool, and sealing of the anal canal. These processes depend on various sensory and motor pathways.

Textbook: Pages 976–977 ANSWER: C, D, E.

105. Which of the following statements about diagnostic studies for the colon and rectum is/are true?

A. Acetylcholinesterase staining of rectal biopsies is unreliable for the diagnosis of Hirschsprung's disease.
B. Cinedefecography is useful for detecting "hidden" prolapse or rectal intussusception.
C. A negative osmotic gap in stool is indicative of secretory diarrhea.
D. A colonic transit time study involves serial abdominal x-rays after ingestion of radiopaque markers.
E. Carcinoembryonic antigen (CEA) is useful for monitoring patients after resection for colon cancer.

DISCUSSION: Rectal biopsy should be performed in all patients with Hirschsprung's disease. The biposy specimen is examined for ganglion cells, but a much more reliable method is staining acetylcholinesterase, which has an accuracy rate of 99%. Cinedefecography involves instilling contrast medium into the rectum and recording the act of defecation with static radiographs and videofluoroscopy videotape. While the static radiographs allow measurement of the anorectal angle and the relationship between the anus and the coccyx/pubis plane, the videotape is used to detect rectal intussusception, which can be missed in static radiographs. In equivocal cases differentiation between malabsorptive and secretory diarrhea can be made by measurement of electrolytes and osmolality in stool. The osmotic gap is calculated by subtracting $2 \times (Na + K)$ from the measured osmolality. A negative osmotic gap is indicative of secretory diarrhea, whereas a positive osmotic gap indicates malabsorptive diarrhea. In a colonic transit study, 20 radiopaque barium-impregnated markers are ingested before breakfast and plain films of the abdomen are obtained on days 4 and 6. The value of CEA is controversial, but most surgeons agree that it is helpful in monitoring following resection for colon cancer.

Textbook: Pages 977–979 ANSWER: B, C, D, E.

106. Which of the following statements about anorectal functional testing is/are true?

A. Anorectal manometry is often performed through open-tipped multilumen catheters perfused with fluid.
B. Anorectal manometry can differentiate between segmental and global defects of the anal sphincter in patients with incontinence.
C. Electromyography can demonstrate persistent contraction of the pubis rectalis muscle during defecation, which is diagnostic of paradoxical pelvic floor contraction.
D. Measurement of sensory thresholds may reveal insensitivity in patients with chronic constipation.

DISCUSSION: Anorectal manometry is most commonly performed through open-tipped multilumen catheters perfused with fluid. These catheters are connected to a transducer and register internal and external sphincter pressures and presence of the anorectal inhibitory reflex. Anorectal manometry is particularly useful in patients with fecal incontinence since it can differentiate between segmental and global defects of the anal sphincter. Electromyography records the action potential derived from the different muscles involved in defecation through endoscopically placed mucosal electrodes along the colon. Electromyography can demonstrate persistent contraction of the pubis rectalis muscle during defecation, which is diagnostic of paradoxical pelvic floor contraction. Sensory threshold measurements may disclose a high rectal threshold (insensitivity) in patients with idiopathic constipation, extent of denervation, or myopathy in the colon wall.

Textbook: Pages 978–979 ANSWER: A, B, C, D.

107. Which of the following statements about the microbiology of the colon is/are true?

A. The colon contains no more bacteria than the stomach.
B. The predominant bacteria in the colon are aerobic.
C. Nearly one third of the dry weight of feces is bacteria.
D. Common bacteria in the colon are *Bacteroides, Bifidobacterium,* and *Enterobacterium* species.
E. The colonic microflora is relatively stable.

DISCUSSION: The number of bacteria in the colon approaches 10^{12} colony-forming units per ml., which is as many as the space in the colonic lumen allows and many more than in the stomach. The colonic microflora is relatively stable with a predominance of anaerobic bacteria. Typical species are *Bacteroides, Bifidobacterium,* and *Enterobacterium.* Depending on the fiber content of the diet, bacteria make up a significant proportion of the dry weight of feces. In the western world this can be as much as one third of the dry weight of feces.

Textbook: Page 979 ANSWER: C, D, E.

108. Which of the following statements about bowel preparation for colon surgery is/are true?

A. Bowel preparation is accomplished by a combination of mechanical cleansing and nonabsorbable antibiotics.
B. Three days of clear liquids provides sufficient mechanical cleansing.
C. Commercial electrolyte-polyethylene glycol solutions provide mechanical cleansing without inducing electrolyte imbalance.
D. Nonabsorbable antibiotics such as neomycin and erythromycin base are administered the day before the operation in three doses.
E. Intravenous antibiotics are also administered the day before surgery.

DISCUSSION: Bowel preparation is accomplished by a combination of mechanical cleansing and nonabsorbable antibiotics. In the past, 3 days of clear liquids was used as a means of mechanical cleansing; this was neither sufficient nor practical. Presently, an electrolyte-polyethylene glycol solution is commercially available that provides effective mechanical cleansing without inducing electrolyte imbalance. Nonabsorbable antibiotics such as neomycin and erythromycin base are administered the day before the operation, usually at 1 P.M., 2 P.M., and 11 P.M. Intravenous antibiotics are administered within hours of surgery to achieve maximal levels in the tissues during the operation.

Textbook: Page 980 ANSWER: A, C, D.

109. Which of the following patients generally does not require surgical intervention as a consequence of acute diverticulitis?

A. A 35-year-old man with no history of diverticulitis.
B. A 68-year-old man status 2 weeks post–renal transplantation.
C. A 55-year-old woman with hypertension and diabetes mellitus.
D. A 50-year-old man with pneumaturia.
E. A 46-year-old man with right-sided diverticulitis.

DISCUSSION: The majority of patients with diverticular disease are elderly and often have comorbid illnesses. The prognosis in these patients depends on the severity of the underlying inflammatory lesion. Certain subsets of patients, however, have been identified whose overall prognosis is worse. Patients younger than 40 years have a higher incidence of complications, as about 70% eventually require surgical intervention. Patients undergoing renal transplantation are routinely immunosuppressed. Such patients do not manifest the usual signs and symptoms of an inflammatory response. Delays in diagnosis and failure of the normal immune response mandates surgical intervention in virtually all of these patients. The presence of pneumaturia is strongly suggestive of a colovesical fistula. All such fistulas require resection of the diseased colon and repair the involved bladder. Patients with right-sided diverticulitis are usually misdiagnosed as acute appendicitis and, therefore, often are not diagnosed until laparotomy.

Textbook: Pages 987–988, 991–992 ANSWER: C.

110. The test with the highest diagnostic yield for detecting a colovesical fistula is:

A. Barium enema.
B. Colonoscopy.
C. Computed tomography (CT).
D. Cystography.
E. Cystoscopy.

DISCUSSION: Of the tests listed above, cystoscopy provides the highest diagnostic yield, between 80% and 95%. The most common finding on cystoscopy is localized inflammation and bullous edema of the bladder mucosa. Actual demonstration of the fistula is unusual, no matter which test is utilized. Barium enema usually demonstrates some abnormality; however, precise delineation of the fistula occurs in only 30% of cases. Recently, CT has been shown to be useful in diagnosing colovesical fistula with accuracy approaching that of cystoscopy. The low diagnostic yields (20%) of cystography and colonoscopy have limited their use.

Textbook: Page 991 ANSWER: E.

111. Which of the following is *not* true of diverticular disease:

A. It is more common in the United States and Western Europe than in Asia and Africa.
B. A low-fiber diet may predispose to development of diverticulosis.
C. It involves sigmoid colon in more than 90% of patients.

D. Sixty per cent develop diverticulitis sometime during their lifetime.
E. It is the most common cause of massive lower gastrointestinal hemorrhage.

DISCUSSION: Among all patients with diverticular disease only 20% can be expected ever to develop symptoms related to their disease. The development of diverticular disease has been linked to low-fiber diets, a type of diet more common in industrialized countries such as the United States and Western Europe. This correlates with the increased prevalence of diverticular disease in these regions. Diverticular hemorrhage accounts for 50% to 60% of all cases of massive lower gastrointestinal hemorrhage.

Textbook: Pages 982–983 ANSWER: D.

112. The most common indication for surgery secondary to acute diverticulitis is:

A. Abscess.
B. Colonic obstruction.
C. Colovesical fistula.
D. Free perforation.
E. Hemorrhage.

DISCUSSION: Complications of diverticular disease include obstruction, fistulization, hemorrhage, and infection. By far, the most common indication for surgery is intra-abdominal abscess formation, accounting for 40% to 50% of all complications of diverticulitis. Intestinal obstruction accounts for another 10% to 30%, while free perforation can be expected in 10% to 15% of complicated cases of diverticulitis. Fistulization is the least common problem, occurring in only 4% to 10% of complicated cases. Bleeding from diverticula occurs in the complete absence of inflammation.

Textbook: Page 987 ANSWER: A.

113. Which of the following is/are true about colorectal polyps?

A. Familial juvenile polyposis is associated with an increased incidence of colon cancer.
B. Although the propensity for development of malignancy is related to the size of a neoplastic polyp, those with mixed tubulovillous histologic appearance are most likely to develop malignant changes.
C. The loss of a single tumor suppressor gene such as *p53* is sufficient to lead to the development of malignancy in colorectal neoplastic polyps.
D. Endoscopic polypectomy results in a decreased incidence of carcinomas of the colon and rectum.

DISCUSSION: Juvenile polyps are hamartomas, and can cause symptoms in children such as bleeding, obstruction, and intussusception. Familial juvenile polyposis is associated with increased risk of colon carcinoma. Polyps with mixed tubular and villous appearance (tubulovillous adenomas) have an intermediate risk of malignancy; villous adenomas are the most likely to contain malignancy in each size range. While *p53* and other tumor suppressor genes may be associated with the adenoma-to-carcinoma transition, it appears likely that multiple genetic defects are involved in this transformation. Alterations in *p53* appear to be among the last, as changes are uncommon in adenomas but very common in carcinomas. The National Polyp Study Group (USA) demonstrated that colonoscopic polypectomy does in fact reduce the incidence of subsequent colorectal carcinomas, which supports the concept that most carcinomas begin as polyps and supports aggressive endoscopic removal.

Textbook: Pages 995–997, 999 ANSWER: A, D.

114. Which of the following statements about familial adenomatous polyposis (FAP) is/are true?

A. Inherited in an autosomal-dominant manner, this genetic defect is of variable penetrance, some patients having only a few polyps whereas others develop thousands.
B. The phenotypic expression of the disease depends mostly on the genotype.
C. Appropriate surgical therapy includes total abdominal colectomy with ileorectal anastomosis and ileoanal pull-through with rectal mucosectomy.
D. Panproctocolectomy with ileostomy is not appropriate therapy for this disease.
E. Pharmacologic management of this disease may be appropriate in some instances.

DISCUSSION: The genetic defect is of high penetrance: nearly all affected patients develop hundreds to thousands of polyps. By definition, at least 100 polyps must be present. Recent studies have shown that even patients with the identical point mutation can exhibit variability in the phenotypic expression, suggesting that environmental or other genetic factors play a significant role. The phenotypic variations concern age at onset, size of polyps, density of polyps, and extracolonic manifestations of the disease. Although panproctocolectomy with ileostomy is not well-accepted by patients because of the stoma, acceptable surgical options include panproctocolectomy with ileostomy, total colectomy with ileorectal anastomosis, and ileoanal anastomosis with rectal mucosectomy. No pharmacologic agents have been demonstrated to be efficacious in this condition, though several have been tried.

Textbook: Pages 997–998 ANSWER: C.

115. Which of the following statements about the etiology of chronic ulcerative colitis are true?

A. Ulcerative colitis is 50% less frequent in nonwhite than in white populations.
B. Psychosomatic factors play a major causative role in the development of ulcerative colitis.
C. Cytokines are integrally involved in the pathogenesis of ulcerative colitis.
D. Ulcerative colitis has been identified with a greater frequency in family members of

patients with confirmed inflammatory bowel disease.

E. Ulcerative colitis is two to four times more common in Jewish than in non-Jewish populations.

DISCUSSION: Despite intensive investigation, the specific cause of ulcerative colitis remains unknown. There appears to be a clear genetic component involved in the etiology and distribution of ulcerative colitis. It is significantly less frequent in nonwhite than in white populations and significantly more frequent among Jews than among other populations. There is a strong familial concordance by disease category: the prevalence of inflammatory bowel disease is 10% to 25% in relatives of patients with confirmed Crohn's disease or ulcerative colitis. There is considerable uncertainty about the fundamental role of infectious agents in the primary pathogenesis of ulcerative colitis. Psychological factors may play a role in exacerbations of the disease, but they are not of primary importance in its pathogenesis. Recent studies have suggested that cytokines and other immunoregulatory substances are integrally involved in the pathogenesis of inflammatory bowel disease.

Textbook: Pages 1001–1002 ANSWER: A, C, D, E.

116. Surgical alternatives for the treatment of ulcerative colitis include all of the following except:

A. Colectomy with ileal pouch–anal anastomosis.
B. Left colectomy with colorectal anastomosis.
C. Proctocolectomy with Brooke ileostomy or continent ileostomy.
D. Subtotal colectomy with ileostomy and Hartmann closure of the rectum.

DISCUSSION: Ulcerative colitis is a mucosal inflammatory disease confined to the rectum and colon. It can thus be cured by total proctocolectomy. For that reason, the standard of therapy for many years was total proctocolectomy and ileostomy. In an effort to avoid permanent ileostomy a number of other alternatives have been evaluated, including subtotal colectomy with ileorectal anastomosis, proctocolectomy with continent ileostomy, and colectomy with endorectal ileal pouch–anal anastomosis. In the past, subtotal colectomy with ileorectal anastomosis was accepted as a compromise operation, with the knowledge that disease-bearing rectal tissue was retained. Because other definitive alternatives are currently available, ileorectal anastomosis is no longer appropriate for elective surgical treatment of ulcerative colitis. In an acutely ill patient or when the diagnosis is in question, subtotal colectomy with ileostomy and Hartmann closure of the rectum is the most expeditious choice and allows later restorative surgery. Partial colectomy has never been an acceptable alternative for elective operative management of ulcerative colitis; thus, left colectomy with colorectal anastomosis would not be an appropriate alternative.

Textbook: Pages 1009–1013 ANSWER: B.

117. The initial management of toxic ulcerative colitis should include:

A. Broad-spectrum antibiotics.
B. 6-Mercaptopurine.
C. Intravenous fluid and electrolyte resuscitation.
D. Opioid antidiarrheals.
E. Colonoscopic decompression.

DISCUSSION: Toxic colitis is a potentially life-threatening complication of chronic ulcerative colitis. Typically it manifests clinically with the onset of abdominal pain and severe diarrhea, followed by abdominal distention and generalized tenderness. Once megacolon and toxicity develop, fever, leukocytosis, pallor, tachycardia, lethargy, and shock set in. The initial treatment for toxic megacolon thus includes intravenous fluid and electrolyte resuscitation, nasogastric suction, broad-spectrum antibiotics to provide anaerobic and aerobic gram-negative coverage, and total parenteral nutrition to improve nutritional status. Large intravenous doses of corticosteroids are generally administered to treat the colitis. In addition, many patients with toxic megacolon are already receiving steroid therapy and, so, need stress doses of steroids to prevent adrenal crisis. The immunosuppressive drugs 6-mercaptopurine and azathioprine may play a role in the management of refractory ulcerative colitis; however, these drugs are not indicated in the acute management of toxicity. Cyclosporine was shown to be effective in treating acute refractory ulcerative colitis in a single controlled trial, but this has not yet been confirmed by other prospective studies, and it remains a potentially dangerous drug. Opioid antidiarrheals should be avoided since they may exacerbate the colonic dilatation and increase the possibility of perforation. Limited proctoscopy may be helpful in determining the cause of the attack, but colonoscopy may be dangerous and is contraindicated in the face of acute toxic megacolon. If toxic colitis, with or without megacolon, does not improve within 48 hours, emergency surgery is warranted.

Textbook: Pages 1008–1009 ANSWER: A, C.

118. Which finding(s) suggest(s) the diagnosis of chronic ulcerative colitis as opposed to Crohn's colitis?

A. Endoscopic evidence of backwash ileitis.
B. Granulomas on biopsy.
C. Anal fistula.
D. Rectal sparing.
E. Cobblestone appearance on barium enema.

DISCUSSION: It has become increasingly important to distinguish between ulcerative colitis and Crohn's colitis, since the operative therapy for the two disease processes is quite different. Patients with ulcerative colitis are candidates for colectomy with ileoanal anastomosis, whereas Crohn's disease is a clear contraindication to this operation. Clinical findings suggestive of Crohn's disease include anal fistula or other perianal disease, though it must be kept in mind that approximately 10% of patients with ulcerative colitis may also develop perianal problems secondary to their chronic diarrhea. Endoscopic or radiographic evidence of rectal sparing is powerful evidence *against* a diagnosis of ulcerative colitis. However, if patients have been treated with steroid or salicylate enemas, they may have less active disease in the rectum than in the more proximal colon, a finding that could mislead the clinician about the presence or degree of rectal involvement. The deep linear ulcers that lead to a cobblestone appearance on barium enema are strongly suggestive of Crohn's disease. Typically, ulcerative colitis is confined to the rectum and colon. Frank small bowel involvement is suggestive of Crohn's disease; however, patients with active pancolitis may have secondary inflammation of the ileum, which has been called *backwash ileitis*. This clears after colectomy. The differential diagnosis may ultimately rely on histologic evaluation. Endoscopic biopsies are not generally useful since they only sample 3-mm. deep segments of mucosa and submucosa. Transmural inflammation and granulomas on surgical pathologic specimens are pathognomonic of Crohn's disease.

Textbook: Pages 928, 1006–1007 ANSWER: A.

119. An 80-year-old man who has been bedridden for many years following a stroke presents with acute onset of abdominal distention, obstipation, and colicky abdominal pain. Abdominal x-rays reveal dilated loops of small bowel and a dilated sigmoid colon resembling a bent inner tube. Examination reveals distention with mild direct tenderness but no rigidity or rebound tenderness. Initial management should consist of:

A. Barium enema examination.
B. Laparotomy with resection of descending colon and descending colostomy.
C. Multiple cleansing enemas to remove impacted feces.
D. Rigid sigmoidoscopy and decompression of the sigmoid colon.

DISCUSSION: This patient appears to have presented with the classic signs and symptoms of acute sigmoid volvulus. The majority of patients with colonic volvulus are elderly men with underlying neurologic dysfunction. They are commonly referred from a chronic care facility. The patient's condition should be assessed immediately. In the absence of peritonitis the preferred initial management consists of urgent endoscopic detorsion of the volvulus. In most patients this can be easily accomplished with a rigid 25-cm. sigmoidoscope or a flexible fiberoptic colonoscope. Often detorsion of the sigmoid colon results in a dramatic expulsion of gas and feces. A rectal tube should be introduced into the sigmoid and then taped to the thigh or buttock and left in place to prevent immediate recurrence of the volvulus.

Textbook: Pages 1016–1017 ANSWER: D.

120. Axial twisting of the right colon or cecal volvulus has been shown to be associated with each of the following except:

A. A history of abdominal operation.
B. A mobile cecum.
C. An obstructing lesion in the transverse or left colon.
D. Inflammatory bowel disease.

DISCUSSION: Volvulus of the right colon is less common than sigmoid volvulus and may involve either an axial twist of the right colon or a cephalad fold of the cecum (cecal bascule). A mobile cecum is a prerequisite for cecal volvulus and may occur in up to one third of individuals. Cecal volvulus has also been called *postoperative volvulus* because of its tendency to follow abdominal surgical procedures. Obstructing lesions in the distal colon may lead to distention and torsion of the right colon in patients with abnormalities of cecal fixation.

Textbook: Pages 1017–1019 ANSWER: D.

121. Sigmoid volvulus has been associated with each of the following *except:*

A. Chronic constipation and laxative abuse.
B. Chronic rectal proplapse.
C. Chronic traumatic paralysis.
D. Medical management of Parkinson's disease.

DISCUSSION: The development of sigmoid volvulus depends on the presence of a dilated, redundant sigmoid colon. This acquired redundancy may be secondary to long-term ingestion of a high-residue diet, particularly in parts of the world where the disease is common. In the United States, the most prominent association is chronic constipation and excessive reliance on laxatives or enemas. Other contributing factors include neurologic or psychiatric conditions such as Parkinson's disease, Alzheimer's disease, multiple sclerosis, traumatic paralysis, chronic schizophrenia, pseudobulbar palsy, and senility. Patients are frequently bedridden and are being managed with various neuropsychotropic drugs, both of which may alter bowel motility.

Textbook: Page 1016 ANSWER: B.

122. Which of the following statements is not true about inhereted susceptibility to colon cancer?

A. There is no known genetic susceptibility to colon cancer.
B. There are known genetic susceptibilities to colon cancer, but they are always associated with multiple adenomatous polyps.
C. There are known genetic susceptibilities to colon cancer, but they are always associated with specific ethnic or racial groups.
D. None of the above.

DISCUSSION: In addition to familial polyposis syndrome, hereditary nonpolyposis colorectal cancer (HNPCC) includes site-specific colorectal cancer and cancer family syndrome, which are synonymous with

Lynch syndromes I and II, respectively. Autosomal-dominant inheritance of colorectal cancer is observed in both syndromes, and the average patient age at cancer diagnosis is 45 years. Persons with HNPCC have a high occurrence of synchronous and proximal colon malignancies. Affected persons usually exhibit one or several adenomatous polyps. The polyps on average are larger, have more villous histology, and occur at a younger age than adenomas in the general population. Cancer family syndrome also includes other malignancies, especially endometrial lesions but also ovarian, gastric, small intestinal, and renal cancer.

Textbook: Pages 1022–1024 ANSWER: D.

123. Which of the following recommendations for adjuvant chemotherapy of colorectal carcinoma are true?

A. Patients with Stage I or Dukes A and B1 disease should receive adjuvant treatment for 1 year with levamisole combined with 5-FU.
B. Patients with Stage III or Dukes C disease should receive adjuvant treatment for 1 year with levamisole combined with 5-FU.
C. There is no role for adjuvant therapy for colon cancer at any stage.
D. Adjuvant chemotherapy is active in colon cancer only when combined with radiotherapy.

DISCUSSION: Some 50% to 60% of patients with colorectal cancer have tumors that penetrate the serosa or involve the regional lymph nodes, eventually recur, and end fatally. Therefore, adjuvant therapy to improve the mortality was sought for this group of patients. *5-Fluorouracil* (5-FU) is the most active drug used against colon cancer, but it achieves only a 10% to 20% response in patients with advanced disease. Levamisole is thought to be an immunomodulating agent in advanced colorectal carcinoma. Randomized controlled trials of 5-FU with levamisole, levamisole alone, and surgery in patients with Dukes B2 or C colon cancer were performed and demonstrated that levamisole plus 5-FU and levamisole improve disease-free survival for patients with Dukes B and C lesions. Subsequent analysis demonstrated that Dukes C patients receiving levamisole and 5-FU also had slightly prolonged survival.

A larger, confirmatory intergroup trial was launched that demonstrated that in patients with Dukes C carcinomas of the colon, adjuvant treatment for 1 year with levamisole combined with 5-FU reduced the risk of cancer recurrence by 41% and reduced mortality overall by 33%, but the results in patients with Dukes B2 disease was equivocal.

Textbook: Pages 1030–1031 ANSWER: B.

124. Optimal front-line treatment of squamous cell carcinoma of the rectum includes:

A. Abdominal perineal resection.
B. Low anterior resection when technically feasible.
C. Radiation therapy.
D. Chemotherapy.
E. Combined radiation and chemotherapy.

DISCUSSION: Combination radiation therapy and chemotherapy is now the treatment of choice for squamous cell carcinoma of the anus. The area of the primary lesion is biopsied, and the patient begins radiotherapy to the pelvis. If inguinal lymph nodes are enlarged, they are also biopsied, usually by fine-needle aspiration, and if positive, they are included in the field of radiation.

Following radiation therapy, patients receive intravenous 5-FU and mitomycin C. Patients who fail therapy have limited options, including additional chemotherapy or radiotherapy. Salvage therapy may also include abdominoperineal resection (APR), lymphadenectomy, or a diverting colostomy, depending on the nature of the recurrence.

Textbook: Pages 1041–1042 ANSWER: E.

125. Which of the following statement(s) is/are true about the maintenance of continence?

A. It depends on both the internal and external sphincters as well as the puborectalis.
B. Resting pressure offers a high-pressure zone that increases resistance to the passage of stools.
C. Maximal squeeze pressure can last no more than 1 minute.

DISCUSSION: Continence depends on numerous complex and interrelated anal, rectal, pelvic floor, and colon factors. Resting pressure depends primarily on the internal sphincter and serves to increase resistance to the passage of stool. Squeeze pressure, generated by contraction of the external sphincter, increases anal canal resting pressure and helps prevent leakage when the rectal contents are presented to the proximal anal canal at inopportune times. It lasts but a minute before fatiguing. The anorectal angle produced by anterior pull of the puborectalis encircles the rectum at the level of the anorectal ring and helps to maintain continence.

Textbook: Pages 1034–1035 ANSWER: A, B, C.

126. Which of the following statement(s) about complete rectal prolapse, or procidentia is/are true?

A. Rectal prolapse results from intussusception of the rectum and rectosigmoid.
B. The disorder is more common in men than in women.
C. Continence nearly always is recovered after correction of the prolapse.
D. All of the above are true.

DISCUSSION: Rectal prolapse is believed to be the result of intussusception of the rectum and rectosigmoid. The condition predominates in women, in those who strain excessively, and in those suffering from mental disorders. Pregnancy and delivery are not implicated, as the condition can be observed in men and in nulliparous women. By the time the diagnosis is established, 50% of patients are incontinent, and continence improves in only half of the patients after surgical correction of the prolapse.

Textbook: Pages 1035–1036 ANSWER: A.

127. Which of the following statements about hemorrhoids is/are *not* true?

A. Hemorrhoids are specialized "cushions" present in everyone that aid continence.
B. External hemorrhoids are covered by skin whereas internal hemorrhoids are covered by mucosa.
C. Pain is often associated with uncomplicated hemorrhoids.
D. Hemorrhoidectomy is reserved for third- and fourth-degree hemorrhoids.

DISCUSSION: Hemorrhoids are specialized, highly vascularized cushions in the anal canal that aid continence. The cause of hemorrhoids is unknown, but they may represent nothing more than the downward sliding of anal cushions associated with straining and irregular bowel habits. They are classified and treated according to the severity of symptoms. External hemorrhoids are covered with anoderm and are distal to the dentate line. Internal hemorrhoids are covered by the mucosal lining of the anal canal proximal to the dentate line. They can cause painless bleeding, usually in association with defecation. Uncomplicated hemorrhoids usually are not associated with pain, but fissures more often are. Hemorrhoidectomy is reserved for third-degree (bleeding with prolapse requiring manual reduction) and fourth-degree (permanently prolapsed with or without bleeding) hemorrhoids.

Textbook: Pages 1036–1037 ANSWER: C.

128. The widely accepted treatment of most localized epidermoid, cloacogenic, or transitional cell carcinoma of the anal canal is:

A. Surgical resection.
B. Chemotherapy alone.
C. Radiotherapy alone.
D. Combined chemoradiation.

DISCUSSION: Tumors arising in the anal canal or in the transitional zone that have squamous, basaloid, cloacogenic, or mucoepidermoid epithelium are similar in their clinical presentation and response to treatment. Combined chemoradiation (the so-called Nigro protocol) promises to preserve continence, avoid colostomy, and offer a similar survival rate. Local excision is reserved for the few very small and superficial lesions. For most lesions, chemoradiation—external-beam radiation, 5-fluorouracil, and mitomycin C—is the treatment of choice.

Textbook: Page 1042 ANSWER: D.

129. Which statement(s) is/are true about hidradenitis suppurativa?

A. It is a disease of the apocrine sweat glands.
B. It causes multiple perianal and perineal sinuses that drain watery pus.
C. The sinuses do not communicate with the dentate line.
D. The treatment is surgical.
E. All of the above.

DISCUSSION: Hidradenitis suppurativa is an inflammatory process of the sweat glands characterized by abscess and sinus formation. The disease may involve other areas where apocrine glands are present, such as the axilla, mammary, inguinal, and genital regions. The affected areas have a blotchy, purplish appearance with numerous sinuses draining watery pus. The condition must be differentiated from cryptoglandular fistulas, which communicate with the dentate line, and Crohn's disease, which may track to the anorectum proximal to the dentate line. Treatment consists of unroofing sinuses for limited disease and wide local excision for more advanced disease.

Textbook: Page 1043 ANSWER: E.

NOTES

NOTES

CHAPTER 11

LIVER, BILIARY SYSTEM, AND PANCREAS

1. Which of the following statements about the *segmental* anatomy of the liver are not true?

A. Segments are subdivisions in both the French and American systems.
B. Segments are determined primarily by the hepatic venous drainage.
C. The French anatomic system is more applicable than the American system to clinical hepatic resection.
D. Segments are important to the understanding of the topographic anatomy of the liver.

DISCUSSION: Segments are the major subdivision of the right and left lobes of the liver. In either the classic lobar (American) or the segmental (French) system, the most variable aspect is the biliary system. Therefore the hepatic venous or portal system defines most segments. The French system depicts eight segments, with the caudate lobe as segment I and the other seven segments defined primarily by the hepatic venous system. Segments are not well-depicted by topography.
Textbook: Page 1048 ANSWER: D.

2. Which of the following anatomic features of the biliary system are important considerations in operative cholangiography?

A. The left hepatic duct comes off farther anterior than the right one.
B. At the confluence there may be more than just a right and a left hepatic duct.
C. Dissection of the triangle of Calot is more important than cholangiography in preventing bile duct injury.
D. Segments V, VII, or VIII sometimes join the biliary system below the confluence.

DISCUSSION: All of these features are important. The angle of takeoff of the left hepatic duct may make operative visualization difficult with the patient in the supine position. Because there may be more than two major hepatic ducts, visualization of two large ducts does not ensure that the system is normal. Ducts from any of the right-side segments can join below the confluence. Dissecting one superior edge of the gallbladder before it joins the cystic duct is particularly important in preventing injury.
Textbook: Pages 1050–1051 ANSWER: A, B, C, D.

3. The hepatic artery:

A. Supplies the same amount of blood to the liver as the portal vein.
B. Provides more blood to the bile ducts than the portal vein.
C. Is autoregulated just as the portal vein is.
D. Supplies most of the blood to hepatic metastases.

DISCUSSION: The portal vein provides two thirds to three quarters of the total hepatic blood flow. The portal vein is incapable of direct autoregulation. The hepatic artery after transplantation classically infarcts portions of the biliary system, whereas hepatic metastases often arrive there via the portal vein. Most of their blood supply comes from the hepatic artery.
Textbook: Pages 1049–1050 ANSWER: B, D.

4. Bile formation is:

A. An active secretory process.
B. Determined at two sites principally.
C. Regulated physiologically by hormones.
D. Largely determined by the intactness of the enterohepatic circulation (EHC).

DISCUSSION: Bile formation is an active process at both the canalicular and ductular sites. The paracellular pathway probably plays a minor physiologic role. Secretin and glucagon are likely physiologic regulators of biliary secretion. Bile salts are extremely important and are probably the most important agent in the changes that occur when enterohepatic circulation is interrupted.
Textbook: Pages 1055–1056 ANSWER: A, B, C, D.

5. Generally, the two most important hepatic functions to consider after hepatic resection are:

A. Hepatic synthetic function.
B. Glucose metabolism.
C. The liver's role in lipid metabolism.
D. The liver's role in vitamin metabolism.

DISCUSSION: While other functions undoubtedly may be important postoperatively, the most common abnormalities occurring after a major hepatic resection are related to loss of protein synthesis and consequences of glucose metabolism. Therefore, it is usually advisable to administer supplemental amounts of protein and sugar postoperatively.

Textbook: Pages 1057–1058 ANSWER: A, B.

6. Which of the following statements about pyogenic abscess of the liver are true?

A. The right lobe is more commonly involved than the left lobe.
B. Appendicitis with perforation and abscess is the most common underlying cause of hepatic abscess.
C. Mortality is largely determined by the underlying disease.
D. Mortality from hepatic abscess is currently greater than 40%.

DISCUSSION: Involvement of the right lobe with abscess formation approximates 70% of pyogenic abscesses. This is thought to be due to the *streaming* effect of superior mesenteric venous inflow to the right lobe. In addition, the greater volume of the right lobe predisposes more tissue to seeding by bacterial organisms. While appendicitis comprised 25% to 40% of cases in early series, early recognition and operative therapy for appendicitis have reduced its importance significantly. In current series, malignant or benign biliary obstruction is the underlying cause of 35% to 50% of cases. Recent studies have shown that the underlying disease or an immunocompromised host is more important prognostically than solitary versus multiple abscesses.

Textbook: Pages 1063, 1066 ANSWER: A, C.

7. Which of the following statements most accurately describes the current therapy for pyogenic hepatic abscess?

A. Antibiotics alone are adequate for the treatment of most cases.
B. All patients require open surgical drainage for optimal management.
C. Optimal treatment involves treatment of not only the abscess but the underlying source as well.
D. Percutaneous drainage is more successful for multiple lesions than for solitary ones.

DISCUSSION: The development of ultrasonography and computed tomography (CT) in the past two decades has enabled earlier diagnosis and advances in treatment of hepatic abscess. Formerly, open surgical drainage was considered necessary in essentially all cases of pyogenic abscess. Numerous recent series, however, have reported high success rates and low mortality from the percutaneous catheter drainage of abscesses under CT or ultrasonographic guidance. Optimal management of pyogenic abscess, however, involves not only treatment of the abscess, whether by percutaneous or surgical methods, but correction of the underlying source as well. All modes of therapy are more successful in treating solitary lesions than multiple ones.

Textbook: Pages 1066–1067 ANSWER: C.

8. Which of the following statements characterize amebic abscess?

A. Mortality is higher than that for similarly located pyogenic abscesses.
B. The diagnosis of amebic abscess may be based on serologic tests and resolution of symptoms.
C. In contrast to pyogenic abscess, the treatment of amebic abscess is primarily medical.
D. Patients with amebic abscess tend to be older than those with pyogenic abscess.

DISCUSSION: Mortality for uncomplicated amebic abscess should be less than 5%, in contrast to the 15% to 20% rate for pyogenic abscess. After the demonstration by radiologic examination of an abscess, appropriate serologic tests and resolution of symptoms after a course of treatment with an antiamebic agent such as metronidazole constitute presumptive diagnosis of amebic abscess. Aspiration of abscess contents rarely yields amebic organisms. In contrast to pyogenic abscess, amebic abscess rarely requires surgical or percutaneous drainage, except in the case of an extremely large abscess or bacterial superinfection. Amebic abscess affects males in a 9:1 to 10:1 ratio and generally affects a younger population than pyogenic abscess. Additionally, in the United States the populations most affected are immigrants from endemic areas such as Mexico or Latin America and American tourists to those regions.

Textbook: Pages 1062, 1064–1065, 1067 ANSWER: B, C.

9. Which of the following statement(s) is/are true about benign lesions of the liver?

A. Adenomas are true neoplasms with a predisposition for complications and should usually be resected.
B. Focal nodular hyperplasia (FNH) is a neoplasm related to birth control pills (BCPs) and usually requires resection.
C. Hemangiomas are the most common benign lesions of the liver that come to the surgeon's attention.
D. Nodular regenerative hyperplasia does not usually accompany cirrhosis.

DISCUSSION: Adenomas typically enlarge and cause symptoms, may rupture, and have a definite malignant potential. Therefore they should generally be resected when found. FNH is not a true neoplasm and generally has an uneventful course. Both are related to BCPs, although the relationship of adenoma is more firmly established. While small bile duct hamartomas are much more common, hemangiomas are the most common lesion to come to the attention of surgeons. They should not generally be biopsied because of possible hemorrhage. By definition, nodular regenerative hyperplasia occurs in the absence of cirrhosis.

Textbook: Pages 1079–1080 ANSWER: A.

10. Which of the following statement(s) about malignant neoplasms of the liver is/are true?

A. Hepatocellular carcinoma is probably the number 1 cause of death from cancers worldwide.
B. The most common resectable hepatic malignant neoplasm in the United States is colorectal metastasis.
C. Hepatoma has at least one variant that has a much more benign course than hepatomas in general.
D. Hepatomas are generally slower growing than was formerly believed

DISCUSSION: Although exact comparisons are impossible, hepatoma seems to be the most common cause of cancer death worldwide, despite its relative infrequency in the United States. Colorectal metastasis is a more common indication for surgical treatment in the United States. The fibrolamellar variant and possibly the very well-differentiated tumor probably have a better prognosis than hepatomas in general. Previous studies from Africa in which there was a high incidence of rupture account for the poor prognosis that was generally attributed to hepatoma. Recent studies from Europe and the United States have shown that survival after presentation is usually measured in years.

Textbook: Pages 1069, 1072–1073, 1079 ANSWER: A, B, C, D.

11. Which of the following statement(s) is/are true about bile duct cancers?

A. If resected, proximal lesions are usually curable.
B. The more proximal the lesion, the more likely is resection to be curative.
C. Radiation clearly prolongs survival.
D. Transplantation is usually successful if the lesion seems confined to the liver.
E. None of the above is true.

DISCUSSION: Most bile duct cancers are discovered after they are incurable, and only a tiny subset of resected proximal lesions are cured. The more distal the lesion, the more likely is resection to achieve cure (e.g., approximately 30% 5-year survival for periampullary lesions as compared with 0% to 10% for hilar lesions). The use of adjuvant or primary radiation remains controversial because of the heterogeneity of the patient populations on which this modality has been used. Because of the localized nature of this disease it would seem that transplantation would produce favorable results; however, this has not been the case.

Textbook: Page 1074 ANSWER: E.

12. Echinococcosis liver disease caused by *Echinococcus granulosus:*

A. Is not a neoplasm.
B. Is endemic to parts of Europe, but not the United States.
C. Is usually curable by resection.
D. Is more deadly than in its *Echinococcus multilocularis* form.

DISCUSSION: The parasitic infection is fairly common in certain parts of Europe but very rare in the United States. Resection without peritoneal soilage is the treatment of choice. The *E. multilocularis* form, which is endemic to parts of the United States, is more likely to be fatal because it is rarely resectable. This form is more likely to resemble a malignancy than *E. granulosus*, although the natural course of the disease usually spans many years.

Textbook: Pages 1081–1082 ANSWER: A, B, C.

13. Which of the following statements about hemobilia are true?

A. Tumors are the most common cause.
B. The primary treatment of severe hemobilia is an operation.
C. Percutaneous cholangiographic hemobilia is usually minor.
D. Ultrasonography usually reveals a specific diagnosis.

DISCUSSION: By far the most common cause of hemobilia is trauma. Tumors also may cause the syndrome but are relatively uncommon causes. For severe hemobilia the best therapy is arteriographic embolization. Usually the site of bleeding or a false aneurysm can be identified. Operation should be reserved as a last resort or when the condition is recognized intraoperatively. Percutaneous cholangiography–associated intrabiliary hemorrhage is usually, but not always, minor and self-limiting. Ultrasonography is a very nonspecific diagnostic technique for hemobilia. Arteriography remains the best diagnostic method.

Textbook: Pages 1084, 1086–1087 ANSWER: C.

14. Ligation of all of the following arteries usually causes significant hepatic enzyme abnormalities except:

A. Ligation of the right hepatic artery.
B. Ligation of the left hepatic artery.
C. Ligation of the hepatic artery distal to the gastroduodenal branch.
D. Ligation of the hepatic artery proximal to the gastroduodenal artery.

DISCUSSION: Ligation of the right or left hepatic artery frequently causes enzyme elevation but is usually tolerated by the patient, particularly when this is a life-saving maneuver. Ligation of the hepatic artery distal to the gastroduodenal branch is more risky but is also usually tolerated. Ligation of the hepatic artery proximal to the gastroduodenal one does not normally cause enzyme abnormalities because of abundant collateral flow through that branch.

Textbook: Page 1087 ANSWER: D.

15. Which of the following is the most common acid-base disturbance in patients with cirrhosis and portal hypertension?

A. Metabolic acidosis.
B. Respiratory alkalosis.

C. Metabolic alkalosis.
D. Respiratory acidosis.

DISCUSSION: Metabolic alkalosis and hypokalemia are common in patients with cirrhosis because they often have associated secondary hyperaldosteronism (especially those with ascites), diarrhea, and frequent emesis. Hyperaldosteronism enhances H^+ and K^+ exchange for Na^+ in the distal tubule of the kidney. The cause of diarrhea in patients with cirrhosis is unknown, but malabsorption secondary to splanchnic venous hypertension may be a contributing factor. Emesis is common in alcoholic cirrhotics and patients with tense ascites. Deleterious effects of metabolic alkalosis include impaired tissue oxygen delivery secondary to shift of the oxyhemoglobin dissociation curve to the left and conversion of ammonium chloride to ammonia, which may contribute to encephalopathy.

Textbook: Page 1090 ANSWER: C.

16. A portal venous pressure of 30 mm. Hg (elevated) and a hepatic venous wedge pressure of 5 mm. Hg (normal) may be associated with which of the following causes of portal hypertension?

A. Portal vein thrombosis.
B. Alcoholic cirrhosis.
C. Schistosomiasis.
D. Alcoholic hepatitis.

DISCUSSION: Pressure measured by wedging a catheter into a hepatic vein (hepatic venous wedge pressure) closely correlates with directly measured portal venous pressure in patients with portal hypertension when the site of elevated resistance is at the sinusoidal or postsinusoidal level. Such is the case in alcoholic cirrhosis and alcoholic hepatitis. When the site of increased resistance is at the presinusoidal level, either within (schistosomiasis) or outside (portal vein thrombosis) the liver, the hepatic venous wedge pressure is normal despite markedly elevated portal vein pressure. Although schistosomiasis is one of the more frequent causes of portal hypertension worldwide, in North America presinusoidal portal hypertension is considerably less common than alcoholic liver disease. A normal hepatic venous wedge pressure in a patient who has bled from varices should lead one to suspect a presinusoidal cause. A specific diagnosis can often be made by visceral angiography or liver biopsy.

Textbook: Pages 1089, 1090–1091 ANSWER: A, C.

17. Which of the following is the most effective definitive therapy for both prevention of recurrent variceal hemorrhage and control of ascites?

A. Endoscopic sclerotherapy.
B. Distal splenorenal shunt.
C. Esophagogastric devascularization (Sugiura procedure).
D. Side-to-side portacaval shunt.
E. End-to-side portacaval shunt.

DISCUSSION: Shunt operations are the most effective means of preventing recurrent variceal hemorrhage. Rebleeding rates after endoscopic sclerotherapy range from 40% to 60%. Although extensive esophagogastric devascularization has effectively prevented recurrent bleeding in Japanese series, these operations have been followed by rebleeding rates in excess of 25% in most Western series. Although one controlled trial has shown more frequent recurrent hemorrhage following the distal splenorenal shunt than after the portacaval shunt, most series have reported rebleeding rates of less than 10% for both of these operations. Both the liver and the splanchnic viscera are important sites of ascites formation. Since the distal splenorenal shunt maintains sinusoidal and mesenteric venous hypertension and requires interruption of important retroperitoneal lymphatics, it tends to aggravate rather than relieve ascites. Hepatic sinusoidal pressure may be unchanged or even increased after an end-to-side portacaval shunt. Only side-to-side portal-systemic shunts, such as the side-to-side portacaval shunt, reliably decompress both the liver and splanchnic viscera, thus preventing ascites formation.

Textbook: Pages 1096–1101 ANSWER: D.

18. Which of the following treatments most effectively preserves hepatic portal perfusion?

A. Distal splenorenal shunt.
B. Conventional splenorenal shunt.
C. Endoscopic sclerotherapy.
D. Side-to-side portacaval shunt.

DISCUSSION: The conventional splenorenal shunt and side-to-side portacaval shunts completely divert portal flow away from the liver (nonselective shunts). The distal splenorenal shunt is a selective shunt that preserves hepatic portal perfusion in the majority of patients; however, the magnitude of portal flow is decreased because the gastrosplenic component is diverted into the renal vein. Additionally, many patients (especially alcoholic cirrhotics) develop collaterals between the mesenteric venous circulation and the shunt, resulting in gradual attrition of the remaining portal flow. Although there have been anecdotal reports of portal vein thrombosis after endoscopic sclerotherapy, two controlled trials have demonstrated better preservation of hepatic portal perfusion in sclerotherapy patients than in persons who receive the distal splenorenal shunt.

Textbook: Pages 1096–1101 ANSWER: C.

19. Which of the following veins is preserved in performing the extensive esophagogastric devascularization procedure described by Sugiura?

A. Left gastric (coronary) vein.
B. Short gastric vein.
C. Splenic vein.
D. Left gastroepiploic vein.

DISCUSSION: The Sugiura procedure consists of devascularization of the esophagus to the inferior pulmonary vein and the proximal two thirds of the stomach, splenectomy, and distal esophageal transection. The devascularization component should be done as close to the esophagus and stomach as possible. The coronary vein and paraesophageal collaterals are preserved to maintain an effective portal-systemic collateral pathway and thereby discourage reformation of varices.

Textbook: Pages 1100–1101 ANSWER: A.

20. Which of the following complications of portal hypertension often require surgical intervention (for more than 25% of patients)?

A. Hypersplenism.
B. Variceal hemorrhage.
C. Ascites.
D. Encephalopathy.

DISCUSSION: While many patients with portal hypertension develop hypersplenism, it is rarely clinically significant. A splenectomy should not be performed unless platelet counts are persistently less than 20,000 per cu. mm. or white blood cell counts are less than 1200 per cu. mm. Unfortunately, splenectomy is sometimes done for clinically insignificant hypersplenism, thus obviating a distal splenorenal shunt if the patient should subsequently bleed from varices. The initial treatment for most patients with bleeding esophageal varices should be endoscopic sclerotherapy; however, operation is required for the approximately one third of patients who fail sclerotherapy and for noncompliant persons, those living in remote geographic locations, and patients bleeding from gastric varices. Ascites can be controlled by a medical regimen of dietary salt restriction and diuretic therapy in more than 95% of patients. When ascites is intractable to medical management, either intermittent large-volume paracenteses or a surgical peritoneovenous shunt should be done With rare exceptions, encephalopathy should be treated medically. Most important is elimination of any precipitating factors that led to the neuropsychological disturbance. Lactulose, neomycin, and dietary protein restriction may also be components of the medical treatment regimen.

Textbook: Pages 1096, 1098, 1101–1102 ANSWER: B.

21. Which of the following effects are advantages of combined vasopressin and nitroglycerin intravenous infusion, as compared with vasopressin infusion alone, in controlling acute variceal bleeding?

A. Lower frequency of encephalopathy.
B. Lower incidence of vasopressin side effects.
C. More effective control of bleeding.
D. Less "rebound effect" when discontinuing the infusion.

DISCUSSION: Vasopressin acts through vasoconstriction of splanchnic arterioles. Both portal venous inflow and portal venous pressure are reduced, resulting in control of acute variceal bleeding in approximately 50% of patients. However, the adverse side effects of systemic hypertension, bradycardia, decreased cardiac output, and coronary vasoconstriction are quite common during vasopressin infusion. Simultaneous administration of nitroglycerin or nitroprusside eliminates these side effects—and in one controlled trial enhanced therapeutic effectiveness. Although the mechanism of action of this combined infusion is not clear, vasodilation of portal-systemic collaterals, resulting in a further reduction in portal pressure, may be responsible.

Textbook: Pages 1093–1094 ANSWER: B, C.

22. Which of the following statements about the peritoneovenous shunt (PVS) is/are correct?

A. For cirrhotic patients with intractable ascites, the LeVeen shunt is an effective "bridge" to liver transplantation.
B. Replacement of ascites with saline or lactated Ringer's solution reduces the coagulopathy following PVS.
C. For patients with cirrhotic ascites, the survival using repeated paracentesis with 5% albumin infusion is equivalent to that with the PVS.
D. Oliguria (less than 25 ml. per hour) in the immediate postoperative period following PVS should be treated with a 5% albumin infusion.
E. The transjugular intrahepatic portacaval shunt with stent (TIPSS) works on the same principle as the PVS.

DISCUSSION: The PVS is a palliative procedure that does not prolong life. In comparing the early risks of the procedure with those of repeated paracentesis, the shunt cannot be justified as a temporizing procedure to facilitate ascites control in the patient awaiting liver transplantation. Oliguria is common in the first 24 hours after shunt insertion. A correctly placed PVS (patency confirmed using an intraoperative "shuntogram") expands the intravascular volume with a continuous reinfusion of ascites. Inspection should identify elevation of the jugular venous pressure, and a diuretic (usually furosemide) is needed. The mechanisms of action of the two shunts are very different. TIPSS reduces portal pressure and controls ascites by reducing the rate of ascites formation. PVS reinfuses the ascites fluid, thereby reducing the prerenal stimulus to sodium retention and making the patient more responsive to diuretic therapy.

Textbook: Pages 1108–1109 ANSWER: B, C.

23. Which of the following clinical situations are considered good indications for PVS?

A. A 50-year-old cirrhotic man had an emergency portacaval shunt for bleeding varices and postoperatively had an ascites leak and mild superficial wound infection.
B. A 57-year-old woman with primary biliary cirrhosis (PBC) has difficult to control ascites and diuretic-induced encephalopathy.
C. A 46-year-old resistant alcoholic has chronic ascites uncontrolled by diuretics combined with repeat paracentesis.
D. A 34-year-old woman taking BCPs had rapid onset of ascites and is found to have hepatic

vein thrombosis causing the Budd-Chiari syndrome.

DISCUSSION: Because of the high complication rate and the long-term failure rate, the PVS is used only when other, more lasting options for therapy either are not available or are contraindicated. The chronic alcoholic patient may benefit from a peritoneovenous shunt because his ascites is the dominant problem related to his chronic liver disease, and persistent alcoholism is a contraindication to liver replacement in most centers. PVS may be quite effective for the temporary management of acute intractable postoperative ascites, such as in patient *A*; however, it is absolutely contraindicated in the presence of infection. Patient *B* has ascites as her dominant problem as well; however, with PBC as the underlying liver disease, she is an excellent candidate for transplantation. Patient *D* also has ascites as the major problem; however, the side-to-side portosystemic shunt is a far better long-term treatment option than PVS.

Textbook: Pages 1105–1108 ANSWER: C.

24. Which of the following explanations account(s) for the fact that hepatitis C is the most common cause of posttransfusion hepatitis?

A. There are more carriers of hepatitis C virus (HCV) in the normal population who serve as blood donors.
B. Blood infected with hepatitis B virus (HBV) is eliminated through routine testing, leaving only HCV as the other blood-borne pathogen.
C. Current serologic tests for HCV antigen do not exclude carriers.
D. Questions designed to eliminate risk groups for HCV from the normal donor population may not be as specific as would be desirable.
E. Hepatitis C is a more virulent form of viral hepatitis, so it is expected that more cases of posttransfusion hepatitis would occur.

DISCUSSION: The ability to specifically identify persons infected with HCV has only recently become available. Therefore, data about epidemiology are less than complete. It is very likely **not** true that more blood donors carry HCV because of the large preponderance of HBV in the United States. It is true, however, that successful elimination of most of the HBV carriers occurs through routine testing. Although serologic tests are available for HCV, they are tests, not of antigen, but of antibody. Therefore, this test alone may not screen out persons who are infected but have not yet developed or may never develop antibody. Risk groups for the relatively newly defined HCV may well not be comprehensively established, and therefore this explanation may be a contributor. There are no differences in virulence between these classes of hepatitis virus.

Textbook: Pages 1113–1114 ANSWER: B, D.

25. True or false: HBV infections:

A. Are usually asymptomatic.
B. May not be clinically recognized but may lead to chronic hepatitis.
C. Reliably protect against subsequent HBV infection regardless of the measured antibody titer to hepatitis B surface antigen (HBsAg).
D. Are completely prevented by postexposure administration of HBIg hepatitis B immunoglobulin (HBIg).
E. Preclude subsequent infection with HDV.

DISCUSSION: Although some types of hepatitis are more often asymptomatic than symptomatic, that is not the case for hepatitis B. Further, even if the HBV infection is asymptomatic, serious long-term side effects may occur. A prior infection with hepatitis B confers lifelong immunity even if the antibody titer wanes below the protective level of 10 mIU. HBIg is useful in reducing the incidence of postexposure HBV infection from around 30% with no intervention, to 15% with standard immune globulin, to about 5% to 7% with HBIg. HBV infection is required for infection with HDV and is therefore an essential step toward, rather than preventive of, HBV infection.

Textbook: Pages 1113–1114 ANSWER: True: B, C. False: A, D, E.

26. Which of the following statements about choledocholithiasis are correct?

A. Common duct stones can originate in the gallbladder and migrate to the common duct, and stones can form *de novo* in the duct system.
B. Calcium bilirubinate stones are associated with the presence of bacteria in the duct system.
C. Common duct stones discovered at laparoscopic cholecystectomy should be treated by postoperative endoscopic extraction.
D. The serum bilirubin value is usually greater than 15 mg. per dl. in the patient with a symptomatic common duct stone.

DISCUSSION: Most common duct stones originate in the gallbladder and migrate to the common duct, where they may become larger. These stones tend to consist predominantly of cholesterol (about 80% of gallbladder stones are predominantly cholesterol). Stones found in the bile ducts after cholecystectomy may have been overlooked, but *de novo* stone formation does occur. Arbitrarily, stones found 2 years after cholecystectomy are assumed to have formed within the duct system. Calcium bilirubinate stones are thought to result from precipitation of insoluble bilirubin monoglucuronide formed by deconjugation of bilirubin diglucuronide, a reaction promoted by the enzyme beta-glucuronidase, which is produced by bacteria in the biliary tract. Calcium bilirubinate stones are found almost exclusively in patients who have some form of biliary tract lesion that causes partial obstruction, and these patients tend to have bactibilia. Stones smaller than approximately 5 mm. often can be extracted through a dilated cystic duct or pushed into the duodenum. Larger stones are best left for postoperative endoscopic sphincterotomy and extraction. Patients with more than five stones or stones larger than 1.5 cm. should be treated by open choledocholithotomy or, when indicated, a biliary-enteric anastomosis. Not all patients with symptomatic common duct stones have elevated serum bilirubin, but when jaundice is present the bilirubin is only rarely greater than 15 mg. per dl.

Textbook: Pages 1119–1121 ANSWER: A, B, C.

27. A benign biliary duct stricture:

A. Need not be treated unless it causes clinical jaundice.
B. Should always be treated by percutaneous balloon drainage.
C. Is prone to recur after treatment with biliary-enteric anastomosis.
D. When due to chronic pancreatitis should be treated by side-to-side choledochoduodenostomy.

DISCUSSION: Even a minor obstructing lesion in the extrahepatic duct system can produce cirrhosis over time; and the development of portal hypertension, ascites, and esophageal varices. Therefore, all biliary strictures should be treated unless this is not possible or there is no chance for success. The presence or absence of jaundice is of no significance. Often, the only biochemical abnormality is mild elevation of alkaline phosphatase. The long-term results of percutaneous balloon dilatation are not yet known, but short-term results are good. Although some argue that balloon dilatation should be the initial treatment, its role is ill-defined, and it should not be viewed as standard therapy at this time. Biliary-enteric anastomoses are predisposed to stricture, for reasons that are ill-understood. A mucosa-to-mucosa anastomosis, large size of the anastomosis, a normal duct at the point of anastomosis, and stenting appear to be elements that work against stricture. About 70% of anastomoses are not complicated by strictures. Common duct strictures caused by chronic pancreatitis are located in the distal portion of the duct and are easily treated by side-to-side choledochoduodenostomy. A wide anastomosis is usually possible, and because of this stenting often is not necessary. Although a Roux-en-Y biliary-enteric reconstruction is acceptable treatment, no advantage over choledochoduodenostomy has been demonstrated.

Textbook: Pages 1122–1123 ANSWER: C, D.

28. Which statements about extrahepatic bile duct cancer are correct?

A. Cholangiography is essential in evaluating patients for resectability.
B. The prognosis is excellent when appropriate surgical and adjuvant therapy are given.
C. The location of the tumor determines the type of surgical procedure.
D. The disease usually becomes manifest by moderate to severe right-side upper quadrant pain.

DISCUSSION: Cholangiography is essential for both diagnosis and evaluation of resectability. Brushings of the lesion for diagnosis and temporary stenting, done percutaneously or endoscopically, are often done at the time of cholangiography. Angiography and CT are helpful, but in the absence of hepatic artery or portal vein occlusion these tests are not accurate predictors of resectability. The primary obstacles to complete resection are invasion of the portal vein or the hepatic artery and proximal extension of the tumor into the liver. The long-range prognosis for patients who undergo treatment for extrahepatic bile duct cancer is poor, even when the lesion is surgically resectable and adjuvant therapy is given. Only about 10% of patients are alive without disease at 10 years. Nevertheless, bile duct cancer tends not to metastasize to distant sites, so resection and radiation therapy are useful in prolonging symptom-free life. Tumors in the proximal third of the extrahepatic bile duct system are treated by a Roux-en-Y biliary-enteric anastomosis. To ensure excision of the entire tumor this anastomosis usually must be made to the individual hepatic ducts, which must be stented individually. Tumors of the middle third usually require anastomosis to the proximal hepatic duct. In contrast, lesions of the distal third require Whipple's procedure with appropriate reconstruction. Thus, the treatment of extrahepatic bile duct cancer depends on the location of the tumor. Pain is not a prominent feature of bile duct cancer. Most cases become manifest by the insidious development of jaundice.

Textbook: Pages 1123–1124 ANSWER: A, C.

29. Which of the following statements about biliary tract problems are correct?

A. Choledochal cyst should be treated by Roux-en-Y cystojejunostomy.
B. Sclerosing cholangitis is characterized by long, narrow strictures in the extrahepatic biliary duct system.
C. Operative (needle) cholangiography is indicated in patients who at operation appear to have no gallbladder.
D. The long cystic duct, which appears to be fused with the common duct and enters it distally, should be dissected free and ligated at its entrance into the common duct.

DISCUSSION: In the past, choledochal cyst was treated by Roux-en-Y cystojejunostomy, but long-term results were poor. Excision of the cyst is essential to prevent recurrent pancreatitis. In addition, the development of carcinoma in about 25% of patients mandates cyst excision. Accordingly, excision of the cyst with biliary reconstruction by Roux-en-Y hepaticojejunostomy and diversion of the flow of pancreatic juice through the ampulla of Vater is currently the standard treatment. Sclerosing cholangitis causes fibrosis of bile ducts both within and outside the liver. This process, which is poorly understood, causes strictures in the duct system, characteristically with normal or dilated segments between strictures. Unfortunately, this anatomic arrangement does not lend itself to biliary reconstructive procedures. Each case must be analyzed, however, because in some patients the anatomic situation may lend itself to balloon dilatation or reconstruction. When the gallbladder appears to be absent, a search should be made for an ectopically located organ in the retroduodenal area, within the falciform ligament, and within the substance of the right lobe of the liver. With true gallbladder agenesis the common duct may be dilated, and choledocholithiasis is present in about one fourth of those who undergo operation. Therefore, operative needle cholangiography should always be done. Dissection of a long, fused cystic duct is fraught with hazard because the cystic and common ducts may share a common wall and serious duct damage may occur. The cystic duct should be ligated and divided immediately proximal to the area of fusion.

Textbook: Pages 1119, 1124 ANSWER: C.

30. Which of the following statements about the diagnosis of acute calculous cholecystitis are true?

A. Pain is so frequent that its absence almost precludes the diagnosis.
B. Jaundice is present in a majority of patients.
C. Ultrasonography is the definitive diagnostic test.
D. Cholescintigraphy is the definitive diagnostic test.

DISCUSSION: The presence of pain is the *sine qua non* of acute calculous cholecystitis. Chronic cholecystitis associated with cholelithiasis may develop in the absence of pain, and in critically ill patients pain may not be a prominent feature of acute acalculous cholecystitis. Only about 10% of patients with acute cholecystitis are jaundiced. Although an occasional patient may have concomitant bile duct obstruction, the jaundice associated with acute cholecystitis is probably due to absorption of bile pigments from the diseased gallbladder. The presence of jaundice in a patient with right-side upper quadrant pain should also suggest the possibility of acute cholangitis secondary to bile duct obstruction. Ultrasonography is very accurate in the detection of gallstones, but stones may be present in the absence of acute cholecystitis. Thickening of the gallbladder wall and a collection of fluid around the gallbladder are ultrasonographic findings in some patients with acute cholecystitis, but they are not always present and are not specific. Ultrasonography may be useful when the diagnosis is obscure because other conditions in the liver, pancreas, and kidney can be detected; however, it is not the definitive test for acute cholecystitis. Cholescintigraphy is specific for the diagnosis of acute calculous cholecystitis (accuracy over 95% in experienced hands). The rapidity, simplicity, and accuracy make cholescintigraphy the definitive diagnostic test in acute calculous cholecystitis; however, it must be interpreted cautiously in the context of another critical illness or recent surgery or trauma, because false-positives are not unusual in these situations.

Textbook: Pages 1126–1128 ANSWER: A, D.

31. Which statements about acute acalculous cholecystitis are correct?

A. The disease is often accompanied by or associated with other conditions.
B. The diagnosis is often difficult.
C. The mortality rate is higher than that for acute calculous cholecystitis.
D. The disease has been treated successfully by percutaneous cholecystostomy.

DISCUSSION: About half of the cases of acute acalculous cholecystitis are associated with other conditions, including sepsis, sarcoidosis, polyarteritis nodosa, and systemic lupus erythematosus. A majority of cases occur after trauma, burns, or major surgical procedures performed for other conditions. The precise pathogenesis has not been determined. The diagnosis of acute acalculous cholecystitis is often difficult because symptoms may be masked by another illness, injury, or the postoperative state. Unlike acute calculous cholecystitis, in which pain is always present, pain occurs in only about 70% of cases. In addition, cholescintigraphy is sometimes inaccurate. These factors make the diagnosis difficult, and a high index of suspicion is necessary, especially in patients who have had operations or trauma. Unexplained abdominal pain, sepsis, and ileus should prompt a thorough investigation. The mortality rate for acute acalculous cholecystitis is higher than that of the calculous type. The incidence of gangrene and perforation of the gallbladder is higher. The accompanying illnesses and conditions and the frequent delays in diagnosis undoubtedly contribute to the higher death rate. Percutaneous cholecystostomy has been used as a diagnostic and therapeutic maneuver in patients who are thought to have acute acalculous cholecystitis. Aspiration and culture of bile assist in confirming the diagnosis, and continuous drainage successfully treats the acute condition. Surprisingly, persistent gangrene and subsequent complications have been infrequent. Immediate cholecystectomy should be done if significant improvement does not take place within 12 hours of percutaneous cholecystostomy. Long-term management of the tube and the need for elective cholecystectomy must be individualized. The experience with percutaneous cholecystostomy is too small to determine whether this technique reduces the mortality rate.

Textbook: Pages 1129–1130 ANSWER: A, B, C, D.

32. True statements about the surgical management of patients with acute calculous cholecystitis include:

A. Operation should be performed in all patients as soon as the diagnosis is made.
B. Antibiotic therapy should be initiated as soon as the diagnosis is made.
C. Dissection of the gallbladder is facilitated by decompression of the organ with the use of a trocar.
D. An operative cholangiogram should be done in every patient.

DISCUSSION: Cholecystectomy should be done in an otherwise healthy patient as soon as the diagnosis is made and the patient is properly prepared for surgery. However, patients who have one or more significant risk factors such as a recent myocardial infarction, unstable angina, clinically significant coronary artery disease, or cirrhosis should not have immediate cholecystectomy unless they do not improve within 24 to 36 hours in response to antibiotic administration and supportive care. Antibiotic administration should commence as soon as the diagnosis is made and should be continued for 24 hours postoperatively—or for 7 days if significant peritonitis is present. This use of antibiotics has significantly reduced septic complications after cholecystectomy for acute cholecystitis. In most cases the gallbladder is tensely distended, making visualization and dissection of the cystic duct area difficult and perhaps dangerous. Decompression of the gallbladder by insertion of a needle facilitates retraction and dissection of the gallbladder. Although some advise that operative cholangiography be done only on a selective basis, its routine use helps to delineate anatomy and facilitates detection of an occasionally unsuspected bile duct stone. Accordingly, it is used routinely in elective cases. In acute cholecystitis, however, the biliary duct system may be very friable, and operative cholangiography should be done only when it is safe to do so.

Textbook: Page 1129 ANSWER: B, C.

33. Which of the following are indications for cholecystectomy?

A. The presence of gallstones in a patient with intermittent episodes of right-side upper quadrant pain.
B. The presence of gallstones in an asymptomatic patient.
C. The presence of symptomatic gallstones in a patient with angina pectoris.
D. The presence of asymptomatic gallstones in a patient who has insulin-dependent diabetes.

DISCUSSION: Cholecystectomy (and concomitant operative cholangiography) are indicated for symptomatic patients to relieve pain and to prevent the development of acute cholecystitis and its complications. Morbidity and expense are not as great for elective cholecystectomy as they are for cholecystectomy for acute cholelithiasis. The risk of the development of symptoms in patients who have asymptomatic stones is approximately 2% per year, a rate associated with mortality and morbidity that do not exceed those of elective cholecystectomy. Therefore, cholecystectomy is not indicated for asymptomatic patients. Patients who have angina pectoris should not have cholecystectomy until their coronary artery disease has been treated adequately, even if this requires a coronary artery bypass procedure. Heart disease is the most frequent cause of death after cholecystectomy. Prophylactic cholecystectomy, formerly recommended for insulin-dependent diabetics, is not indicated because several studies have shown that the mortality rate from acute cholecystitis is no higher for diabetics than for nondiabetics.

Textbook: Page 1134 ANSWER: A.

34. Which of the following statements about laparoscopic cholecystectomy are correct?

A. The procedure is associated with less postoperative pain and earlier return to normal activity.
B. The incidence of bile duct injury is higher than for open cholecystectomy.
C. Laparoscopic cholecystectomy should be used in asymptomatic patients because it is safer than open cholecystectomy.
D. Pregnancy is a contraindication.

DISCUSSION: Studies have clearly documented that postoperative pain following laparoscopic cholecystectomy is less than that experienced after open cholecystectomy and that patients can resume normal activity sooner. This appears to be related to the reduced trauma to the abdominal wall by virtue of the very small incisions used in laparoscopic procedures. The best evidence is that the bile duct injury rate (0.4%) is approximately double that for open cholecystectomy. The incidence of this serious complication will probably decrease with improved techniques, better training, and more advanced instrumentation. Only symptomatic patients should have cholecystectomy. Prophylactic removal of the gallbladder is not cost effective. All elective operations are contraindicated in the first trimester, so as to prevent fetal anomalies and spontaneous abortion. The laparoscopic technique is not contraindicated thereafter except in patients in whom peritoneal access cannot safely be established. This is rarely a problem. Premature labor is a risk in the third trimester. Thus, unless cholecystectomy can be avoided altogether during pregnancy, the second trimester is the most propitious time.

Textbook: Page 1135 ANSWER: A, B.

35. Which of the following statements about cholangitis are correct?

A. Charcot's triad is always present.
B. Associated biliary tract disease is always present.
C. Chills and fever are due to the presence of bacteria in the bile duct system.
D. The most common cause of cholangitis is choledocholithiasis.

DISCUSSION: Although Charcot's triad (pain, chills and fever, jaundice) is diagnostic of cholangitis, the complete triad occurs only in 50% to 70% of patients. Fever is the most common symptom; therefore, cholangitis should be considered in all patients who have unexplained fever. Episodes of pain, chills, and fever are often so brief as not to concern the patient. Cholangitis does not occur in the absence of partial or complete bile duct obstruction. All patients diagnosed as having cholangitis should have appropriate diagnostic studies to determine the cause. This usually involves cholangiography. The presence of bacteria in bile does not produce symptoms in the absence of partial or complete obstruction of the bile duct system. When obstruction is present, pressure within the system increases, giving rise to reflux of bacteria or their toxic products into the hepatic venous circulation. This cholangiovenous reflux produces chills, fever, and the hemodynamic changes of sepsis. Death may ensue if treatment is not instituted promptly. Choledocholithiasis, the most commonly associated problem, may produce partial or complete obstruction. When bacteria are not present in the bile duct system, choledocholithiasis may go undetected unless the degree of obstruction is sufficient to cause jaundice. Other causes of cholangitis are benign and malignant strictures, biliary-enteric anastomoses, invasive procedures, foreign bodies, and parasitic infestation of the bile ducts.

Textbook: Pages 1140–1142 ANSWER: B, C, D.

36. Recurrent episodes of cholangitis:

A. Suggest the presence of undetected or overlooked bile duct pathology.
B. Occur frequently in patients who have indwelling biliary tubes or stents.
C. May be ameliorated by long-term administration of antibiotics.
D. May be associated with the development of secondary biliary cirrhosis.

DISCUSSION: Cholangitis does not occur in the presence of a normal bile duct system, and all patients with cholangitis have an abnormality. Thus, recurrent episodes of cholangitis signal the need for diagnostic studies. Cholangiography usually will be necessary. The presence of any foreign body in the biliary tract is frequently associated with bactibilia and recurrent episodes of cholangitis. Even a silk suture exposed to the lumen of a bile duct has been known to cause cholangitis. Pigment stone and sludge formation may result from the bacterial deconjugation of bilirubin diglucuronide to bilirubin monoglucuronide, which precipitates as calcium bilirubinate. This material can occlude indwelling tubes and predispose to more frequent episodes of cholangitis. Long-term administration of an oral antibiotic may reduce the frequency and severity of attacks of cholangitis; however, this method of management should not be routine. Correction of the underlying problem is essential. Chronic obstruction and recurrent infection eventually lead to secondary biliary cirrhosis and its complications of portal hypertension, ascites, and bleeding esophageal varices. Once this stage of the disease is reached, correction of the underlying biliary tract problem does not reverse the changes in the liver. Once again, every effort should be made to eliminate the cause of the cholangitis early in the course of disease. The only effective treatment for end-stage liver disease is hepatic transplantation.

Textbook: Pages 1141–1144 ANSWER: A, B, C, D.

37. The initial goal of therapy for acute toxic cholangitis is to:

A. Prevent cholangiovenous reflux by decompressing the duct system.
B. Remove the obstructing stone, if one is present.
C. Alleviate jaundice and prevent permanent liver damage.
D. Prevent the development of gallstone pancreatitis.

DISCUSSION: Uncontrolled sepsis and the consequent multisystem organ failure are the life-threatening sequelae of acute toxic cholangitis. Thus, the initial goal of treatment is to decompress the biliary duct system to prevent reflux of bacteria and their toxic products into the circulation. This can be done by intubating the duct system through the percutaneous, transhepatic, or the endoscopic route or by insertion of a T tube in the common duct at operation. Removal of the stone causing the obstruction is not necessary to stabilize the patient. Only after the duct is decompressed should the cause of the obstruction be addressed. When transhepatic biliary drainage has been used, endoscopic or surgical removal of the stone can be carried out after the patient has recovered completely. When initial therapy is sphincterotomy, the stone should be removed as part of the procedure. Often the stone falls out without manipulation. If surgical placement of a T tube is the initial treatment, the stone should be removed only if it is convenient to do so. The long-range goal of treatment of patients with bile duct obstruction is to prevent cirrhosis, ascites, portal hypertension, and hemorrhage from esophageal varices; however, death from sepsis is the immediate threat in acute toxic cholangitis. Gallstone pancreatitis may occur in patients who have an impacted stone in the distal duct, independent of the presence or absence of acute toxic cholangitis; however, gallstone pancreatitis is more often associated with the passage of a stone into the duodenum.

Textbook: Pages 1143–1144 ANSWER: A.

38. The clinical picture of gallstone ileus includes which of the following?

A. Air in the biliary tree.
B. Small bowel obstruction.
C. A stone at the site of obstruction.
D. Acholic stools.
E. Associated bouts of cholangitis.

DISCUSSION: An antecedent biliary-enteric fistula is necessary to allow stone migration into the intestinal tract, and this results in air entering the biliary tree (pneumobilia). It also allows contamination of the bile ducts with intestinal bacteria, which in fact occurs in only a minority of such cases. The stone obstructs the narrower distal bowel, producing small bowel obstruction. Such a stone, if opaque, can be seen on plain radiography and, if not, can be appreciated by sonography. Stools are *not* acholic, since the cholecystoenteric fistula allows bile access to the intestinal lumen.

Textbook: Page 1147 ANSWER: A, B, C, E.

39. Which of the following statement(s) about gallstone ileus is/are not true?

A. The condition is seen most frequently in women older than 70.
B. Concomitant with the bowel obstruction, air is seen in the biliary tree.
C. The usual fistula underlying the problem is between the gallbladder and the ileum.
D. When possible, relief of small bowel obstruction should be accompanied by definitive repair of the fistula since there is a significant incidence of recurrence if the fistula is left in place.
E. Ultrasound studies may be of help in identifying a gallstone as the obstructing agent.

DISCUSSION: It is true that gallstone ileus occurs mostly in elderly women and should always be suspect when small bowel obstruction presents in this age group. The great majority of cases of gallstone ileus are preceded by a spontaneous fistula occurring between the gallbladder and duodenum, allowing gallstones to enter the intestinal tract, which can potentially block the terminal ileum. Finding air within the biliary tree should always arouse suspicion of the possibility of this diagnosis when it is associated with a radiographic pattern of small bowel obstruction. The initial part of the operative approach to this disease is to relieve the bowel obstruction by performing an enterotomy just proximal to the point of obstruction to remove the stone. Where possible, definitive repair of the fistula should be undertaken to avoid recurrent obstruction and to obviate the possible recurring complications of cholangitis. Percutaneous drainage of bile collections combined with endoscopic papillotomy may be sufficient treatment for external and internal biliary fistulas but is never an allowable approach in the presence of gallstone ileus with small bowel obstruction. Relief of the obstruction is mandated in this setting.

Textbook: Page 1147 ANSWER: C.

40. Which of the following lesions are believed to be associated with the development of carcinoma of the gallbladder?

A. Cholecystoenteric fistula.
B. A calcified gallbladder.
C. Adenoma of the gallbladder.
D. Xanthogranulomatous cholecystitis.
E. All of the above.

DISCUSSION: The prevalence of carcinoma of the gallbladder in patients who have or have had a cholecystoenteric fistula is believed to be 15%. The prevalence of carcinoma in a calcified, or "porcelain," gallbladder is reported to range from 12.5% to 61%. It is generally accepted that adenoma of the gallbladder is a precancerous lesion that presents as a polypoid lesion. Xanthogranulomatous cholecystitis is a rare form of chronic cholecystitis believed to be associated with a higher incidence of cancer. This form of cholecystitis is also important because, grossly, it may mimic cancer of the gallbladder.

Textbook: Pages 1148–1149 ANSWER: E.

41. The preferred treatment for carcinoma of the gallbladder is:

A. Radical resection that includes gallbladder in continuity with the right hepatic lobe and regional lymph node dissection.
B. Radiation therapy.
C. Chemotherapy.
D. Combined treatment involving surgical therapy, chemotherapy, and radiation.
E. None of the above.

DISCUSSION: Radical resection, radiation therapy, and chemotherapy have been effective only anecdotally. Most believe that the dismal prognosis of carcinoma of the gallbladder does not justify anything more than palliative treatment. About 88% of patients are dead within a year of diagnosis, and only about 4% are alive after 5 years, regardless of the type of treatment. Those whose surgeon was unaware of the presence of the tumor at the time of cholecystectomy (approximately 12% of cases) are most likely to survive long term. There are insufficient data to support conclusively the proposition that the patient with unexpected carcinoma found on histologic examination should undergo reoperation with intent for radical excision. There also are indirect suggestions that the prognosis of gallbladder carcinoma may be improving, but it is not clear if this is spontaneous or due to either earlier diagnosis or surgical management.

Textbook: Pages 1150–1151 ANSWER: E.

42. Which of the following statement(s) about pancreatic embryonic malformations is/are correct?

A. Pancreas divisum can be a cause of gastrointestinal bleeding.
B. Heterotopic pancreatic tissue predisposes to pancreatic adenocarcinoma.
C. Annular pancreas may cause gastrointestinal obstruction in children or in adults.
D. Relative obstruction to the flow of pancreatic juice through the minor papilla appears to be the cause of pancreatitis in some patients with pancreas divisum.

DISCUSSION: The clinically recognized embryonic malformations of the pancreas include heterotopic pancreas, pancreas divisum, and annular pancreas. Heterotopic pancreatic tissue most often takes the form of a firm nodule of variable size in the stomach, duodenum, small bowel, or Meckel's diverticulum. The typical complications of heterotopic pancreas include intestinal obstruction, ulceration, or hemorrhage. Pancreas divisum is an anatomic variant that results from failure of fusion of the two primordial pancreatic duct systems. In pancreas divisum the major portion of the pancreas is drained via the duct of Santorini through the minor duodenal papilla. Relative stenosis of the minor duodenal papilla can cause pancreatitis. Pancreas divisum is not associated with gastrointestinal bleeding. Annular pancreas results when histologically normal pancreatic tissue completely or partially encircles the second portion of the duodenum. Varying degrees of duodenal obstructive symptoms may be observed in both children and adults with this condition.

Textbook: Pages 1152–1153 ANSWER: C, D.

43. The pancreas occupies a retroperitoneal position in the upper abdomen. Which statement(s) is/are correct?

A. The superior mesenteric vein and the splenic vein join to form the portal vein posterior to the neck of the pancreas.
B. The uncinate process of the pancreas extends posterior to the inferior vena cava.
C. The tail of the pancreas extends to the left of the aorta, toward the splenic hilum.
D. The head of the pancreas is jointly supplied by arterial blood from the celiac axis and the superior mesenteric artery.

DISCUSSION: The pancreas occupies a retroperitoneal position in the upper abdomen, extending obliquely from the duodenal C loop to a more cephalad position where the pancreatic tail abuts the hilum of the spleen. The portion of the pancreas anterior to the confluence of the superior mesenteric vein, splenic vein, and portal vein is designated the neck of the gland. The uncinate process extends posterior to the superior mesenteric vein and approaches the superior mesenteric artery. The head of the pancreas is intimately associated with the second portion of the duodenum, and these two structures are jointly supplied by two arterial arcades known as the anterior and posterior pancreaticoduodenal arteries, which originate as branches of the celiac axis and superior mesenteric artery.

Textbook: Pages 1153–1154 ANSWER: A, C, D.

44. Both endocrine and exocrine tissue comprise the pancreas. Which statement(s) is/are true?

A. The islets of Langerhans total 1 million per gland and drain their secretions via intercalated duct cells through the ampulla of Vater.
B. Islet alpha cells produce glucagon.
C. Islet sigma cells produce somatostatin.
D. The acini and ductal systems constitute the exocrine portion of the pancreas.

DISCUSSION: The endocrine portion of the pancreas is served by the islets of Langerhans, which number 1 million islets per gland. The islets of Langerhans drain their endocrine secretions into the bloodstream. Insulin-producing beta cells comprise the majority of the islet population. Alpha cells produce glucagon and constitute approximately 20% to 25% of the total islet cell number. Delta cells of the islets produce somatostatin. The acini and ductal systems constitute the exocrine portion of the pancreas. The acinar cells contain zymogen granules in their narrow, centrally located apical portion. The pancreatic duct system includes intercalated duct cells along the ductal pathway, terminating in the main excretory duct of the pancreas.

Textbook: Page 1154 ANSWER: B, D.

45. Pancreatic exocrine secretory products include a bicarbonate-rich electrolyte solution as well as digestive enzymes. Which of the following statement(s) is/are true?

A. Cholecystokinin (CCK) is the most potent endogenous stimulant of pancreatic enzyme secretion.
B. The chloride and bicarbonate concentrations of pancreatic juice vary and depend on the secretory flow rate.
C. Secretin is the most potent endogenous stimulant of pancreatic water and electrolyte secretion.
D. The peptidases synthesized by acinar cells are released into the pancreatic duct system in active form.

DISCUSSION: CCK is the most potent endogenous stimulant of pancreatic enzyme secretion. The pancreatic acinar cells respond to CCK with release of their zymogen granules into the ductal system. Peptidases are released in inactive form, later to be activated by contact with duodenal enterokinase and activated trypsin. Secretin is the most potent endogenous stimulant of pancreatic water and electrolyte secretion. The concentrations of the anions bicarbonate and chloride vary and are largely dependent on the secretory flow rate stimulated by secretin.

Textbook: Pages 1155–1156 ANSWER: A, B, C.

46. Which of the following parameters is/are *not* included in the Ranson's prognostic signs useful in the early evaluation of a patient with acute pancreatitis?

A. Elevated blood glucose.
B. Leukocytosis.
C. Amylase value greater than 1000 U per dl.
D. Serum lactic dehydrogenase (LDH) greater than 350 IU per dl.
E. Alanine aminotransferase greater than 250 U per dl.

DISCUSSION: Several prognostic systems have been demonstrated to predict the severity of pancreatitis accurately. Two Ranson prognostic criteria have been developed: one each, for pancreatitis that is not due to gallstones and pancreatitis that is. The systems have minor differences. In both of the Ranson systems elevated blood glucose, leukocytosis, and elevations of serum LDH have proved to have prognostic importance. The degree of amylase elevation is not one of the parameters, nor is the degree of ALT elevation.

Textbook: Page 1161 ANSWER: C, E.

47. Standard supportive measures for patients with mild pancreatitis include the following:

A. Intravenous fluid and electrolyte therapy.
B. Withholding of analgesics to allow serial abdominal examinations.
C. Subcutaneous octreotide therapy.
D. Nasogastric decompression.
E. Prophylactic antibiotics.

DISCUSSION: Standard therapy for all patients with mild acute pancreatitis should include intravenous fluid resuscitation, electrolyte replacement, and analgesics. Nasogastric decompression is typically reserved for patients with significant ileus who are at risk for emesis and aspiration. Subcutaneous therapy with octreotide, the octapeptide analog of somatostatin, has not been proven to influence the outcome in patients with mild pancreatitis. Prophylactic antibiotics are not used for mild pancreatitis. Antibiotics are reserved for patients with severe pancreatitis (defined as greater than three Ranson prognostic signs with associated CT evidence of pancreatic or peripancreatic necrosis).

Textbook: Pages 1161–1162 ANSWER: A.

48. Which of the following statements about chronic pancreatitis is/are correct?

A. Chronic pancreatitis is the inevitable result after repeated episodes of acute pancreatitis.
B. Patients with chronic pancreatitis commonly present with jaundice, pruritus, and fever.
C. Mesenteric angiography is useful in the evaluation of many patients with chronic pancreatitis.
D. Total pancreatectomy usually offers the best outcome in patients with chronic pancreatitis.
E. For patients with disabling chronic pancreatitis and a dilated pancreatic duct with associated stricture formation, a longitudinal pancreaticojejunostomy (Peustow procedure) is an appropriate surgical option.

DISCUSSION: Chronic pancreatitis is a clinical entity that includes recurrent or persistent abdominal pain with evidence of exocrine and endocrine pancreatic insufficiency. While chronic pancreatitis may result from repeated episodes of acute pancreatitis, not all patients with recurring acute pancreatitis progress to chronic pancreatitis. The most common causes of chronic pancreatitis include alcohol abuse, hyperparathyroidism, congenital anomalies of the pancreatic duct, pancreatic trauma, and cystic fibrosis. The most useful radiographic tests in patients with suspected chronic pancreatitis are CT and endoscopic retrograde cholangiopancreatography (ERCP). Mesenteric angiography has no role in the evaluation of most patients with chronic pancreatitis. Patients with disabling chronic pancreatitis who require operative intervention are candidates for a longitudinal pancreaticojejunostomy (Peustow procedure) if pancreatography demonstrates a dilated pancreatic duct. Total pancreatectomy is rarely performed because of the significant problems associated with labile insulin sensitivity, steatorrhea, and weight loss.

Textbook: Pages 1165–1167 ANSWER: E.

49. Which of the following statements about pancreatic ascites is/are correct?

A. Patients typically present with painful ascites, reflecting the release of toxic pancreatic enzymes into the peritoneal cavity.
B. The standard evaluation of a patient with new-onset ascites includes abdominal paracentesis. In cases of pancreatic ascites, the peritoneal fluid contains high concentrations of both amylase and protein.
C. Pancreatic ascites can follow an episode of acute pancreatitis.
D. Patients with pancreatic ascites may fail to improve with nonoperative therapy and require surgical procedures. At abdominal exploration an acceptable approach to the pancreatic duct disruption involves suture ligation with omental patching.

DISCUSSION: Pancreatic ascites typically occurs because of a pancreatic duct disruption, most commonly involving alcohol abuse and resultant acute pancreatitis. In pancreatic ascites, pancreatic exocrine secretions exit a pancreatic duct disruption and drain anteriorly into the peritoneal cavity. Patients typically present with painless massive ascites, as the pancreatic enzymes that extravasate into the peritoneal cavity are typically nonactivated. The diagnosis of pancreatic ascites is best made by paracentesis, in which the analysis of the ascites fluid reveals it to be high in amylase (more than 1000 U. per dl.) and high in albumin (more than 3 gm. per dl.). Nonoperative treatment is initially indicated in most patients with pancreatic ascites. Should nonoperative therapy fail, surgical therapy is directed to closure of the pancreatic duct disruption. Preoperative pancreatography is useful in directing surgical therapy. Distal pancreatic duct disruption may be treated with distal pancreatectomy or with Roux-en-Y pancreaticojejunostomy. Pancreatic leaks in the more proximal aspects of the gland are treated with Roux-en-Y pancreaticojejunostomy. Suture ligation of the pancreatic duct with omental patching is not considered appropriate therapy for pancreatic duct disruptions.

Textbook: Pages 1170–1171 ANSWER: B, C.

50. Which of the following statements about adenocarcinoma of the pancreas is/are correct?

A. It is the fifth most common cause of cancer death in the U.S.
B. Most cases occur in the body and tail of the pancreas, making distal pancreatectomy the most commonly performed resectional therapy.
C. For cancers of the head of the pancreas

resected by pancreaticoduodenectomy, prognosis appears to be independent of nodal status, margin status, or tumor diameter.

D. The most accurate screening test involves surveillance of stool for carbohydrate antigen (CA 19–9).

DISCUSSION: Adenocarcinoma of the pancreas is newly diagnosed in approximately 28,000 patients in the United States every year. It is the fifth most common cause of cancer death in the United States, exceeded only by lung, colorectal, breast, and prostate cancer. The majority of cases of adenocarcinoma of the pancreas occur in the head of the gland, and if resectable, are treated via pancreaticoduodenectomy. Recent studies have shown that factors favoring long-term survival after pancreaticoduodenectomy for adenocarcinoma of the head of the pancreas include negative nodal status, negative margin status, small tumor diameter, and diploid DNA content. No accurate screening tests for adenocarcinoma of the pancreas are currently available. The best serologic test appears to be the CA 19–9, which is elevated in the majority of patients with adenocarcinoma of the head of the pancreas. Unfortunately, the test is not sufficiently sensitive or specific, and further screening tests are needed.

Textbook: Pages 1171–1174 ANSWER: A.

51. A 35-year-old woman presents with episodes of obtundation, somnolence, and tachycardia. An insulinoma is suspected based on a random serum glucose test value of 38 mg. per dl. Which of the following statements is/are true?

A. The most important diagnostic study for insulinoma is an oral glucose tolerance test.
B. It may be helpful to perform ERCP in an effort to localize the tumor.
C. Most patients with insulinoma present with extensive disease, rendering them only rarely resectable or curable.
D. An important component of the preoperative evaluation in patients with presumed insulinoma involves confirming elevated C-peptide or proinsulin levels and screening for anti-insulin antibodies.

DISCUSSION: Insulinoma is the most common endocrine tumor of the pancreas. Insulinoma is associated with Whipple's triad, which consists of (1) symptoms of hypoglycemia at fasting; (2) documentation of blood glucose levels of less than 50 mg. per dl.; and (3) relief of symptoms following administration of glucose. The most reliable method for diagnosing insulinomas is a monitored fast. Neither an oral or an intravenous glucose tolerance test is indicated in the majority of patients being evaluated for insulinoma. Support for the diagnosis of insulinoma can come from documenting elevated C peptide and proinsulin levels. Screening for anti-insulin antibodies is indicated to rule out the possibility of surreptitious insulin administration. Tumor localization is typically performed with CT, endoscopic ultrasonography, or angiography. ERCP is not indicated for evaluation of most pancreatic endocrine tumors, as the tumors only rarely communicate with the main pancreatic duct system. As many as 90% of patients with insulinoma have benign solitary pancreatic adenomas amenable to surgical cure.

Textbook: Page 1177 ANSWER: D.

52. Which of the following statements about gastrinoma (Zollinger-Ellison syndrome) is/are correct?

A. As many as 75% of gastrinoma patients have sporadic disease; 25% have gastrinoma associated with multiple endocrine neoplasia type 1 (MEN 1).
B. Extrapancreatic gastrinomas are common, and exploration should include careful assessment of the duodenum and peripancreatic lymph nodes.
C. Diarrhea may be a prominent presenting feature of some patients with gastrinoma.
D. Before elective operation acid-reducing medications such as omeprazole should be administered.

DISCUSSION: Gastrinoma patients typically present with peptic ulceration of the upper gastrointestinal tract and abdominal pain. As many as 50% of patients may have diarrhea, which may be a prominent feature in some cases. Approximately 25% of gastrinoma patients have the disease associated with the MEN-1 syndrome, whereas 75% have a sporadic variety of the disease. Recent evidence indicates that extrapancreatic gastrinomas are common. Careful attention must be paid to the duodenum and peripancreatic lymph nodes at the time of abdominal exploration. Before elective operation it is imperative that the gastric acid hypersecretion be controlled. The control of gastric hypersecretion is best performed by the administration of one of the substituted benzimidazoles, such as omeprazole or lansoprazole.

Textbook: Pages 1177–1180 ANSWER: A, B, C, D.

NOTES

NOTES

CHAPTER 12

SPLEEN AND LYMPHATIC SYSTEM

1. As the functional anatomy of the spleen is divided into red pulp, white pulp, and marginal zone, what function is incorporated into the anatomy of the cortical zone that relates to infection control?

A. Filtration of red cells, encapsulated bacteria, and other foreign material.
B. Red pulp for formation of red cells.
C. White pulp for its role in formation of granulocytes.
D. Gray areas, so formed because of the production of platelets.
E. Fibrous trabeculae.

DISCUSSION: The cortical networks described by Billroth are lined with B-, T-, and other lymphocyte subpopulations. The open zones, called by some *the cords of Billroth,* serve as an anatomic microfilter as well as a functional mechanism for removing foreign materials. For example, immature red cells with retained nuclei are "pitted" by these cords and removed from circulation. Pneumococcal and other bacteria (encapsulated and nonencapsulated) can be removed by the spleen. The filter mechanism of the spleen, combined with this immune capacity, is what is mainly lost in splenectomy that exposes the asplenic patient to overwhelming postsplenectomy sepsis syndrome (OPSS).

Textbook: Pages 1187–1188 ANSWER: A.

2. During the evolution of the understanding of hematologic diseases, the indications for splenectomy have changed. The most common indications for splenectomy are, in descending order of frequency:

A. Traumatic injury, immune thrombocytopenia, hypersplenism.
B. Immune thrombocytopenic purpura, traumatic injury, hypersplenism.
C. Hypersplenism, traumatic injury, immune thrombocytopenia.
D. Immune thrombocytopenia, hypersplenism, traumatic injury.
E. None of the above.

DISCUSSION: Over the years, the indications for splenectomy have varied as better understanding and altered therapy for immune system diseases have occurred. Whereas in the past splenectomy was the available therapy for hypersplenism, better understanding of the diseases causing hypersplenism (which is a syndrome) has allowed other therapies to emerge. Splenectomy, therefore, is less often required for the treatment of hypersplenism associated with some types of hematologic malignancies. Traumatic injury remains the most common indication for splenectomy, although this situation may change as conservative management of splenic injuries continues to increase. Moreover, immune thrombocytopenia is increasing in frequency and is definitively cured by splenectomy.

Textbook: Pages 1189–1190 ANSWER: A.

3. Useful methods for detection of splenic injury, in descending order of sensitivity, are:

A. Diagnostic peritoneal lavage.
B. CT.
C. Ultrasonography.
D. Isotope scan.
E. Magnetic resonance imaging (MRI).

DISCUSSION: Diagnosis of splenic injury is most specifically made and quantitated by CT. Diagnostic peritoneal lavage is useful for detecting intra-abdominal bleeding, but not specific to splenic injury. Isotope scans are useful to a point but do not delineate the anatomy of the spleen that is injured. Classifications of splenic injury are currently being developed based on the images provided by CT scans and are evolving into prospective decision trees for operation or conservative management.

Textbook: Pages 1190–1191 ANSWER: B.

4. The following statements about splenosis are correct:

A. Autotransplantation of splenic tissue is an etiology.
B. May protect against OPSS.
C. May over time be "born again" and regain some immune function.
D. May produce tuftsin and properdin.
E. All of the above.

DISCUSSION: Splenosis or autotransplantation of splenic tissue, which may follow splenic injury, can result in the return of some types of immune function. The "born again" spleen refers to the detection in blood samples of the opsonin tuftsin and properdin, which have been observed to occur in the occasional patient at a period of time remote from splenic injury. The supposition is that as the splenic implants grow and multiply in time, they reach a critical mass whereby opsonins may be formed and presumably the implants can provide some of the host defense mechanisms that were lost with splenectomy.

Textbook: Pages 1192–1193 ANSWER: E.

5. The following comments about immune thrombocytopenic purpura (ITP) are accurate:

A. Platelet count is low.
B. Circulating antiplatelet factor is present.
C. Antiplatelet factor is immunoglobulin G (IgG) antibody.
D. Purpura is directed against a platelet-associated antigen.
E. May be fatal.
F. All of the above.

DISCUSSION: ITP is a disease characterized by low platelet counts and a bone marrow with proliferative megakaryocytes. The disease is usually diagnosed by abnormal episodes of bleeding, which may occur from trauma, menses, etc. The causative event by which sensitized platelet-associated antibodies are developed is probably multiple. The effect of the platelet-associated antibodies, which is usually IgG, is directed against a platelet-associated antigen and, when coating of normal platelets occurs, results in the platelets being sequestered from the system by the reticuloendothelial system with resultant thrombocytopenia.

Textbook: Pages 1193–1196 ANSWER: A.

6. ITP:

A. Is most common in men in their 20s.
B. Is frequently cured in adults by corticosteroid administration.
C. Usually requires splenectomy in children.
D. Is most common in the sixth decade of life.
E. Is in remission in more than 80% of patients with splenectomy.

DISCUSSION: ITP is characterized by a low platelet count and is definitively diagnosed by low platelet count in association with bone marrow that shows thrombasthenia. Patients with this illness experience abnormal bleeding during menstruation or nosebleeds or in response to minor insults. Occasionally, a patient who bleeds excessively after an auto accident is found to have undiagnosed ITP. The usual therapy is initiated with prednisone, and some believe that the prednisone response is predictive of success after splenectomy. Approximately 80% of patients, however, require increasing doses of steroids to maintain satisfactory platelet counts and ultimately require splenectomy. Similarly, approximately 80% of patients achieve normal platelet counts within 3 months after splenectomy, whereas more than 90% are remitted from further bleeding episodes.

Textbook: Pages 1193–1196 ANSWER: E.

7. Splenectomy and perioperative therapy for ITP:

A. Follow successful steroid therapy.
B. Respond permanently to high-dose intravenous gamma globulin.
C. Are best preceded by polyvalent vaccines for *Pneumococcus, Haemophilus influenzae*, and *Neisseria meningitidis*.
D. Cannot be done laparoscopically.
E. Are associated with splenomegaly.

Textbook: Pages 1195–1196 ANSWER: C.

8. Thrombotic thrombocytopenic purpura (TTP) is a syndrome characterized by all of the following except:

A. Thrombocytopenia.
B. Microangiopathic hemolytic anemia.
C. Deposition of platelet microthrombi.
D. Fluctuating neurologic abnormalities.
E. Renal failure.
F. Afebrile.

DISCUSSION: This disease, sometimes called Moschcowitz's syndrome, is characterized by thrombocytopenia, microangiopathy, chemolytic anemia, fluctuating neurologic abnormalities, progressive renal failure, and fever. Platelet deposits, with hyaline material composed of aggregated platelets and fibrin, occur. The cause is unknown, and the prognosis is very poor: survival is less than 10%. A combined approach using antiplatelet drugs and corticosteroids can be effective and sometimes has improved results if done with splenectomy.

Textbook: Page 1196 ANSWER: F.

9. Which of the following comments does not describe hypersplenism?

A. It may occur without underlying disease identification.
B. It may be secondary to many hematologic illnesses.
C. It is associated with work hypertrophy from immune response.
D. It requires evaluation of the myeloproliferation.
E. It is associated with antibodies against platelets.

DISCUSSION: Hypersplenism was described by Chauffard in 1907 and initially was mostly associated with the syndrome in which a variety of hematologic illnesses, ranging from sickle cell disease to the leukemias, could be found to have improved circulating blood elements if the spleen were removed. Diagnosis of these illnesses has improved, and illnesses once classified as primary hypersplenism now are frequently classified as secondary, as the primary mechanism involved is known. The spleen may enlarge owing to differing pathophysiologic mechanisms, but when it achieves a certain size, it removes all of the main circulating cellular blood elements (red blood cells, white blood cells, platelets). One element may be more deficient than others.

Textbook: Pages 1196–1197 ANSWER: E.

10. Hyposplenism is a potentially lethal syndrome. Which of the following statements is incorrect?

A. It is confirmed by isotope scan.
B. It is always associated with an atrophic spleen.
C. It may be associated with overwhelming postsplenectomy sepsis syndrome (OPSS).
D. It is associated with thyrotoxicosis, corticosteroid administration, and some contrast agents.
E. It may be associated with ulcerative colitis or sickle cell anemia.

Textbook: Pages 1197–1198 ANSWER: B.

11. Hodgkin's disease is a malignant lymphoma with four histologic subtypes. Which of the following is not one of the subtypes?

A. Lymphocyte predominance.
B. Nodular sclerosis.
C. Mixed cellularity.
D. Lymphocyte depletion.
E. Leukocyte-lymphocyte dominance.

DISCUSSION: A variety of histologic conventions for the major subtypes of Hodgkin's disease have been derived over the years. They are useful in identifying the prognosis and predictions for morbity and mortality. The subtypes are further subdivided to provide more precise association with therapeutic approaches, with identification with various staging levels, etc.

Textbook: Pages 1198–1200 ANSWER: E.

12. Which of the following statements about lymphatic capillaries are true?

A. These vessels have delicate tricuspid valves every 2 to 3 mm.
B. Lymphatic capillaries are more permeable than blood capillaries.
C. Lymphatic capillaries are less permeable than blood capillaries.
D. Lymphatic capillaries contain gaps large enough to admit particles as large as lymphocytes.

DISCUSSION: The transporting lymphatic vessels have valves but lymphatic capillaries do not. The lymphatic capillaries will accept particles including bacteria, red blood cells, and lymphocytes and transport them to regional lymph nodes.

Textbook: Page 1573 ANSWER: C, D.

13. Which of the following forces do not promote the formation of interstitial fluid?

A. Increased venous pressure.
B. Constrictive pericarditis.
C. Hypernatremia.
D. Hypoproteinemia.

DISCUSSION: Interstitial fluid production is a function of the hydrostatic and colloid osmotic pressures across the capillary membrane. Forces tending to increase interstitial fluid flux across the capillary membrane include obstruction to outflow of the capillary due to structural or functional obstruction in the venous system or increase in venous pressure from any cause, reduction in osmotic pressure due to hypoproteinemia, and increase in pore size due to local mediators of inflammation.

Textbook: Page 1574 ANSWER: C.

14. The most frequent cause of primary lymphedema is:

A. A deficiency of transporting lymphatic channels.
B. Valvular incompetence in lymphatic channels.
C. Obstruction or removal of regional lymph nodes.
D. Thrombosis of lymphatic channels.

DISCUSSION: Primary lymphedema is most frequently due to hypoplasia or aplasia of extremity transporting lymphatic channels.

Textbook: Page 1575 ANSWER: A.

15. Most patients with lymphedema can be managed by:

A. Pedicle transfer of lymphatic bearing tissue into the affected area.
B. Elevation, elastic support garments, and massage therapy or mechanical pneumatic compression.
C. Lymphatic bypass using an autogenous vein graft.
D. Excision of hypertrophic scarred fibrotic skin and subcutaneous tissue down to muscle fascia and coverage with split-thickness skin grafts.

DISCUSSION: The vast majority of patients with mild to moderate lymphedema can be managed with leg elevation and elastic support garments, and some will require mechanical pneumatic compression or massage therapy. Only patients with very severe deforming elephantiasis require operative therapy.

Textbook: Pages 1576–1577 ANSWER: B.

16. Which statements about lymphangiomas are true?

A. Most lesions appear during puberty.
B. These lesions frequently respond to small doses of radiation therapy.
C. The lesions usually grow slowly but may infiltrate local tissues.
D. Malignant transformation is frequent.

DISCUSSION: Lymphangiomas are congenital malformations of the lymphatic vessels. Most appear at birth or during early infancy. The lesions grow slowly and infiltrate local tissues, but actual malignant degeneration is exceedingly rare. The lesions are not responsive to radiation therapy.

Textbook: Page 1577 ANSWER: C.

NOTES

NOTES

NOTES

CHAPTER 13

HERNIAS

1. The most common hernia in females is:

A. Femoral hernia.
B. Direct inguinal hernia.
C. Indirect inguinal hernia.
D. Obturator hernia.
E. Umbilical hernia.

DISCUSSION: Indirect inguinal hernias are the most common hernia in both females and males. Femoral hernias are more common in females than in males.

Textbook: Page 1219 ANSWER: C.

2. Which of the following statements regarding unusual hernias is incorrect?

A. An obturator hernia may produce nerve compression diagnosed by a positive Howship-Romberg sign.
B. Grynfeltt's hernia appears through the superior lumbar triangle, whereas Petit's hernia occurs through the inferior lumbar triangle.
C. Sciatic hernias usually present with a painful groin mass below the inguinal ligament.
D. Littre's hernia is defined by a Meckel's diverticulum presenting as the sole component of the hernia sac.
E. Richter's hernia involves the antimesenteric surface of the intestine within the hernia sac and may present with partial intestinal obstruction.

DISCUSSION: Sciatic hernias usually present with intestinal obstruction or a mass in the gluteal or infragluteal region.

Textbook: Pages 1230–1231 ANSWER: C.

3. Staples may safely be placed during laparoscopic hernia repair in each of the following structures except:

A. Cooper's ligament.
B. Tissues superior to the lateral iliopubic tract.
C. The transversus abdominis aponeurotic arch.
D. Tissues inferior to the lateral iliopubic tract.
E. The iliopubic tract at its insertion onto Cooper's ligament.

DISCUSSION: Placement of staples inferior to (below) the lateral iliopubic tract may result in injury to the lateral femoral cutaneous nerve or the genitofemoral nerve. Staples should also not be placed within the *triangle of doom,* owing to the risk of major vascular injury.

Textbook: Pages 1224–1225 ANSWER: D.

4. The following Nyhus classification of hernias is correct except for:

A. Recurrent direct inguinal hernia—Type IVa.
B. Indirect inguinal hernia with a normal internal inguinal ring—Type I.
C. Femoral hernia—Type IIIc.
D. Direct inguinal hernia—Type IIIa.
E. Indirect inguinal hernia with destruction of the transversalis fascia of Hesselbach's triangle—Type II.

DISCUSSION: An indirect inguinal hernia with destruction of the transversalis fascia of Hesselbach's triangle is classified as a Type IIIb hernia. Also classified as Type IIIb hernias are sliding, pantaloon, and massive scrotal hernias. Type II hernia is an indirect inguinal hernia with a dilated internal ring but without displacement of the inferior deep epigastric vessels or destruction of the transversalis fascia of Hesselbach's triangle.

Textbook: Page 1219 ANSWER: E.

5. Which of the following statements about the causes of inguinal hernia is correct?

A. Excessive hydroxyproline has been demonstrated in the aponeuroses of hernia patients.
B. Obliteration of the processus vaginalis is a contributing factor for the development of an indirect inguinal hernia.
C. Physical activity and athletics have been shown to have a protective effect toward the development of inguinal hernias.
D. Elevated levels of circulating serum elastalytic activity have been demonstrated in patients with direct herniation who smoke.
E. The majority of inguinal hernias are acquired.

DISCUSSION: A correlation between cigarette smoking and an inguinal hernia formation has been demonstrated. Elevated circulating serum elastalytic activity and free active unbound neutrophil elastase has been detected in smokers.

Textbook: Page 1219 ANSWER: D.

6. The following statements about the repair of inguinal hernias are true except:

A. The conjoined tendon is sutured to Cooper's ligament in the Bassini hernia repair.
B. The McVay repair is a suitable option for the repair of femoral hernias.
C. The Shouldice repair involves a multilayer, imbricated repair of the floor of the inguinal canal.
D. The Lichtenstein repair is accomplished by prosthetic mesh repair of the inguinal canal floor in a tension-free manner.
E. The laparoscopic transabdominal preperitoneal (TAPP) and totally extraperitoneal approach (TEPA) repairs are based on the preperitoneal repairs of Cheattle, Henry, Nyhus, and Stoppa.

DISCUSSION: The Bassini repair is accomplished by high ligation of the hernia sac followed by suturing the conjoined tendon and the internal oblique muscle to the inguinal ligament.

Textbook: Pages 1219–1224 ANSWER: A.

NOTES

NOTES

CHAPTER 14

PEDIATRIC SURGERY

1. Polyhydramnios is frequently observed in all of the following conditions except:

A. Esophageal atresia.
B. Duodenal atresia.
C. Pyloric atresia.
D. Hirschsprung's disease.
E. Congenital diaphragmatic hernia.

DISCUSSION: Polyhydramnios is defined as excessive amounts of fluid (>2000 ml.) in the amniotic sac during pregnancy. The amniotic pool is a dynamic pool with a relatively rapid turnover. In the fourth intrauterine month the fetus begins to swallow amniotic fluid (25% to 40% of the volume) and absorbs the fluid from the upper gastrointestinal tract. The fluid is urinated back out into the amniotic pool by the fetal kidneys and a functioning bladder. Although there are maternal causes of polyhydramnios (cardiac failure, renal failure, other causes of fluid retention) and some idiopathic cases, many instances are related to the presence of fetal anomalies. These include central nervous system problems such as anencephaly, which prevents normal swallowing, and any high alimentary tract obstruction that blocks the passage of the amniotic fluid and prevents its absorption (including esophageal atresia, pyloric atresia, and duodenal atresia). In addition, infants with congenital diaphragmatic hernia have obstructions due to herniation of the stomach and bowel into the thoracic cavity. This is a poor prognostic finding in these infants. Hirschsprung's disease is a form of low intestinal obstruction, and therefore an adequate length of proximal patent intestine is available for absorption of the swallowed amniotic fluid and polyhydramnios is usually not present.

Textbook: Pages 1236–1237 ANSWER: D.

2. Which of the following statements about Hirschsprung's disease is/are true?

A. There are no ganglion cells seen in Auerbach's plexus.
B. There is an increased incidence of Down syndrome.
C. It is more common in girls.
D. It may be associated with enterocolitis.
E. It may involve the small intestine.

DISCUSSION: The affected segment of bowel in patients with Hirschsprung's disease has hypertrophic nerves in Auerbach's intermyenteric plexus, but no ganglion cells are present. Ganglion cells are also absent in Meissner's submucosal plexus. Some 3% to 5% of babies with Hirschsprung's disease also have Down syndrome. Hirschsprung's disease should be suspected in infants with Down syndrome that manifest evidence of abdominal distension and constipation. Hirschsprung's disease is much more common in boys (4:1). The enterocolitis of Hirschsprung's disease is a condition associated with delay in diagnosis, low bowel obstruction, severe abdominal distension, explosive diarrhea, and colonic mucosal ulceration. The course may be fulminant. This complication is associated with increased morbidity and mortality. Bacterial translocation and endotoxemia may complicate the condition. Treatment includes nasogastric suction, intravenous fluids, antibiotics, and rectal tube decompression of the obstructed rectosigmoid segment. In approximately 10% of cases aganglionosis extends into varying lengths of small bowel. In rare instances, the entire small bowel and colon may be aganglionic.

Textbook: Pages 1243–1244 ANSWER: A, B, D, E.

3. Which of the following statements is/are true of infants with gastroschisis?

A. It is associated with malrotation.
B. There is a high incidence of associated anomalies.
C. There is prolonged adynamic ileus following repair.
D. It is complicated by intestinal atresia in 10% to 12% of cases.
E. It is associated with chromosomal syndromes.

DISCUSSION: Because of intrauterine herniation of bowel to an extra-abdominal location, normal intestinal rotation and fixation do not occur. Most infants with gastroschisis have nonrotation. In contrast to infants with omphalocele, in which a high incidence of associated anomalies coexist, babies with gastroschisis have little else wrong. Following repair of the abdominal wall defect, infants with gastroschisis have a long delay in return of intestinal function. They usually require total parenteral nutrition to supply adequate caloric intake until gut function returns (3 to 4 weeks). Intestinal atresia is observed in 10% to 12% of neonates with gastroschisis. This is caused by bowel ischemia due to intrauterine volvulus or compression of the herniated viscera in a small, tight defect in the abdominal wall. Although infants with omphalocele frequently have chromosomal syndromes such as Beckwith syndrome or trisomy 13 to 15 or 16 to 18, babies with gastroschisis do not.

Textbook: Pages 1248–1249 ANSWER: A, C, D.

4. In neonates with congenital diaphragmatic hernia, which of the following statements is true?

A. The defect is more common on the right side.
B. Survival is significantly improved by administration of pulmonary vasodilators.
C. An oxygen index of 20 is an indication for extracorporeal membrane oxygenation (ECMO).
D. Oligohydramnios is a frequent occurrence.
E. Mortality is the result of pulmonary hypoplasia.

DISCUSSION: In infants with congenital diaphragmatic hernia the defect is more common on the left side (85%). Polyhydramnios is sometimes noticed and is a poor prognostic indicator of survival. Oligohydramnios is noted in fetuses with urinary tract obstruction and may be associated with pulmonary hypoplasia with an intact diaphragm. Although pulmonary vasodilators were used extensively in babies with congenital diaphragmatic hernia, they have not significantly improved survival. An oxygen index of greater than 40 is the usual indication for ECMO. Pulmonary hypoplasia is the main cause of mortality in babies with congenital diaphragmatic hernia.

Textbook: Pages 1249–1251 ANSWER: E.

5. Which of the following statements are true regarding the premature neonate?

A. A 15% to 20% right-to-left shunt occurs across the foramen ovale and patent ductus arteriosus.
B. Surfactant levels are normal after 30 weeks' gestation.
C. Fluid requirements are higher than in a full-term baby.
D. Rectal temperature is the best indicator of core body temperature.
E. They are more at risk for infection than the full-term infant.

DISCUSSION: The newborn infant has a relatively elevated pulmonary artery pressure and shunts a significant amount of unoxygenated blood through the foramen ovale and patent ductus arteriosus. The normal PaO_2 below the ductus, as measured through an umbilical artery catheter, would be between 60 and 80 mm. Hg. Surfactant levels do not approach normal until after the 34th week of gestation, when enzyme levels in the surfactant pathway mature. Amniocentesis is performed to measure the lethicin-to-sphingomyelin ratio (L:S ratio) and determine whether maturation has occurred. Fluid requirements in the premature infant are between 140 and 150 ml. per kg. per day in comparison with those of the normal neonate in whom 80 ml. per kg. per day would be adequate. Increased insensible losses and the need for overhead warmers play a role in this increase. Axillary or skin probe temperature monitoring is more accurate than the rectal temperature in the neonate. The rectal temperature is not a good indicator of core body temperature until approximately 18 months of age. Premature infants lack immunoglobulin A (IgA) and have low levels of IgM, the C3b component of complement, and decreased opsonins. In addition, the leukocytes have reduced phagocytic ability, creating an increased risk of infection. *Escherichia coli* and beta-hemolytic streptococcus are the two most common infectious agents affecting the neonate.

Textbook: Pages 1234–1236 ANSWER: A, C, E.

6. In neonates with necrotizing enterocolitis, which of the following findings is an indication of significant bowel ischemia?

A. Increased gastric residuals.
B. Septic shock.
C. Cardiac failure due to a patent ductus arteriosus.
D. Elevated platelet count.
E. Erythema of the abdominal wall.

DISCUSSION: Necrotizing enterocolitis (NEC) is a condition that occurs in 2% of babies admitted to neonatal intensive care facilities. Increased gastric residuals can occur for a number of reasons and are seen as an early indicator of NEC, but they may not reflect the presence of ischemic bowel. Septic shock may be due to a wide variety of causes besides NEC. Cardiac failure due to patent ductus arteriosus may predispose to NEC but is not necessarily an indicator of ischemic bowel. Most babies with NEC have a progressive decrease in their platelet count in association with bowel ischemia. Erythema of the abdominal wall is an indication for surgical exploration and is consistent with NEC with perforation and inflammation of the peritoneum and abdominal wall.

Textbook: Pages 1246–1247 ANSWER: E.

7. The treatment of choice for neonates with uncomplicated meconium ileus is:

A. Observation.
B. Emergency laparotomy, bowel resection, and Bishop-Koop enterostomy.
C. Intravenous hydration and a gastrograffin enema.
D. Emergency laparotomy, bowel resection, and anastomosis.
E. Sweat chloride test and pancreatic enzyme therapy.

DISCUSSION: Meconium ileus is a form of intestinal obstruction that occurs in 10% to 15% of neonates with cystic fibrosis. The obstruction is related to intraluminal concretions of abnormal meconium. The treatment of choice is adequate hydration and evacuation with a hypertonic gastrograffin enema. The hyperosmolar contrast material causes an outpouring of fluids into the bowel lumen, which flushes out the obstructing meconium and negates the need for laparotomy. Observation alone is not a useful method of treatment. When gastrograffin evacuation fails, laparotomy, placement of a pursestring suture in the bowel wall, and intraluminal irrigation with saline and gastrograffin (administered through a catheter inserted through a small enterotomy within the pursestring) will often clear the obstructing meconium. This obviates the need for resection or enterostomy in most cases. Postoperatively, a sweat chloride test should be obtained to confirm the diagnosis of cystic fibrosis. Pancreatic enzyme should be given when diet is initiated.

Textbook: Pages 1242–1243 ANSWER: C.

8. The pentalogy of Cantrell includes all of the following except:

A. Epigastric omphalocele.
B. Sternal cleft.
C. Intracardiac defect.
D. Pericardial cyst.
E. Ectopia cordis.

DISCUSSION: The pentalogy of Cantrell includes an epigastric-located omphalocele, ectopia cordis, anterior pleuropericardial defect in the diaphragm, sternal cleft, intracardiac defect (most commonly a ventricular septal defect), and in approximately one third of the cases a diverticulum of the left ventricle. Pericardial cysts are not part of the pentalogy.

Textbook: Page 1248 ANSWER: D.

9. In infants with duodenal atresia all the following statements are true except:

A. There is an increased incidence of Down syndrome.
B. Duodenal atresia can be detected by prenatal ultrasound examination.
C. It may occur in infants with situs inversus, malrotation, annular pancreas, and anterior portal vein.
D. It is best treated by gastroenterostomy.
E. There is a high incidence of associated cardiac defects.

DISCUSSION: The diagnosis of duodenal atresia can be made prior to the infant's birth with a prenatal ultrasound examination. Infants with duodenal atresia are often premature and have a high incidence of associated anomalies, especially congenital heart disease. Duodenal atresia may also coexist in patients with annular pancreas, situs inversus, malrotation, and anterior portal vein. Approximately one third of the cases occur in babies with Down syndrome. The operative treatment of choice is a duodenoduodenostomy. Duodenojejunostomy is an alternative procedure. Gastrojejunostomy is not recommended.

Textbook: Pages 1239–1240 ANSWER: D.

10. The initial treatment of choice for a 2.5-kg. infant with a 20.0-cm. long proximal jejunal atresia and 8.0 cm. of distal ileum is:

A. Laparotomy, nasogastric suction, proximal dilatation to lengthen the atretic jejunum, total parenteral nutrition, and delayed anastomosis.
B. Laparotomy and proximal end-jejunostomy.
C. Laparotomy and immediate small bowel transplantation.
D. Laparotomy and double-barrel enterostomy (jejunum and ileum), with refeeding of jejunal contents into distal ileum and delayed anastomosis.
E. Laparotomy, tapering jejunoplasty, and end-to-oblique jejunoileal anastomosis.

DISCUSSION: The patient has short bowel syndrome with most of the bowel length involving the dilated proximal jejunal atresia. The treatment of choice is to perform a tapering jejunoplasty to preserve bowel length and construct an anastomosis. Early feedings are initiated when bowel function returns in order to stimulate bowel adaptation. Jejunal dilatation will not significantly lengthen the atretic jejunum and will not alter its abnormal motility. End-jejunostomy decompresses the obstruction but produces a high ostomy with excessive loss of succus entericus. A double-barrel enterostomy might allow refeeding of jejunal content into the distal ileum and colon, but the proximal atretic loop may have poor function. Small bowel transplantation is not a feasible alternative in the neonate at the present time.

Textbook: Pages 1240–1241 ANSWER: E.

11. A 2.8-kg. neonate with excessive salivation develops respiratory distress. Attempts to pass an orogastric catheter fail because the catheter coils in the back of the throat. A chest film is obtained and shows right upper lobe atelectasis and a gasless abdomen. The most likely diagnosis is:

A. Proximal esophageal atresia without a fistula.
B. Proximal esophageal atresia with a distal tracheoesophageal (TE) fistula.
C. "H-type" TE fistula.
D. Esophageal atresia with both proximal and distal TE fistula.
E. Congenital esophageal stricture.

DISCUSSION: Proximal esophageal atresia will result in excess salivation and aspiration of saliva. It is often associated with right upper lobe collapse. Infants with a distal TE fistula will have air in the stomach and intestine, as will babies with both proximal and distal fistulas, "H-type" fistula, and an esophageal stricture. Infants with proximal atresia but without a TE fistula will not have air beneath the diaphragm. Attempts at passing an orogastric catheter will be met by an obstruction and coiling of the catheter in the infant's mouth. The catheter will pass into the stomach in infants with "H-type" TE fistula and in most with esophageal stricture.

Textbook: Pages 1237–1239 ANSWER: A.

12. Neonates with NEC may demonstrate all of the following findings on abdominal films except:

A. Pneumatosis intestinalis.

B. Portal vein air.
C. Pneumoperitoneum.
D. Colovesical fistula.
E. Fixed and thickened bowel loops.

DISCUSSION: Infants with NEC do not develop a colovesical fistula as an initial x-ray finding. Pneumatosis, portal vein air, pneumoperitoneum, and fixed intestinal loops with thickened bowel wall are all observed with some regularity in babies with NEC.

Textbook: Pages 1246–1247 ANSWER: D.

13. The most common type of congenital diaphragmatic hernia is caused by:

A. A defect in the central tendon.
B. Eventration of the diaphragm in the fetus.
C. A defect through the space of Larrey.
D. An abnormally wide esophageal hiatus.
E. A defect through the pleuroperitoneal fold.

DISCUSSION: Eventration of the diaphragm is related to phrenic nerve paralysis. It is more commonly observed after a breech delivery and may be associated with torticollis and Erb's palsy. The space of Larrey is located anteriorly just off the midline. A Morgagni hernia passes through this potential space. An abnormally wide esophageal hiatus would most likely create a sliding hiatal hernia. The most common type of congenital diaphragmatic hernia in the neonate is the posterolateral Bochdalek hernia, which passes through a defect in the developing pleuroperitoneal fold.

Textbook: Pages 1249–1251 ANSWER: E.

14. The calorie-nitrogen ratio for an infant should be maintained at:

A. 75:1.
B. 100:1.
C. 50:1.
D. 150:1.
E. 25:1.

DISCUSSION: The calorie-nitrogen ratio should be maintained at 150:1 for most infants. Fever, major illness, sepsis, or trauma may increase the caloric requirements significantly.

Textbook: Page 1236 ANSWER: D.

15. All of the following conditions are derived from the primitive embryonic foregut except:

A. Bronchogenic cyst.
B. Cystic adenomatoid malformation.
C. Gastric duplication.
D. Mesenteric cyst.
E. Pulmonary sequestration.

DISCUSSION: Mesenteric cysts are derived from lymphatic anlage in the abdomen and are unassociated with foregut development. The lung buds arise from the primitive foregut and anomalies associated with tracheopulmonary development are therefore all derived from foregut. These include tracheoesophageal fistula, congenital lobar emphysema, enteric cysts (which may communicate to the normal esophagus, lung, or spinal canal; e.g., neurenteric cyst), cystic adenomatoid malformations, solitary lung cysts, intra- and extralobar sequestrations, and bronchogenic cysts. The stomach and first part of the duodenum are also of foregut origin, and thus a gastric duplication is by definition derived from foregut.

Textbook: Pages 1255–1256 ANSWER: D.

NOTES

NOTES

CHAPTER 15

OTOLARYNGOLOGY

1. Which of the following statements about foreign bodies of the ear canal is/are correct?

A. In general, grasping smooth foreign bodies with forceps is more effective than raking them out with a blunt hook.
B. Insects are more easily removed after they have been asphyxiated.
C. Metal and glass beads can be removed with irrigation.
D. A general anesthetic is good management in any difficult-to-remove foreign body.
E. Complications of removal of foreign bodies of the ear canal include perforation of the tympanic membrane and dislocation of the ossicles.

DISCUSSION: Foreign bodies of the ear canal that are smooth are likely to be forced deeper into the ear canal as forceps are closed, while a blunt hook can be effectively passed deep to the foreign body so that it can be raked out. Until asphyxiated with mineral oil, insects cling to the walls of the ear canal with barbed limbs. Once killed, they are easily removed with forceps. Metal and glass beads may be irrigated from the ear canal, but hygroscopic foreign bodies such as beans, kernels of corn, etc., swell with the addition of water and become more difficult to remove. Once a foreign body lies close to the tympanic membrane, its removal is likely to be painful and, in children, a general anesthetic is good management for this problem. Movement of the patient during removal of a foreign body can result in perforation of the tympanic membrane and dislocation of the ossicles.

Textbook: Pages 1277–1278 ANSWER: B, C, D, E.

2. Which of the following statements about basal skull fractures is/are correct?

A. Basal skull fractures can result in nystagmus, hearing loss, and facial paralysis.
B. Sensorineural hearing loss is the only type of hearing loss likely to be caused by a basal skull fracture.
C. Hemotympanum or bleeding from the ear canal secondary to a blow to the head remote from the ear is pathognomonic of a basal skull fracture.
D. Meningitis is a complication of a basal skull fracture.

DISCUSSION: Basal skull fractures may traverse the inner ear and the fallopian canal resulting in hearing loss, vestibular disturbances, and facial paralysis. Hearing loss may result from injury to the inner ear, which would produce sensorineural hearing loss, or from blood in the middle ear or dislocation of an ossicle, which would result in conductive hearing loss. In a transverse fracture of the temporal bone hemotympanum occurs and, with a longitudinal fracture bleeding comes through the perforated tympanic membrane or the fracture in the ear canal. Both are pathognomonic of a basal skull fracture if the blow to the head is remote from the ear. With fractures of the temporal bone, there is a communication between the middle ear and the subarachnoid space. Bacteria that reach the middle ear through the perforated tympanic membrane or the eustachian tube may initiate meningitis through the communication with the subarachnoid space.

Textbook: Page 1278 ANSWER: A, C, D.

3. Which of the following statements about middle ear effusions is/are correct?

A. Middle ear effusions frequently result from eustachian tube obstruction.
B. Middle ear effusions cause conductive hearing loss.
C. Chronic middle ear effusions frequently respond to antibiotic therapy.
D. Chronic middle ear effusions regularly resolve with myringotomy and insertion of a tympanostomy tube.

DISCUSSION: Eustachian tube obstruction due to nasopharyngeal infection, allergy, or adenoid hypertrophy prevents ventilation of the middle ear, and fluid accumulates in the middle ear. The fluid in the middle ear damps the movement of the tympanic membrane and ossicles, resulting in conductive hearing loss. Pathogenic bacteria can be cultured from half of the chronic middle ear effusions that occur in children, and antibiotic therapy produces resolution in one third to one half of effusions. Myringotomy and insertion of a tympanostomy tube regularly reventilates the middle ear, regardless of the cause of the eustachian tube obstruction.

Textbook: Pages 1278–1281 ANSWER: A, B, C, D.

4. Which of the following statements about chronic otitis media is/are correct?

A. If chronic otitis media is complicated by

cholesteatoma, the purpose of mastoidectomy is to improve hearing.

B. The objectives of tympanoplasty are to improve sound pressure transmission to the oval window and to provide sound protection to the round window.

C. The middle ear ossicle most frequently destroyed in chronic otitis media is the stapes.

D. Complications of chronic otitis media include meningitis, brain abscess, lateral sinus thrombosis, and epidural abscess.

DISCUSSION: The purpose of mastoidectomy in chronic otitis media complicated by cholesteatoma is to make the ear safe; that is, to prevent intracranial infections such as meningitis, brain abscess, lateral sinus thrombosis, and epidural abscess. The long process of the incus is the most vulnerable part of the ossicular chain in chronic otitis media. The objectives of tympanoplasty are to restore sound pressure transmission to the oval window and to provide sound protection to the round window by repairing the tympanic membrane or creating a closed space in the middle ear that communicates with the eustachian tube.

Textbook: Pages 1279–1281 ANSWER: B, D.

5. Which of the following statements about acoustic neurinomas is/are correct?

A. Initial symptoms of acoustic neurinomas are usually hearing loss and tinnitus.

B. Among audiologic tests, auditory brain stem responses are the most effective means of differentiating neural from sensory hearing loss.

C. Until the acoustic neurinoma exceeds 1 cm. in diameter it cannot be detected with magnetic resonance imaging (MRI).

D. Patients with acoustic neurinomas are more likely to complain of unsteadiness than vertigo.

DISCUSSION: Although acoustic neurinomas arise from Schwann's cells of the vestibular division of the eighth cranial nerve, the first symptoms are likely to be related to the auditory system, namely hearing loss and tinnitus. The vestibular disturbance is more likely to be described as unsteadiness rather than a spinning sensation. Absence of some or all of the brain stem auditory waveforms and prolonged interwave and interaural latencies are the most reliable indicators of neural hearing loss. Acoustic neurinomas as small as 0.5 cm. can be detected with MRI using gadolinium enhancement.

Textbook: Page 1283 ANSWER: A, B, D.

6. Which of the following statements about sinusitis is/are correct?

A. Maxillary sinusitis can result from a dental infection.

B. Inflammatory tissue in the ostiomeatal complex may be a contributing factor to the development of maxillary, frontal and sphenoid sinusitis.

C. In children ethmoid sinusitis can cause orbital cellulitis and orbital abscess.

D. Frontal sinusitis is more likely than maxillary sinusitis to cause an intracranial complication.

DISCUSSION: Periapical abscesses of the canine, premolar, and molar teeth may cause destruction of the bone between the tooth socket and the maxillary sinus, causing chronic maxillary sinusitis. Inflammatory tissue in the ostiomeatal complex, which is in the middle meatus, can obstruct the ostia of the maxillary, anterior ethmoid, and frontal sinuses. Ethmoiditis is the most frequent cause of orbital cellulitis and abscess in children and adults. Maxillary sinusitis rarely results in intracranial infections. Intracranial infections secondary to sinusitis are most frequently associated with frontal sinusitis.

Textbook: Pages 1285–1286 ANSWER: A, C, D.

7. Which of the following statements about epistaxis is/are correct?

A. Most epistaxis occurs from vessels of the nasal septum that are visible with a nasal speculum.

B. Bleeding from branches of the internal maxillary artery far posterior in the inferior meatus is associated with hypertension and arteriosclerosis.

C. Bleeding from the nasal septum can be effectively controlled with cautery or packing.

D. Bleeding from the sphenopalatine artery can be controlled with packing or ligation or embolization of the internal maxillary artery.

DISCUSSION: Ninety percent of epistaxis requiring professional care arises from the anterior and inferior portion of the nasal septum. It can be controlled by mild cautery with a silver nitrate applicator or easily applied packing with petrolatum gauze strips. The more serious bleeding associated with hypertension and arteriosclerosis occurs from the sphenopalatine artery, a branch of the internal maxillary artery, in the inferior meatus. This site of bleeding requires posterior nasal packing with choanal obstruction with a Foley catheter or gauze pack and firm packing with petrolatum gauze in the posterior part of the inferior meatus, ligation of the internal maxillary artery through the posterior wall of the maxillary sinus or transfemoral embolization of the internal maxillary artery with polyvinyl alcohol particles.

Textbook: Pages 1286–1287 ANSWER: A, B, C, D.

8. Which of the following statements about abscesses resulting from pharyngitis and breakdown of lymphadenitis is/are correct?

A. Young children with retropharyngeal abscesses may demonstrate opisthotonos.

B. Fluctuance is apparent on physical examination before computed tomography shows evidence of pus formation.

C. Parapharyngeal abscesses should be drained through a transverse incision in the neck.
D. Retropharyngeal abscesses should be drained through a vertical incision in the posterior pharyngeal wall.

DISCUSSION: Retropharyngeal abscesses lie between the prevertebral fascia and the superior constrictor muscle of the pharynx and cause the child to hyperextend the neck. Pus formation is difficult to demonstrate on physical examination in these abscesses, but computed tomography or magnetic resonance imaging readily demonstrates liquefaction when it is present. Parapharyngeal abscesses lie along the carotid sheath and should be drained through the neck. Incisions through the lateral pharyngeal wall place the internal carotid artery and internal jugular vein at risk. A retropharyngeal abscess cannot satisfactorily be reached through a cervical incision but may safely be approached through an incision in the posterior pharyngeal wall.

Textbook: Page 1290 ANSWER: A, C, D.

9. Which of the following statements about aspiration of a peanut into the tracheobronchial tree is/are true?

A. The peanut is more likely to be in the left lower lobe bronchus.
B. After aspirating the peanut the patient coughs for 30 minutes; then the coughing is likely to subside for several hours.
C. On auscultation of the chest, the most likely finding is an expiratory wheeze.
D. One hour after aspiration flouroscopic evidence of the peanut is most likely to be obstructive emphysema distal to the foreign body.
E. The peanut should be removed with the patient under general anesthesia through an open bronchoscope with forceps designed to grasp peanuts.

DISCUSSION: A foreign body of the bronchus is more likely to enter the right bronchus because it is larger than the left one, its angle with the long axis of the trachea is less acute, and the carina is to the left of the midline of the tracheal lumen. At first, the peanut is likely to be moved from one site to another, producing coughing. After a while it comes to rest, and the coughing subsides until the purulent bronchitis begins. As soon as the initial coughing subsides one can hear a localized expiratory wheeze and demonstrate obstructive emphysema distal to the foreign body on inspiratory and expiratory chest radiography and flouroscopy. Both findings result from the one-way valve produced by the foreign body that allows air to enter the lung on inspiration owing to dilatation of the bronchus and limits escape of air on expiration. Tracheobronchial foreign bodies are most safely removed through an open bronchoscope under general anesthesia with forceps especially designed for the particular foreign body.

Textbook: Pages 1293–1294 ANSWER: B, C, D, E.

10. Which of the following statements about epiglottitis (supraglottic laryngitis) is/are correct?

A. In a young child with inspiratory stridor the differentiation of epiglottitis and laryngotracheobronchitis should be made with computed tomography.
B. Epiglottitis is most commonly caused by *Haemophilus influenzae* type b.
C. Once the diagnosis of epiglottitis is made in a young child, the safer course of management is nasotracheal intubation.
D. The *H. influenzae* type b vaccine against meningitis has not reduced the incidence of epiglottitis in the United States.

DISCUSSION: Supraglottic swelling in epiglottitis can be adequately demonstrated on a lateral neck radiograph. Epiglottitis is most commonly caused by *H. influenzae* type b and, fortunately, the vaccine does reduce the incidence of epiglottitis. Since the upper airway obstruction can abruptly become worse in epiglottitis in children, nasotracheal intubation for 48 hours until the supraglottic swelling subsides is the management of choice, along with antibiotic therapy for the *H. influenzae* infection.

Textbook: Pages 1294–1295 ANSWER: B, C.

11. Which of the following statements about squamous cell carcinoma of the larynx is/are correct?

A. Twelve thousand new cases of laryngeal cancer are expected each year in the United States.
B. The male-female ratio is 10:1.
C. Hoarseness lasting 2 weeks or longer should be managed with visualization of the larynx and biopsy of any discrete lesion.
D. Early cordal carcinoma can be effectively managed with radiation therapy.
E. Advanced laryngeal cancer is treated more effectively by a combination of operation and radiation therapy.

DISCUSSION: The number of new cases of laryngeal cancer in the United States continues to increase and now approximates 12,000 per year. Twenty years ago the male-female ratio was 8:1. Now it is 5:1. Hoarseness lasting 2 weeks is one of the important warning symptoms of cancer, and all discrete lesions of the larynx should be biopsied. Radiation therapy achieves 85% to 95% 5-year disease-free survival for early cordal carcinoma. Once the cartilage of the larynx is invaded the cure rate with radiation therapy declines, and operation is required to yield the highest survival rate.

Textbook: Pages 1296–1297 ANSWER: A, C, D, E.

NOTES

NOTES

NOTES

CHAPTER 16

PLASTIC AND MAXILLOFACIAL SURGERY

1. A 65-year-old male with a low-grade fibrosarcoma on the proximal tibia undergoes wide local resection followed by postoperative radiation. Resection of the lesion results in a 10-cm. by 8-cm. defect with exposed bone devoid of periosteum. The best method of closure is:

A. Split-thickness skin graft.
B. Local myocutaneous or muscle flap.
C. Free muscle flap using microvascular technique for immediate vascularization.
D. Full-thickness skin graft.

DISCUSSION: A wound of the upper third of the leg with exposed bone and no viable underlying periosteum should be covered, when possible, with a local muscle, myocutaneous, or fasciocutaneous flap. Typically, the medial or lateral gastrocnemius muscle flap is used as the first choice for coverage of proximal tibial defects. Free flaps are reserved for situations when a local flap is not available, for they involve a more extensive operative procedure. Skin grafts will not survive over bare bone.

Textbook: Pages 1306–1309 ANSWER: B.

2. A 55-year-old man has a moderate-sized basal cell carcinoma excised from the dorsum of his nose. The defect is 1.5 cm. in diameter and has a well-vascularized underlying bed and no exposed cartilage. The most appropriate management of this wound would involve:

A. Full-thickness skin graft from the antecubital fossa.
B. Full-thickness skin graft from the postauricular area.
C. Split-thickness skin graft from the supraclavicular area.
D. A forehead rotational flap.
E. Primary closure of the defect.

DISCUSSION: The most appropriate management of this defect would involve coverage with a full-thickness skin graft taken from an area of the body of similar skin color and texture. The most common site for limited nasal defects is the postauricular skin. The scar is hidden and the site can easily provide more than 2 cm. of skin. A split-thickness skin graft would not give as good a cosmetic result as a full-thickness graft. Flaps are reserved for deeper, more demanding reconstructive situations. Primary closure would likely result in a cosmetic deformity secondary to tension at the closure site and leave a depressed scar.

Textbook: Pages 1304–1306 ANSWER: B.

3. A 6-year-old child is bitten on the face by a dog. She sustains several facial lacerations with minimal skin loss over one of the lacerations. The best management of the facial wounds is:

A. Débridement, wound irrigation, antibiotics, and primary closure.
B. Débridement, wound irrigation, antibiotics, and closure by secondary intention.
C. No débridement, antibiotics, and closure by secondary intention.
D. Débridement, wound irrigation, antibiotics, and closure with a full-thickness skin graft.
E. Débridement, wound irrigation, antibiotics, and closure with a local flap.

DISCUSSION: Bites of the face are very common among children and are of special concern because of the profuse bacterial contamination in the wound. The risk of infection is 15 times higher in these wounds than in simple lacerations. These wounds require copious irrigation and aggressive débridement before closure. Most wounds can be closed primarily after débridement and irrigation if they can be safely monitored for the first week following closure. If extensive cellulitis develops or pus drains from the wound sutures should be removed and the wound opened.

Textbook: Page 1299 ANSWER: A.

4. Advantages of a full-thickness skin graft over a split-thickness skin graft include all the following except:

A. They tend to undergo less primary contraction.
B. They are especially useful in closing defects of the face.
C. Typical donor sites can be closed primarily.
D. They maintain their normal pigmentation.
E. They result in less secondary wound contraction.

DISCUSSION: Full-thickness skin grafts tend to undergo greater primary contraction owing to the elasticity of the underlying dermis. As compared with split-thickness skin grafts they result in less secondary contraction of the wound bed into which they are placed.

Textbook: Page 1304 ANSWER: A.

5. The incidence of cleft lip in neonates is:

A. 1 in 100.
B. 1 in 700.
C. 1 in 5000.
D. 1 in 7000.
E. 1 in 10,000.

DISCUSSION: Cleft lip and palate is the most common of the major craniofacial deformities. The overall incidence of clefting is approximately 1 per 700 births. Eighty-five percent of cleft lips are nonsyndromal, (i.e., they are not associated with other congenital deformities or with known genetic aberrations). Risk factors for clefting include maternal diabetes, increased paternal age, and smoking during pregnancy. A number of drugs, including dilantin, vitamin A, and corticosteroids, have also been associated with development of cleft lip and palate.

Textbook: Pages 1309–1310 ANSWER: B.

6. A 35-year-old male is involved in an altercation and sustains a blow to his right orbit from an unknown blunt object. He presents to the emergency room with ecchymosis and swelling of the right periorbital area. Appropriate evaluation and management of this injury include all of the following except:

A. Visual acuity examination.
B. Examination of extraocular movement to test for limitation of upward and downward gaze.
C. Standard facial radiographs to evaluate for fractures.
D. Computed tomography (CT) of the face and orbits with axial and coronal views.
E. Panorex.

DISCUSSION: The most common orbital fracture is the so-called blowout fracture of the orbital floor. The mechanism of injury is usually a direct blow to the orbit that rapidly increases orbital pressure. This pressure is then released through a fracture in the orbital floor. Orbital fat and inferior rectus muscle may become entrapped in this fracture, causing gaze restriction. Standard facial radiographs should be obtained for facial bone evaluation. If an orbital fracture is noted on the plain radiograph or is strongly suspected, CT is the most sensitive technique for imaging facial fractures. A panorex, a panoramic radiograph of the entire mandible, is not indicated unless mandibular or maxillary trauma is suspected.

Textbook: Pages 1315–1317 ANSWER: E.

7. A 35-year-old right hand–dominant male printing machine operator gets his left thumb caught in the press, and it is amputated just above the level of the metacarpophalangeal joint. The severed thumb was brought to the emergency room with the patient by a friend. At this point you should:

A. Place the amputated thumb in a sterile container of iced saline, irrigate the wound, close the stump, and refer the patient for reimplantation.
B. Discard the thumb and irrigate and close the wound.
C. Place the amputated thumb in a plastic bag of iced saline, place a bulky dressing on the hand, and refer the patient for reimplantation.
D. Discard the thumb, complete the amputation to the level of the metacarpophalangeal joint, and close the stump.

DISCUSSION: Amputated digits and particularly the thumb should be preserved for possible replantation whenever possible. The most effective means of preservation of the amputated digit is to place it in a plastic bag in iced saline. The stump wound should be irrigated and wrapped once any bleeding is controlled and a microsurgical specialist consulted immediately.

Textbook: Page 1299 ANSWER: C.

8. Squamous cell cancer of the head and neck is associated with all the following except:

A. Male-female incidence ratio of 2:1.
B. Increased incidence with alcohol consumption.
C. Increased risk in occupational workers in the nickel-refining, woodworking, and textile fiber industries.
D. Development of metachronous cancers in 30% to 40% of patients who continue to smoke.
E. Vague symptoms and minimal physical findings in 35% to 45% of patients with early-stage disease.

DISCUSSION: The majority of head and neck cancers are squamous cell lesions. It is generally a disease of males in the fifth or sixth decade, accounting for 8.5% of all malignancies in this age group. The male-female ratio is 4:1 but is decreasing because of an increase in tobacco use among women. Alcohol consumption potentiates tobacco-related carcinogenesis and is an independent risk factor. Occupational risk factors, including nickel refining, woodworking, and exposure to textile fibers, may predispose to cancers of the nasal cavity and paranasal sinuses. Metachronous cancers develop in 30% to 40% of patients who continue to smoke, but the risk decreases to 6% in those who quit.

Textbook: Page 1317 ANSWER: A.

9. Squamous cell cancer of the lip is:

A. The most common cancer of the oral cavity.
B. Is most commonly found on the lower lip in males with a history of smoking and prolonged sun exposure.
C. Treated by V surgical excision and primary closure if the cancer is a primary lesion.

D. Frequently associated with lymph node metastasis requiring modified neck dissection.
E. Treated with radiation therapy, particularly if the lesion involves the oral commissure.

DISCUSSION: The lip is the most common site of cancer in the oral cavity. The 5-year survival for all stages is 70% to 90%. Primary lesions are usually treated by "V" surgical excision and primary closure after repair of the orbicularis muscle. Lesions of the oral commissure can be treated with radiation therapy to reduce morbidity. Lymph node metastasis is uncommon and elective node dissection is not indicated in the majority of SCC of the lip.
Textbook: Page 1321 ANSWER: D.

10. All of the following are true concerning parotid gland tumors except:

A. 75% of all salivary gland tumors involve the parotid.
B. Parotid tumors arise deep to the plane of the facial nerve in 10% of cases.
C. Preoperative CT/MRI is indicated for parotid tumors when deep lobe involvement is suspected or when facial nerve involvement or cervical lymphadenopathy is present.
D. There is a greater than 90% correlation between fine-needle aspiration (FNA) and parotid malignancy.
E. The malignant mixed tumor is the most common parotid malignancy.

DISCUSSION: Malignant mixed tumor or carcinoma ex pleomorphic adenoma is the second most common parotid malignancy. Mucoepidermoid carcinoma is the most common malignancy of the parotid. It has three histologic grades, which correspond to increasing proportions of epidermoid components and decreased cell differentiation. The 10-year survival rate for all grades is 50%.
Textbook: Pages 1322–1324 ANSWER: E.

11. Concerning the nature of pilonidal cysts and sinuses, the evidence weighs most heavily in favor of their being:

A. Congential lesions in all but the rare case.
B. Acquired in all but the rare case.
C. A disease (jeep disease) of army personnel.
D. All of the above.

DISCUSSION: Evidence weighs heavily in favor of an acquired nature for all but the rare case of pilonidal disease. Stretching of the integument at puberty, associated with rapid growth, particularly of the gluteal muscles, produces distention of hair follicles, sebaceous glands, and apocrine glands, and sufficient spreading of their cutaneous orifices to allow insinuation of foreign matter. Thus, the tiny midline holes or pits (sinuses), which are seen in the sacrococcygeal cleft of almost all patients with pilonidal disease, represent distorted hair follicles that may ingest hair or become filled with keratin and other debris. The cavity becomes infected and ruptures into the deeper fat. That hair ingestion by some of the existing pilonidal cavities occurs secondarily offers a reasonable explanation for the fact that hair, until now considered the single source of pilonidal disease, is found in only half of the patients. Formerly thought to be common among army personnel (hence the name *jeep disease*), such a predilection has not been demonstrated with certainty in recent literature.
Textbook: Page 1330 ANSWER: B.

12. Concerning the definitive surgical treatment of chronic sacrococcygeal pilonidal disease:

A. Treatment is now widely practiced in an outpatient setting.
B. Treatment should be started by the administration of pain medication and an antibiotic regimen directed against *Staphylococcus aureus* and *Bacteroides* species.
C. Surgical evacuation of hair and debris should be accomplished through an incision that avoids the midline *ditch* containing the pits and sinuses.
D. All of the above are true.

DISCUSSION: Antibiotics are rarely indicated for the treatment of acute pilonidal abscesses unless the patient has a medical condition such as rheumatic heart disease or is immunosuppressed. However, because of the central role of bacterial infection in the perpetuation of chronic pilonidal disease, treatment of these patients is started with oral pain medication and an antibiotic regimen directed specifically against *S. aureus* and *Bacteroides* species. The chronic abscess is opened widely by a long incision that lies parallel to and 2 cm. to one side of the midline. Avoidance of the midline containing the pits and sinuses is increasingly advocated. The abscess cavity is scrubbed free of hair and debris and the visible holes excised from the midline skin with minimal tissue loss. Antibiotics are continued for 24 hours, and the patient is instructed in local care of the wound, including tub baths and Water Pik irrigation. Consensus is building that pilonidal disease should be managed conservatively. Treatment in an outpatient setting has gained acceptance and is widely practiced.
Textbook: Pages 1332–1333 ANSWER: D.

NOTES

NOTES

NOTES

CHAPTER 17

NEUROSURGERY

1. Which of the following are true about the history of neurosurgery?

A. The history of trepanation dates back to the Neolithic period.
B. The earliest known writing dealing with surgical topics is the Ebers papyrus.
C. The writings of Hippocrates contain the first recorded descriptions of trepanation.
D. The three key developments that were necessary to permit successful intracranial and intraspinal surgery were anesthesia, asepsis, and the concept of localization of different functions in different areas of the nervous system.
E. Victor Horsely of London was the first surgeon to specialize in neurosurgery.

DISCUSSION: Many skulls from the Neolithic period have been found, some of which contain cranial defects with evidence of bone healing, indicating that these individuals underwent trepanation during life and survived the operation. The earliest known writing dealing with surgical topics is the Edwin Smith papyrus. In the works of Hippocrates is the first written account of trepanation. During the second half of the nineteenth century, general anesthesia was introduced and the principles of asepsis were developed. These steps were important for all areas of surgery, including neurosurgery. In addition, it became recognized that certain areas of the nervous system were especially important for certain neurologic functions and that intracranial and intraspinal abnormalities might be localized by the history and neurologic examination findings, thus providing a more specific target for neurosurgical exploration through the small bony openings to which surgeons were restricted at the time. Victor Horsley of London was the first surgeon to prepare himself specifically for surgery of the nervous system and to concentrate his efforts in that area.

Textbook: Pages 1335–1336 ANSWER: A, C, D, E.

2. The neurosurgeon who has had the most profound influence on the development of neurosurgery is:

A. Fedor Krause of Germany.
B. William Macewen of Scotland.
C. Harvey Cushing of the United States.
D. Egas Moniz of Portugal.
E. Goeffrey Jefferson of England.

DISCUSSION: Harvey Cushing (1869–1939) laid the groundwork for much of what is done in neurosurgery. For example, he standardized operative procedures and introduced many techniques and instruments that are still in use. He also made careful and detailed studies of intracranial tumors and established their classification. By his own multifaceted career and through his many students from around the world he influenced the development of neurosurgery to a degree not equaled before or since.

Textbook: Pages 1335–1336 ANSWER: C.

3. Which of the following conditions can be evaluated by magnetic resonance imaging (MRI)?

A. Stroke is suspected in a patient with a cardiac pacemaker.
B. Computed tomography (CT) shows a skull base tumor.
C. A coma patient with CT-demonstrated subarachnoid hemorrhage and an aneurysmal clip.
D. A patient with intractable complex partial seizure.
E. A lung cancer patient whose plain film of the lumbar spine shows a compression fracture of the L2 vertebral body.

DISCUSSION: MRI has proved to be a better modality than CT for evaluation of disease of the central nervous system (CNS), such as diseases at the base of the skull (particularly the sellar and cerebellopontine angle cistern regions) and for most tumors, white matter disease (e.g., multiple sclerosis), early stroke, congenital abnormalities, vascular malformations, and spinal disease. New techniques of MRI such as fast spin echo (FSE) pulse sequence have been developed to detect mesial temporal sclerosis, which is the most common cause of intractable complex partial seizure. Differentiating pure compression fracture from metastatic disease of the vertebral bodies in a patient with known primary cancer is also possible by new MRI technique; however, for patients with certain types of metal (pacemaker, surgical clip, or foreign body, which may move in the magnetic field and cause injury to the patient or significant artifacts) within the bodies, MRI is contraindicated.

Textbook: Pages 1338–1344 ANSWER: B, D, E.

4. Which of the following statements about neuroradiologic imaging modalities is/are correct?

A. Diffusion-weighted MRI can differentiate tumor from edema and identify the nonenhancing part of the tumor.
B. For evaluating the stenosis of the carotid bifurcation, MR angiography (MRA) is the most accurate imaging modality.
C. Myelography is still useful in detecting some diffuse spinal disease such as cerebrospinal fluid (CSF) seeding.
D. For evaluating the bony detail of patients with facial trauma, CT is a better imaging modality than MRI.
E. Decreased amount of *N*-acetyl aspartate (NAA) and increased amount of lactate can be shown in the MR spectroscopy (MRS) of a patient with acute stroke.

DISCUSSION: Diffusion-weighted MR is a new development in MR applications and is sensitive to microscopic motion of water protons (Brownian motion). Initial applications have involved imaging of early stroke and neoplasia. Early evidence also suggests that diffusion-weighted imaging can differentiate tumoral edema from tumor and identify the nonenhancing part of the tumor. Doppler sonography, MRA, and CT angiography (CTA) are all useful for evaluating the stenotic condition of carotid bifurcation noninvasively. However, sonography is very operator dependent, and MRA commonly overestimates the degree of carotid stenosis resulting from the turbulence, dephasing at points of stenosis or irregularity. CTA obtained by spiral or helical CT has a good correlation rate with carotid angiography (92%). Conventional carotid angiography remains the most accurate imaging modality for evaluation of the stenosis of carotid bifurcation. Although CT and MRI have taken the place of myelography in evaluating neurologic diseases, it is still useful in detecting diffuse subarachnoid seeding, which may be difficult to identify on MRI. The bone detail and calcification are poorly identified on MR, so in a patient with facial trauma, CT is a better modality than MR. With MRS, metabolites within a selected region of interest (ROI) can be investigated, and spectral peaks that reflect the concentrations of the metabolite within the ROI can be obtained. The metabolites include lactate, neuronal marker (NAA), phosphorus metabolites, creatine, and choline. Reduction in the NAA level and elevation in lactate level could be noted in acute stroke.

Textbook: Pages 1337–1343 ANSWER: A, C, D, E.

5. Which of the following are true about intracranial tumors?

A. The most common location of brain tumors of childhood is the posterior cranial fossa.
B. With few exceptions, examination of the CSF is of no value in the diagnosis of an intracranial tumor.
C. Even the most malignant of primary brain tumors seldom spread outside the confines of the central nervous system (CNS).
D. The majority of astrocytomas can be cured surgically.
E. Primary neoplasms of astrocytic, oligodendroglial, or ependymal origin represent gradations of a spectrum from slowly growing to rapidly growing neoplasms.

DISCUSSION: In children, brain tumors are more commonly situated below the tentorium than above it. In adults, the reverse is true. Cytologic examination of CSF may provide critical diagnostic information in a patient with meningeal carcinomatosis or subarachnoid spread of a primary brain tumor such as a medulloblastoma, but in most instances CSF examination is not of significant value. Furthermore, in a patient with a brain tumor lumbar puncture may be dangerous; it may promote brain herniation. If there has not been a surgical breach of the dura mater, primary brain tumors seldom spread to areas outside the intracranial and intraspinal compartments. Most gliomas, including astrocytomas, cannot be cured by surgical resection. The pilocytic astrocytoma of the cerebellum and the optic nerve glioma are exceptions to that rule. Neoplasms of astrocytic, oligodendroglial, or ependymal origin vary histologically along a spectrum from benign to malignant, with no sharp dividing line. Furthermore, even the most benign-looking ones tend to recur after surgical resection.

Textbook: Pages 1344–1348 ANSWER: A, B, C, E.

6. The intracranial tumor most likely to be encountered in a middle-aged man with the acquired immunodeficiency syndrome (AIDS) is:

A. Glioblastoma multiforme.
B. Ependymoma.
C. Meningioma.
D. Oligodendroglioma.
E. Lymphoma.

DISCUSSION: Primary intracranial lymphomas occur with increased frequency in patients who are immunocompromised, such as recipients of organ transplants and patients with AIDS.

Textbook: Page 1348 ANSWER: E.

7. Patients who have survived a subarachnoid hemorrhage from a ruptured intracranial aneurysm are at risk for:

A. Rehemorrhage.
B. Cerebral artery vasospasm.
C. Ischemic stroke.
D. Hydrocephalus.

DISCUSSION: Twenty percent of patients who suffer a subarachnoid hemorrhage from a ruptured intracranial aneurysm experience a second hemorrhage in the ensuing 2 weeks. Following subarachnoid hemorrhage, the patient is at risk for developing vasospasm, an idiopathic narrowing of the intracranial arteries that reside in the subarachnoid space. Vasospasm manifests clinically as cerebral ischemia or stroke. Blood within the subarachnoid space hinders normal flow and absorption of spinal fluid, frequently resulting in mild hydrocephalus. Although this hydrocephalus usually resolves in the days or weeks following the hemorrhage, in some cases it persists, necessitating a ventricular shunt.

Textbook. Pages 1349–1350 ANSWER: A, B, C, D.

8. Intracranial hemorrhages resulting from chronic arterial hypertension:

A. Most often originate in the basal ganglia.
B. Most often originate in the subarachnoid space.
C. Can present as an enlarging cerebellar mass.
D. Should not be treated surgically when they occur in the cerebellum.

DISCUSSION: The most frequent site of a hypertensive hemorrhage is the basal ganglia. Blood may appear in the spinal fluid after the hemorrhage has dissected through the brain parenchyma into the cerebral ventricles. Approximately 10% of hypertensive hemorrhages originate in the cerebellum. Rapid removal of a cerebellar hemorrhage can be life saving.

Textbook: Page 1352 ANSWER: A, C.

9. The physician is most effective in treating:

A. Cerebral contusions.
B. Epidural hematomas.
C. Cerebral lacerations.
D. Hypoxia.

DISCUSSION: The physician can do very little to repair damage incurred at the time of the head trauma such as cerebral contusions and lacerations. The physician's job is to thwart secondary injuries to the brain. Enlarging intracranial mass lesions, especially hematomas, are a common cause of secondary brain injury. Evacuation of an epidural, subdural, or intracranial hematoma can be life saving. Metabolic insults are another cause of secondary neurologic injury. Hypoxia, hypotension, and hypocapnia are avoidable secondary insults that should be treated at the scene of the accident. Unfortunately, a large percentage of trauma patients still arrive at the emergency room with metabolic abnormalities.

Textbook: Pages 1355–1357 ANSWER: B, D.

10. The evaluation of a comatose patient with a head injury begins with:

A. The cardiovascular system.
B. Pupillary reflexes.
C. Establishment of an airway.
D. Computed tomography (CT) of the brain.

DISCUSSION: The treatment of every comatose patient begins with an assessment of the patient's respiratory system, followed shortly thereafter with an assessment of the patient's cardiovascular system. The unconscious patient's normal protective pharyngeal reflexes are compromised, making mechanical airway obstruction and aspiration pneumonia common events. Hypotension, secondary to intra- or extracorporal hemorrhage, is deleterious to the patient's cerebral injury. Neurologic assessment is undertaken only after the patient's respiratory and cardiovascular status are secured.

Textbook: Page 1356 ANSWER: C.

11. An epidural hematoma:

A. Is usually arterial in origin.
B. Is usually accompanied by a skull fracture.
C. Should be suspected only in comatose patients.
D. Can be diagnosed from a brain CT scan.

DISCUSSION: An epidural hematoma is a blood clot situated between the skull and the dura. Epidural hematomas are usually arterial in origin and most often are secondary to hemorrhage from the middle meningeal artery. Approximately 90% of adult patients with an epidural hematoma have a concomitant skull fracture. Such skull fractures are much less common in children under the age of 2 years. The epidural hematoma is best diagnosed before transtentorial herniation and the development of third cranial nerve palsy ("blown pupil"). The outcome of therapy is directly related to the patient's level of consciousness before surgery. The clinical diagnosis of an epidural hematoma is rarely confirmed by brain CT.

Textbook: Page 1359 ANSWER: A, B.

12. Which of the following statements is/are true?

A. Cranial osteomyelitis most frequently arises from the spread of bacteria through the bloodstream from an infection elsewhere in the body.
B. Subdural empyema is ordinarily treated by administration of antibiotics without the need for surgical drainage.
C. Bacterial meningitis may lead to the development of hydrocephalus.
D. A bacterial brain abscess commonly presents as a mass lesion of the brain, without systemic signs of infection such as fever or leukocytosis.
E. Bacterial brain abscesses are difficult to visualize by CT.

DISCUSSION: Cranial osteomyelitis can arise from hematogenous spread, but more often it results from direct spread from an infected paranasal sinus, inoculation by a penetrating object, or operative infection of a craniotomy bone flap. Subdural empyema ordinarily cannot be brought under control with antibiotics alone, and it does require surgical drainage. One of the sequelae that can follow bacterial meningitis is hydrocephalus, which is usually due to the obliteration of subarachnoid spaces and interference with CSF reabsorption. A brain abscess, per se, is not ordinarily accompanied by systemic signs of infection; these can be present if the patient also has meningitis or an active infection elsewhere. CT, especially after intravenous administration of a contrast agent, is an excellent way to demonstrate a brain abscess.

Textbook: Pages 1358–1359 ANSWER: C, D.

13. Complete excision of a brain abscess used to be the preferred method of treatment, and it is still performed occasionally today. Most commonly, now, a brain abscess is treated by:

A. Systemic antibiotic administration.
B. Aspiration and drainage of the abscess through a small opening in the skull.
C. Injection of antibiotics into the abscess.
D. Aspiration and drainage of the abscess plus systemic antibiotic administration.
E. Marsupialization of the abscess.

DISCUSSION: In the past, the preferred treatment of a brain abscess was total surgical excision. Now that such abscesses can be followed closely by CT, aspiration and drainage is usually employed, at least initially, to reduce the mass effect, provide information about the pathogens, and lower the risk of intraventricular rupture while the abscess is treated by systemic administration of antibiotics.

Textbook: Page 1362 ANSWER: D.

14. Which of the following statements are true?

A. Extradural neoplasms are usually benign.
B. A typical type of intramedullary tumor is a meningioma.
C. An intradural extramedullary neoplasm is ordinarily treated by a combination of surgical resection and radiotherapy.
D. Extradural neoplasms are usually malignant.
E. A hemangioblastoma is a benign intramedullary tumor that has the potential for surgical cure.

DISCUSSION: Extradural neoplasms are usually malignant, the most common type being a metastasis to a vertebra from a primary carcinoma elsewhere in the body. A meningioma is an extramedullary tumor arising from the meninges surrounding the spinal cord rather from within the cord itself. Most intradural extramedullary neoplasms are benign tumors (meningiomas, neurofibromas, schwannomas) that are treated by surgical excision without postoperative radiotherapy. Despite its name, the hemangioblastoma is a benign tumor. It typically arises within the spinal cord and can be cured if it is completely removed surgically.

Textbook: Pages 1363–1364 ANSWER: D, E.

15. Which of the following statements about intraspinal dermoid and epidermoid tumors and lipomas are true?

A. They are benign lesions.
B. They can be found within the spinal subarachnoid space.
C. They can be found within the spinal cord.
D. They are most common in the lumbosacral area.
E. They are at times associated with spinal dysraphism.

DISCUSSION: Intraspinal dermoid and epidermoid tumors and lipomas are benign lesions that can be found within the subarachnoid space or the spinal cord, or both. They are most common in the lumbosacral area. Dermoid and epidermoid tumors can be associated with spinal dysraphism and in particular with a dermal sinus tract that opens onto the back, usually in the lumbosacral region. Lipomas are also associated with spinal dysraphism, at times in the form of a lipomyelomeningocele with a tethered spinal cord.

Textbook: Page 1365 ANSWER: A, B, C, D, E.

16. Which of the following statements are true?

A. The usual symptomatic lumbar disc herniation occurs in a posterolateral direction.
B. Approximately 95% of lumbar disc herniations occur at the L5–S1 or L4–L5 level.
C. *Sciatica* is a term used to denote pain felt along the distribution of the sciatic nerve.
D. Weakness of dorsiflexion of the foot is a mechanical sign of a lumbar disc herniation.
E. X-ray films of the lumbosacral spine are obtained to demonstrate the presence and location of a lumbar disc herniation.

DISCUSSION: Most symptomatic lumbar disc herniations do occur in a posterolateral direction, impinging on the overlying nerve root. About 95% of lumbar disc herniations occur at the L5–S1 or L4–L5 level. Approximately 4% occur at the L3–L4 level, and less than 1% at the L2–L3 or L1–L2 level. *Sciatica* is a term used to refer to pain along the course of the sciatic nerve. A ruptured lumbar disc typically causes low back pain and ipsilateral sciatica. The mechanical signs of a lumbar disc herniation include paravertebral muscle spasm, lumbar scoliosis, tenderness over one or more of the lower lumbar spines, limitation of low back motion, limitation of straight leg raising, and a positive popliteal compression test. Weakness of dorsiflexion of the foot is a neurologic sign, not a mechanical sign. Plain x-ray films of the spine do not demonstrate the presence and location of a lumbar disc herniation except in the rare instance of a calcified disc herniation. Myelography, CT, or MRI is needed to visualize the herniated disc.

Textbook: Pages 1366–1368 ANSWER: A, B, C.

17. A right-sided disc herniation at the L5–S1 level typically may cause:

A. Low back pain and right sciatica.
B. Weakness of dorsiflexion of the right foot.
C. A diminished or absent right ankle jerk.
D. Diminution of sensation over the medial aspect of the right foot, including the great toe.
E. Weakness of dorsiflexion of the left foot.

DISCUSSION: A lumbar disc herniation at the L5–S1 or L4–L5 level typically causes low back pain and ipsilateral sciatica. If a ruptured L5–S1 disc causes weakness, it ordinarily involves plantar flexion of the ipsilateral foot. Although a diminished or absent ankle jerk can be caused by either an L5–S1 or an L4–L5 disc herniation, it is more common with the former. The L5–S1 disc herniation ordinarily affects the S1 nerve root, which supplies the lateral aspect of the foot, including the small toe.

Textbook: Page 1368 ANSWER: A, C.

18. Which of the following statements are true?

A. A symptomatic cervical disc herniation usually occurs in an anterolateral or anterior direction and can be removed by a surgical approach through the front of the neck.
B. Cervical spondylosis represents a combination of degenerative disc disease and osteoarthritis in the cervical spine.
C. The joints of Luschka are the main spinal facet joints.
D. The term *cervical myelopathy* refers to pain and/or neurologic dysfunction in the distribution of one or more cervical nerve roots.
E. Full neck extension frequently accentuates the neck and arm pain of a patient with a cervical disc herniation.

DISCUSSION: A symptomatic cervical disc herniation usually occurs in a posterolateral direction, although a directly posterior (central) herniation may occasionally occur. The posterolateral herniated disc can be removed by either a posterior or an anterior approach, but the anterior approach is preferred for the central herniation because the surgeon can remove the ruptured disc without manipulating (and possibly injuring) an already compromised spinal cord. Cervical spondylosis represents a combination in the cervical spine of degenerative disc disease and osteophyte formation (including that from osteoarthritis of the apophyseal joints and the joints of Luschka). The cervical spine contains the joints of Luschka, which are not present elsewhere in the spine. These joints, one on each side of the disc, are separate from the more posteriorly situated facet joints (apophyseal or interpedicular joints). The term *cervical myelopathy* refers to dysfunction of the cervical portion of the spinal cord. Pain and/or neurologic dysfunction in the distribution of one or more cervical nerve roots is termed *cervical radiculopathy*. Neck movement, especially extension, often intensifies the neck and arm pain of a patient with a cervical disc herniation.

Textbook: Pages 1369–1370 ANSWER: B, E.

19. A 36-year-old man developed neck and left arm pain. He noted paresthesias in the left index and long fingers. He was found to have weakness of the left triceps muscle and a diminished left triceps jerk. His left-sided disc herniation is most likely to be at:

A. C3–C4.
B. C4–C5.
C. C5–C6.
D. C6–C7.
E. C7–T1.

DISCUSSION: This patient has all of the neurologic components of the most common cervical disc syndrome, that caused by a herniation at the C6–C7 level with compression of the C7 nerve root.

Textbook: Pages 1370–1371 ANSWER: D.

20. Which of the following statements are true?

A. The fascicles in a peripheral nerve divide and recombine along their course.
B. Neurapraxia is a type of nerve injury in which the nerve is still in continuity but individual axons are disrupted.
C. Recovery from neurotmesis requires surgical repair.
D. Axonal sprouting begins 1 to 2 months after transection of a peripheral nerve.
E. The patient's age influences the rate and success of nerve regeneration.

DISCUSSION: Fascicles within a peripheral nerve do divide and recombine along their course, forming funicular plexuses. If a segment of a nerve is removed and the remaining ends are reapproximated, the fascicles will not match exactly. In neurapraxia (first-degree nerve injury) anatomic continuity of the axons is preserved, but there is selective demyelination. Surgical repair is not necessary. Recovery does not depend on regeneration and occurs within days or weeks. With neurotmesis there is significant disorganization in the nerve or actual disruption of its continuity, which precludes recovery without surgical repair. Axonal sprouting ordinarily begins 10 to 20 days after transection of a peripheral nerve. The patient's age affects the rate and success of nerve regeneration: the younger the patient is, the faster and more complete is the recovery.

Textbook: Pages 1372–1373 ANSWER: A, C, E.

21. Which of the following statements are true?

A. The Hoffmann-Tinel sign localizes the level of a nerve injury.
B. *Causalgia* is a term used to denote the etiology of pain.
C. Secondary repair of a lacerated nerve 3 to 8 weeks after injury has several advantages.
D. A surgeon who finds at delayed (3 to 8 weeks) exploration that a clinically nonfunctioning nerve is in continuity should resect the injured portion of the nerve and suture together the ends.
E. If a nerve is found to be disrupted at delayed (3 to 8 weeks) exploration, the surgeon should find the two ends of the nerve and suture them together.

DISCUSSION: The Hoffmann-Tinel sign identifies the most distal point of small nerve fiber regeneration. As nerve regeneration progresses, this point moves farther away from the level of the nerve injury. Causalgia is a specific severe pain syndrome that may accompany a partial injury to a mixed peripheral nerve. As compared with primary repair, the extent of damage to a nerve can be better assessed and the correct amount trimmed off, with a secondary repair 3 to 8 weeks after the injury; the epineurium and perineurium are stronger and can be sutured more easily; optimal operating room conditions can be arranged; and there is no time for wallerian degeneration (i.e., the involved neurons are capable immediately of regenerating new distal segments, and the regenerating axons can penetrate the repair site before a significant amount of scar forms). If a clinically nonfunctioning nerve is in continuity when it is explored some weeks after the initial injury the surgeon may find it helpful to stimulate the nerve electrically proximal to the injury and to look distally for evidence of muscle contraction or transmission of nerve action potentials. If there is no evidence of transmission across the area of injury, the injured portion of the nerve should be excised and the cut ends sutured together. If there is transmission across the area of injury, surgical treatment should be limited to external neurolysis. A disrupted nerve should be reapproximated surgically, but only after each end has been trimmed back to healthy fascicles. The trimmed nerve ends must not be under tension when they are sewn together.

Textbook: Pages 1372–1373 ANSWER: C.

22. Which of the following lesions is not one of the cutaneous stigmata of occult spinal dysraphism?

A. Midline lumbar capillary hemangioma.
B. Focal hairy patch over the thoracolumbar spine.
C. Dermal sinus located above the midsacrum.
D. Midline subcutaneous lipoma.
E. *Café-au-lait* spot over the thoracolumbar spine.

DISCUSSION: *Café-au-lait* spots are not a feature of spina bifida occulta. The other four skin features all may be associated with significant intradural pathology and warrant further investigation, most commonly with magnetic resonance imaging (MRI). A dermal sinus tract that overlies the coccyx is a pilonidal sinus and is not likely to be associated with intradural pathology.

Textbook: Page 1377 ANSWER: E.

23. Myelomeningoceles are congenital malformations of the spinal cord. Which of the following findings are not commonly associated?

A. Hydrocephalus.
B. Chiari II malformation.
C. A midline dorsal spinal mass easily noted at birth.
D. Skin, bone, and dural defects superficial to the neural placode.
E. Mandatory urinary incontinence.

DISCUSSION: Myelomeningoceles are usually associated with hydrocephalus and the Chiari II malformation. The myelomeningocele sac is a midline dorsal spinal mass associated with defects in the skin, bone, and dura overlying the neural placode, and the sac is readily apparent at birth. Although the innervation of the bladder is dysmorphic, the majority of patients can achieve social urinary continence through the use of clean intermittent bladder catherization.

Textbook: Pages 1377–1378 ANSWER: E

24. Which of the following signs does Horner's syndrome include?

A. Ptosis.
B. Facial hyperhidrosis.
C. Miosis.
D. Exophthalmos.
E. Mydriasis.

DISCUSSION: Horner's syndrome is due to loss of sympathetic innervation to the head and neck and includes ptosis, anhidrosis, miosis, and the appearance of enophthalmos. The pupil is small owing to loss of the tonic dilating effect of the sympathetics in the presence of continued parasympathetic activity. There is sympathetic innervation to Muller's muscle in the upper lid. Sympathetic nerves supply the sweat glands. It commonly follows stellate ganglion resection and involves removal of the T1 cord level sympathetic outflow.

Textbook: Page 1386 ANSWER: A, C.

25. Cordotomy results in which of the following?

A. Contralateral loss of pin appreciation.
B. Vagal instability.
C. Contralateral loss of temperature appreciation.
D. Ipsilateral loss of pin and temperature appreciation.
E. Contralateral loss of two-point discrimination.

DISCUSSION: Cordotomy results in a lesion of the spinothalamic tract, which is a crossed pathway carrying signals for pain and temperature.

Textbook: Page 1384 ANSWER: A, C.

26. Surgical therapy for epilepsy should be considered in patients with:

A. Seizures poorly controlled with antiepileptic medications.
B. A single epileptic focus.
C. Seizures arising from multiple areas of cerebral cortex.
D. Seizures arising within the cortical motor strip.

DISCUSSION: Because seizure surgical procedures can never be guaranteed to alleviate seizures, it is only undertaken when medical therapy fails to control the patient's seizures at doses that do not produce intolerable side effects. Most surgical procedures are aimed at removing a single epileptogenic area of cerebral cortex and are rarely employed in patients with multiple areas of epileptogenic cortex. Eloquent areas of cerebral cortex such as those subserving speech or hand functions generally are not intentionally resected in an attempt to achieve seizure control.

Textbook: Page 1389 ANSWER: A, B.

27. The epileptogenic area of cerebral cortex is localized by:

A. Direct identification.
B. Observing the patient's seizures.
C. Electroencephalography.
D. Visualizing cortical abnormalities on cerebral imaging studies.

DISCUSSION: Since the exact anatomy of an epileptogenic focus remains obscure, the focus of the patient's seizures is determined by concordance of the clinical manifestations of the seizures, abnormalities demonstrated by cerebral imaging, and abnormalities demonstrated by electroencephalography.

Textbook: Page 1390 ANSWER: B, C, D.

28. Which of the following stereotactic procedures would be performed primarily to alter the function of the brain?

A. Stereotactic biopsy of a brain tumor in the right posterior thalamus.
B. Stereotactic radiotherapy of an arteriovenous malformation in the right ventrolateral thalamus.
C. Stereotactic radiofrequency lesion of the right ventrolateral thalamus for Parkinson's disease.
D. Stereotactic craniotomy for excision of arteriovenous malformation in the right posterior thalamus.

DISCUSSION: The biopsy of a lesion, radiotherapy treatment of an arteriovenous malformation, and excision of an arteriovenous malformation are all procedures for structural lesions of the brain that can be imaged by either CT or MRI. These structural lesions may or may not cause neurologic changes, but the treatment directed at them is intended principally to keep lesion-induced damage from increasing (for example, with the development of hemorrhage). On the other hand, the thalamus is expected to have a normal structural appearance and function in Parkinson's disease, when the neurochemical abnormality is located in the substantia nigra and the striatum (caudate and putamen). Thus, a lesion is made in the thalamus principally to affect the function of the brain, altering a normal component of one of the motor circuits to compensate for the changes in the other parts (i.e., the basal ganglia).

Textbook: Pages 1395–1396 ANSWER: C.

29. What is the critical difference between frame-based and frameless stereotactic procedures?

A. The use of digitized imaging studies such as CT and MRI.
B. The use of rendered three-dimensional images and a three-dimensional digitizer.
C. Rigid fixation of the patient's head to the operating room table.
D. The presence of a lesion in the brain on digitized imaging studies.
E. The absence of a lesion in the brain on digitized imaging studies.

DISCUSSION: Frame-based and frameless procedures both use digitized imaging studies as the basis for converting the scan coordinate system into a treatment coordinate system. Both types of procedures also require rigid fixation of the patient's head to the operating room table and can be performed in the presence or absence of a lesion. The critical difference is the use of a rendered, three-dimensional image and the three-dimensional digitizer, which together allow the alignment to be generated between the patient's imaging studies and the patient; this alignment occurs in frame-based stereotactic procedures because of the imaging study performed after the frame is applied.

Textbook: Pages 1393–1395 ANSWER: B.

NOTES

NOTES

NOTES

CHAPTER 18

ORTHOPEDICS

1. Which of the following statements about open fractures is/are correct?

A. Intravenous antibiotics should be administered as soon as possible.
B. They should be regarded as an emergency.
C. Wound closure is necessary within 8 hours.
D. Systematic wound débridement and irrigation should be performed.
E. They most often result from low-energy injuries.

DISCUSSION: Open fractures represent an orthopedic emergency. They result most frequently from high-energy injuries. Current treatment includes administration of intravenous antibiotics, systematic wound irrigation, and débridement with respect for the neurovascular bundles. Immediate wound closure is rarely indicated and should be performed once the wound contamination is determined to be low.

Textbook: Pages 1398, 1399–1400 ANSWER: A, B, D.

2. The goals of proper fracture reduction include which of the following?

A. Providing patient comfort and analgesia.
B. Allowing for restoration of length of the extremity.
C. Correcting angular deformity and rotation.
D. Enabling immediate motion of all fractured extremities.
E. Providing a foundation for bone healing and union.

DISCUSSION: The goals of fracture reduction include patient comfort and analgesia through stabilization of the bone ends. Furthermore, restoration of the length, angulation, and rotational alignment of the extremity should be achieved to allow proper union. Reduction does not, however, allow immediate motion for all fractures.

Textbook: Page 1399 ANSWER: A, B, C, E.

3. Which statement is true about the "three-column concept" of spinal fracture stability?

A. An unstable spine consists of bone or soft tissue injury in a single column.
B. An unstable spine involves injury to all three columns.
C. Instability results from injury to two columns plus evidence of compression of the dural tube.
D. Instability results from significant bone and/or soft tissue injury in two columns.

DISCUSSION: Denis developed a classification system for a thoracolumbar spine injury based on a three-column concept. In this system, the spine is divided into three longitudinal regions or columns: anterior, middle, and posterior. Although references to such "columns" is anatomically imprecise, the term is clinically useful in assessing the stability of the injured spine. In general, instability results when significant disruption is present in two of the three columns, regardless of the presence or absence of neurologic deficit.

Textbook: Page 1405 ANSWER: D.

4. All of the following statements are true of Jefferson's fracture of the atlas except:

A. The injury results from an axial load to the cervical spine.
B. The fracture fragments characteristically displace into the spinal canal.
C. Neurologic injury is uncommon.
D. Computed tomography (CT) best demonstrates the fracture's configuration.

DISCUSSION: Fracture of the atlas (Jefferson's fracture) occurs from an axial load, usually to the top of the head. The resulting forces fracture the ring of C1 and displace the fragments outward. This results in an increase in the cross-sectional area of the spinal canal at the level of injury. Neurologic injury is, therefore, unusual in this fracture. CT is the best roentgenographic study available to evaluate fractures of the atlas.

Textbook: Page 1402 ANSWER: B.

5. Which of the following statements about burst fractures of the thoracolumbar spine are correct?

A. The injury most often occurs at the thoracolumbar junction.
B. The injury results from axial loading of the spine, often with concomitant flexion.
C. Anterior and middle column failure are always present in this injury.
D. Laminectomy provides satisfactory decompression.

DISCUSSION: Burst fractures result from axial compression of the spine, frequently associated with varying degrees of flexion. These injuries, which most often occur at the thoracolumbar junction, are characterized by circumferential expansion of the entire vertebra with failure of the anterior and middle spinal columns and in some cases, the posterior ones. Middle column failure in burst fractures results in retropulsion of the posterior superior portion of the vertebral body into the spinal canal. With marked retropulsion, compression of the dural tube occurs, often with associated neurologic deficit.

Surgical procedures designed to decompress and stabilize thoracolumbar burst fractures can be performed through anterior or posterior approaches. The major site of compression is anterior, and for this reason laminectomy does little to relieve compression of the spinal cord over an anterior lesion. Indeed, laminectomy further increases the instability of the spine.

Textbook: Pages 1406–1407 ANSWER: A, B, C.

6. The neurovascular structure most commonly injured as a result of an anterior dislocation of the shoulder is the:

A. Musculocutaneous nerve.
B. Axillary nerve.
C. Axillary artery.
D. Median nerve.

DISCUSSION: The axillary nerve is at greatest risk for injury. Occasionally a more severe neurologic deficit can occur as a result of injury to the brachial plexus. Rarely has injury to the axillary artery been reported.

Textbook: Page 1408 ANSWER: B.

7. The classification of fractures of the proximal humerus is based on:

A. The number of fracture segments and amount of displacement.
B. The mechanism of injury.
C. Presence or absence of associated dislocations.

DISCUSSION: The classification is based on fracture patterns involving the four "segments" of the proximal humerus (anatomic neck, surgical neck, and greater and lesser tuberosities). Fractures are one-, two-, three-, or four-part fractures, depending on the number of fracture segments and amount of displacement.

Textbook: Page 1410 ANSWER: A.

8. The radial nerve is at greatest risk for injury with which fracture?

A. Fracture of the surgical neck of the humerus.
B. Fracture of the shaft of the humerus.
C. Supracondylar fracture of the humerus.
D. Olecranon fractures.

DISCUSSION: The radial nerve lies in proximity to the humerus as it courses laterally at the junction of the middle and distal thirds of the shaft of the humerus. Therefore, it is at greatest risk of injury in shaft fractures. If radial nerve paralysis is present in association with this fracture, it is advisable to observe the patient since most nerve injuries recover spontaneously within 6 to 12 weeks.

Textbook: Page 1410 ANSWER: B.

9. The best method of treating a supracondylar fracture of the humerus in a child that is unstable when the elbow is flexed to 90 degrees is:

A. Hyperflexion of the elbow to 130 degrees and casting.
B. Open reduction and internal fixation.
C. Percutaneous pinning.

DISCUSSION: Best results with this fracture are obtained with percutaneous pinning. Hyperflexion of the elbow usually achieves stability but incurs the risk of occluding arterial inflow and may cause permanent neuromuscular deficit. Open reduction is not indicated unless the fracture is irreducible or associated with a vascular injury.

Textbook: Page 1412 ANSWER: C.

10. Both-bone forearm fractures in adults are best managed by:

A. Closed reduction and casting.
B. Closed reduction and application of an external fixator.
C. Open reduction and placement of intramedullary rods.
D. Open reduction and internal fixation with compression plates.

DISCUSSION: Studies have shown that function is best restored with less complications if open reduction and rigid fixation is achieved with compression plates. Closed reduction rarely achieves an anatomic position and some forearm rotation is therefore usually lost. External fixation is occasionally used in severe open fractures.

Textbook: Page 1414 ANSWER: D.

11. The most consistent sign of a fracture of the carpal scaphoid is:

A. Wrist pain during attempted push-ups.
B. Diffuse swelling on the dorsum of the wrist.
C. Localized tenderness in the anatomic snuffbox.
D. Wrist popping on movement.

DISCUSSION: Wrist pain during attempted push-ups or diffuse swelling on the dorsum of the wrist may be caused by a variety of factors. Wrist popping on movement may be the result of carpal instability, subluxation of a tendon on extension and flexion of the wrist, or intra-articular problems such as an articular cartilage flap or a tear of the triangular fibrocartilage. Localized tenderness at the anatomic snuffbox (scaphoid) is the most consistent sign of scaphoid fracture.

Textbook: Page 1416 ANSWER: C.

12. A patient describes a fall on the outstretched hand during sports activities. Multiple radiographic views show no distinct fracture. He is tender to palpation in the anatomic snuffbox. The most suitable method of management is:

A. Diagnose "sprained wrist" and apply an elastic bandage.
B. Diagnose suspected scaphoid fracture and apply a short-arm cast to include the thumb.
C. Apply a canvas wrist splint for immobilization.
D. Prescribe salicylates and permit continued activity.

DISCUSSION: If the patient sustained a fall on the outstretched hand and is tender to palpation in the anatomic snuffbox, fracture of the scaphoid should be suspected. Neither an elastic bandage nor a canvas wrist splint provides adequate immobilization for the scaphoid. A short-arm cast to include the thumb is the most appropriate treatment. Salicylates and continued activity would not treat scaphoid fracture. If no fracture is noted initially, the cast is applied and films are taken at 10 days to 2 weeks since nondisplaced scaphoid fractures are often more easily visualized at that time.

Textbook: Pages 1416–1418 ANSWER: B.

13. Median nerve compression syndrome in which the patient has motor weakness of the flexor pollicis longus and the flexor digitorum profundus of the index finger without alteration in sensibility is due to:

A. Compression of the median nerve at the elbow by the lacertus fibrosus.
B. Compression of the median nerve in the axilla.
C. Compression of the anterior interosseous nerve by the arcade of Frohse.
D. Compression of the anterior interosseous nerve by an aberrant accessory forearm muscle.

DISCUSSION: Compression of the median nerve at the elbow by the lacertus fibrosus causes symptoms at more locations than just the flexor pollicis longus and flexor profundus at the index finger, since the entire median nerve is affected. Compression of the median nerve at the axilla affects both motor and sensory elements diffusely. The arcade of Frohse is a fibrous band at the origin of the supinator muscle. It can compress the posterior interosseous portion of the radial nerve but does not involve the median nerve. The anterior interosseous portion of the median nerve can be compressed by an aberrant accessory forearm muscle (Gantzer's muscle).

Textbook: Pages 1480–1481 ANSWER: D.

14. Total interruption of the radial nerve at midarm produces specific findings on physical examination. The most complete description of the neurologic deficit includes:

A. Paralysis of the thumb extensors, interphalangeal joint extensors, extensor carpi radialis, and extensor carpi ulnaris.
B. Paralysis of the extensor carpi radialis longus and brevis, abductor pollicis longus, extensor pollicis brevis, and extensor pollicis longus.
C. Paralysis of the brachioradialis, extensor carpi radialis longus and brevis, extensor carpi ulnaris, thumb extensors, and metacarpophalangeal (MCP) joint extensors, and loss of cutaneous sensibility at the dorsal aspect of the thumb and index fingers.
D. Paralysis of the brachioradialis, extensor carpi radialis longus and brevis, radialis, thumb extensors, finger MCP joint extensors, and flexor carpi radialis, and loss of sensation in the cutaneous distribution over the dorsal aspect of thumb and index fingers.

DISCUSSION: The extensor carpi radialis, extensor carpi ulnaris, and thumb extensors are innervated by the radial nerve. Although finger MCP joint extension is performed by the extensor digitorum communis muscle, which is innervated by the radial nerve, the interphalangeal joints of the fingers are extended by the intrinsic muscles in the hand, which are innervated by the ulnar and median nerves. The extensor carpi radialis longus and brevis, the abductor pollicis longus, and the extensor pollicis longus and brevis are all innervated by the radial nerve. However, answer *B* is not complete because MCP joint extension of the fingers and radial sensory deficit are not included. The brachioradialis, extensor carpi radialis longus and brevis, extensor carpi ulnaris, thumb extensors, and finger MCP joint extensors are all innervated by the radial nerve. The superficial radial nerve provides sensibility to the dorsal aspect of thumb and index finger in the dorsal radial aspect of the hand. The extensor carpi radialis longus and brevis and thumb extensors are innervated by the radial nerve. The superficial radial nerve provides sensibility at the dorsal aspect of thumb and index. Not included in answer *D* is the extensor carpi ulnaris. It should be remembered that although the extensor ulnaris is on the ulnar aspect of the wrist and uses the term *ulnaris*, it is innervated not by the ulnar nerve but by the radial nerve and would not function with complete interruption of the radial nerve at midarm. In addition, despite the fact that the wrist flexor on the radial aspect of the wrist is termed the flexor carpi radialis, it is not innervated by the radial nerve. It is innervated by the median nerve. Therefore, it should not be included in this list.

Textbook: Page 1484 ANSWER: C.

15. The most common physical findings in a patient with median nerve compression at the wrist (carpal tunnel syndrome) are:

A. Diminished two-point discrimination and dryness of the index and long fingers.
B. Atrophy of the abductor pollicis brevis and opponens pollicis.
C. A positive percussion test at the wrist and a positive wrist flexion test producing paresthesias at the thumb, index, and long fingers.

D. A weak grip in addition to hand cramping and difficulty writing.

DISCUSSION: While patients with carpal tunnel syndrome often complain of subjective symptoms such as numbness of the thumb, index, and long fingers, objective decreased sensibility is not usually present. Testing with von Frey filaments produces the most sensitive results. Decreased light touch is noted before decreased two-point discrimination. Dryness of the skin in the median nerve distribution is evident with severe injury to the nerve but not in the routine carpal tunnel syndrome. Although the abductor pollicis brevis and opponens pollicis are supplied by the motor branch of the median nerve, atrophy of these muscles is not seen until long-term median nerve compression has occurred. Symptomatic carpal tunnel syndrome without evidence of thenar atrophy has a greater frequency than the more severe median nerve compression, with demonstrable thenar atrophy. Percussion over the median nerve at the wrist producing paresthesias distally in the distribution of the median nerve and paresthesias caused by wrist flexion are two of the most common signs of median nerve compression at the wrist. Although patients with carpal tunnel syndrome intermittently complain of weak grip and dropping objects, cramping of the hand while writing and difficulty writing are not routine symptoms of this condition.

Textbook: Pages 1480–1481 ANSWER: C.

16. Which of the following describes the most desirable position in which to immobilize the hand?

A. Wrist is flexed, MCP joints are extended, and IP joints are flexed.
B. Wrist is flexed, MCP joints are flexed, and IP joints are extended.
C. Wrist is extended, MCP joints are extended, and IP joints are flexed.
D. Wrist is extended, MCP joints are flexed, and IP joints are flexed.
E. Wrist is extended, MCP joints are flexed, and IP joints are extended.

DISCUSSION: Plaster splints and dressings should hold the digits in the "intrinsic plus" position. This includes 60 to 80 degrees of flexion at the MCP joints, 10 to 20 degrees of flexion at the proximal interphalangeal (PIP) joints, and 5 to 10 degrees of flexion at the distal interphalangeal (DIP) joints. With the MCP joints in flexion and the PIP joints in extension the collateral ligaments are elongated, thereby decreasing the likelihood of ligament contracture and subsequent joint stiffness. At times, however, the PIP joint is immobilized in greater flexion to correct palmar angulation and to maintain proper rotation of the digit after an unstable fracture.

Textbook: Pages 1419–1420 ANSWER: E.

17. An early sign of compartment syndrome in the hand includes:

A. Pain with passive stretch of the digits.
B. Absent radial pulse.
C. Motor paralysis.
D. Swelling of the digits.
E. Stiffness of the digits.

DISCUSSION: Early sign of compartment syndrome is pain with passive motion. Paralysis occurs later, and absence of the radial pulse is an even later finding.

Textbook: Page 1422 ANSWER: A.

18. Palmar dislocation of the PIP joint with fracture:

A. Is more common than dorsal dislocation.
B. Is treated by splinting with the PIP joint in flexion.
C. Is treated by splinting with the PIP joint and DIP joints in extension.
D. If not splinted properly, will cause a boutonniere deformity.
E. If not splinted properly will cause a swan neck deformity.

DISCUSSION: Palmar dislocation of the PIP joint is much less common than dorsal dislocation. Palmar dislocation of the PIP joint can disrupt the central slip of the extensor mechanism at the proximal part of the middle phalanx and can disrupt the dorsal capsule in addition to the palmar plate. If the joint is stable after reduction it is treated by splinting to immobilize the PIP joint in extension, while the DIP is allowed to actively flex. If not splinted properly, this injury can cause boutonniere deformity with resultant loss of normal PIP extension and hyperextension of the distal joint.

Textbook: Pages 1423–1424 ANSWER: D.

19. Fracture of the fifth metacarpal neck:

A. Usually requires open reduction and internal fixation.
B. Must be reduced anatomically and stabilized with pins.
C. Is called a "boxer's fracture."
D. Will result in significant functional disability if angulated 30 degrees dorsally.
E. Is uncommon.

DISCUSSION: Fifth metacarpal neck fracture is a common injury. It is termed *boxer's fracture* because the mechanism of injury is often that of hitting the fist against a firm object. This fracture does not need to be reduced anatomically and usually does not require open reduction and internal fixation. The relative mobility of the fifth metacarpal (as compared with the relative lack of mobility at the index and long fingers) allows excellent function despite dorsal angulation of 30 degrees.

Textbook: Page 1428 ANSWER: C.

20. A Bennett's fracture is:

A. An extra-articular fracture of the base of the thumb metacarpal.
B. Displaced by the pull of the abductor pollicis longus and adductor pollicis.

C. Displaced by the pull of the abductor pollicis longus and extensor pollicis longus.
D. Usually successfully treated with closed reduction and casting.
E. A comminuted T-type fracture of the base of the thumb metacarpal.

DISCUSSION: A Bennett's fracture is an intra-articular fracture of the proximal end (base) of the thumb metacarpal. The resulting bone fragment is held by the intermetacarpal ligament. The base of the metacarpal is displaced laterally by the pull of the abductor pollicis longus. The adductor pollicis pulls the proximal phalanx and distal metacarpal toward the palm and the proximal metacarpal away from its adjacent fracture fragment. These forces acting on the fracture tend to displace the metacarpal, usually making cast treatment alone ineffective. Treatment is by percutaneous pinning if closed reduction can be achieved, or by open reduction and internal fixation if significant displacement cannot be corrected by closed methods.

A comminuted T-type fracture of the base of the thumb metacarpal was described by Rolando.

Textbook: Pages 1429–1430 ANSWER: B.

21. A 39-year-old male presents in the emergency room after a high-speed motor vehicle accident. The patient has been intubated by paramedics at the scene and is on assisted ventilation. He is unconscious. Physical examination reveals a distended abdomen, and initial screening x-rays reveal a displaced fracture of the pelvic ring. Initial evaluation should include which of the following?

A. Fluid resuscitation and establishment of venous access.
B. Diagnostic peritoneal lavage.
C. Thorough physical examination, including evaluation of the urinary and lower gastrointestinal tract.
D. Emergent application of external fixation.
E. CT of the abdomen.

DISCUSSION: This trauma patient has presented with a displaced pelvic fracture and a distended abdomen. In this setting, it is quite difficult to distinguish intra-abdominal trauma from abdominal distention related to a fracture of the pelvis and secondary bleeding. Diagnostic peritoneal lavage would be indicated as well as physical examination of the genitourinary and lower gastrointestinal tract to rule out an open pelvic fracture. Application of an external fixator for the pelvis would be withheld unless the patient became unstable. Without evidence of intra-abdominal trauma, pelvic bleeding is implicated as the source of instability. Imaging studies of the pelvis and abdomen would be indicated after the initial resuscitation.

Textbook: Pages 1432–1444 ANSWER: A, B, C.

22. A patient sustains a displaced fracture of both columns of the acetabulum with extension into the sciatic notch. The patient is initially placed in traction. After treatment of other associated injuries, pre-operative evaluation should include which of the following?

A. CT evaluation of the acetabular fracture.
B. Aspiration of the hip joint.
C. Pelvic arteriography.
D. Preoperative ventilation-perfusion lung scan.
E. Prolonged bed rest.

DISCUSSION: Treatment of a displaced fracture of both columns of the acetabulum requires careful preoperative evaluation, including CT with three-dimensional reconstruction, if the fracture anatomy is not clear from standard radiographic imaging. If an extended iliofemoral approach is considered, preoperative pelvic angiography should be performed to ascertain patency of the superior gluteal artery. For this approach, the flap is dependent on a superior gluteal artery for survival. Early operative intervention and expeditious mobilization decrease the incidence of pulmonary complications, and preoperative pulmonary evaluation is not indicated unless specific problems arise.

Textbook: Pages 1435–1436 ANSWER: A, C.

23. Which of the following statements about the blood supply to the hip are true?

A. The medial femoral circumflex artery circles around to the posterior aspect of the hip, where it becomes confluent with the retinacular blood vessels.
B. A small portion of the blood supply of the femoral head is provided by the obturator artery via the ligamentum teres.
C. Displacement of a femoral neck fracture can disrupt the branches of the medial femoral circumflex artery.
D. The retinacular vessels are supplied by the lateral femoral circumflex artery, which takes a posterior course.
E. Muscular attachments to the periarticular bone structures provide blood supply to the femoral head.

DISCUSSION: The blood supply to the femoral head is provided predominantly by the branches of the medial femoral circumflex artery, which take a posterior course and are confluent with the retinacular vessels. The lateral femoral circumflex artery runs anteriorly.

Textbook: Page 1439 ANSWER: A, B, C.

24. A 24-year-old woman presents to the emergency room with a dislocated knee. In transferring the patient from stretcher to examining table, the knee is spontaneously reduced. Physical examination reveals no palpable or "Dopplerable" pulses in the foot on the affected side and booming pulses in the foot on the nonaffected side. Proper treatment would include which of the following?

A. Doppler evaluation of the arteries in the lower

extremity followed by arteriography if the Doppler study was abnormal.
B. Magnetic resonance imaging (MRI) of the affected leg.
C. Close follow-up examination.
D. Emergent transfer to the operating room for exploration of the popliteal artery.
E. Immobilization of the knee with gentle warming of the extremity and elevation.

DISCUSSION: An abnormal vascular examination after a documented dislocation of the knee indicates damage to the popliteal artery at the level of the knee dislocation. This is a limb-threatening injury that requires expeditious exploration of the popliteal artery to provide appropriate treatment and decrease the chances of vascular compromise leading to amputation of the extremity.
Textbook: Pages 1442–1443 ANSWER: D.

25. The Ilizarov device aids in management of tibial fractures because of its ability to:

A. Stabilize acute fractures.
B. Correct angular deformities in cases of malunion.
C. Transport bone by distraction callotasis.
D. Noninvasively provide fixation for juxta-articular fractures, such as the tibial plateau and pylon.
E. All of the above.

DISCUSSION: The Ilizarov device is a very useful external fixation device that is versatile and has had a positive impact on the management of tibial fractures.
Textbook: Page 1448 ANSWER: E.

26. An 8 cm. by 10 cm. soft tissue defect over the proximal third of the tibia with exposed bone devoid of periosteum is best treated with:

A. Skin graft.
B. Gastrocnemius rotational myoplasty.
C. Soleus rotational myoplasty.
D. Free tissue transfer.

DISCUSSION: The proximal third of the tibia can be covered effectively with the gastrocnemius rotational flap using the medial hem of the gastrocnemius. The middle third can be successfully covered by the soleus myoplasty. Open fractures with soft tissue defects over the distal third usually require free tissue transfer because of lack of available local tissue coverage.
Textbook: Page 1448 ANSWER: B.

27. Prognosis of healing in tibial fractures correlates best with:

A. Energy absorption at the time of fracture.
B. Amount of soft tissue damage.
C. Location of the fracture (i.e., in the proximal, middle, or distal third).
D. Age of patient.

DISCUSSION: The amount of energy absorption and the degree of bony comminution is the most significant factor in predicting healing of tibial fractures. Location along the tibia and age are not thought of as significant factors in healing. The soft tissue damage may contribute to lack of vascular envelope, but the destruction of soft tissue is based on the amount of energy absorbed.
Textbook: Page 1445 ANSWER: A.

28. Management of a III-b tibia fracture is best treated initially by:

A. Plaster immobilization.
B. Immediate plating.
C. Reamed intramedullary nailing.
D. External fixation.

DISCUSSION: Studies by Hansen and others have demonstrated that open reduction and internal fixation of Grade III-b or Grade III-c fractures are likely to cause more stripping of soft tissue and therefore further devascularize an already devascularized tibia. The external fixator is selected because it is a treatment apparatus that reduces and holds the bone fragments and provides important stability for soft tissue healing. Treatment of open wounds with a plaster cast is impractical and wound care is difficult. Reaming intramedullary nailing further compromises blood supply to the bone by destroying the intramedullary blood supply that may be critical to fracture healing.
Textbook: Pages 1446–1448 ANSWER: D.

29. The most frequent forces acting on the foot that cause ankle fractures are:

A. External rotation.
B. Internal rotation.
C. Plantar flexion.
D. Dorsiflexion.

DISCUSSION: Fractures most frequently involve external rotation of the foot and ankle joint, which is usually due to an internal rotation or twisting of the leg on a foot that is fixed by weight bearing. Axial loading injuries commonly produce distal tibia fractures.
Textbook: Page 1449 ANSWER: A.

30. Patients who have abduction injuries to the foot are prone to injure the following structures:

A. Medial malleolus and deltoid.
B. Lateral malleolus and deltoid ligament.
C. Interosseous ligament.
D. Posterior tibiofibular ligament.

DISCUSSION: If the mechanism of fracture is an abduction force, the medial malleolus fractures below or at the level of the ankle joint, and this may include tears of the deltoid ligament. These are usually accompanied by a fibula fracture as well.
Textbook: Page 1449 ANSWER: A.

31. Of the following bones in the foot, the tarsal bone that is most prone to vascular compromise is the:

A. Calcaneus.

B. Navicular.
C. Talus.
D. Cuboid.

DISCUSSION: The blood supply of the talus is somewhat tenuous because there are no muscles or tendons associated with this bone.

Textbook: Pages 1450–1451 ANSWER: C.

32. A Lisfranc fracture is a fracture-dislocation involving:

A. Calaneocuboid joint.
B. Tarsometarsal joint.
C. Metatarsophalangeal joint.
D. Talocalcaneal dislocation.

DISCUSSION: The fracture can be either divergent, dorsal, or plantar. It usually involves a significant soft tissue injury that, if unrecognized, leads to ischemia of the forefoot and gangrene resulting in amputation.

Textbook: Page 1450 ANSWER: B.

33. The most common reason for surgical amputation in the general population is:

A. Trauma.
B. Tumor.
C. Infection.
D. Congenital deformity.
E. Ischemia.

DISCUSSION: Congenital deformities leading to amputation are relatively rare, as are musculoskeletal tumors. Traumatic amputations are the most common in the younger population, but the majority of amputations are of the lower extremity and are caused by ischemia secondary to peripheral vascular disease. Approximately 50% of the patients suffering from extremity ischemia also suffer from diabetes.

Textbook: Pages 1452–1453 ANSWER: E.

34. The level of amputation in a dysvascular extremity is determined by:

A. Clinical inspection.
B. Xenon skin clearance.
C. Doppler systolic blood pressure ratios.
D. Transcutaneous oxygen measurements.
E. Nutritional competence and immunocompetence.

DISCUSSION: Clinical competence of the extremity with observations of skin turgor, discoloration, perfusion, sensation, and integrity is the mainstay of surgical decision making. This can be complemented by transcutaneous Po_2, ankle-arm systolic pressure ratios, xenon skin clearance, serum albumin levels, and total lymphocyte count.

Textbook: Pages 1453–1454 ANSWER: A, B, C, D, E.

35. Knee disarticulation has the following advantages over above-knee amputation:

A. Longer lever arm.
B. Better cosmetic result.
C. Easier prosthetic fitting.
D. End-bearing stump.
E. Supracondylar suspension.

DISCUSSION: Patients with knee disarticulations have a slightly worse cosmetic appearance due to an inequality of knee heights particularly noticeable when sitting. Additionally, prosthetic fitting is significantly more difficult and requires the involvement of a prosthetist familiar with the specific considerations. On the other hand, the increase in lever arm, the end-bearing stump, and the use of supracondylar suspension far outweigh the disadvantages when such an amputation is possible from an anatomic standpoint.

Textbook: Pages 1456–1457 ANSWER: A, D, E.

36. Hematogenous osteomyelitis most frequently affects:

A. The diaphysis of long bones.
B. The epiphysis.
C. The metaphysis of long bones.
D. Flat bones.
E. Cuboidal bones.

DISCUSSION: Hematogenous osteomyelitis occurs most frequently in children and involves the metaphyseal ends of long bones. The cause is thought to relate to the pattern of blood flow in the metaphysis wherein arterioles empty into numerous sinusoidal veins with sluggish blood flow favoring the lodgement of bacteria.

Textbook: Page 1459 ANSWER: C.

37. A 5-year-old child presents with a 2-day history of the atraumatic onset of pain, erythema, and swelling of the right knee joint. The child is febrile with an elevated white blood cell count. The differential diagnosis includes:

A. Acute rheumatic fever.
B. Leukemia.
C. Scurvy.
D. Acute septic arthritis.
E. Acute juvenile rheumatoid arthritis.

DISCUSSION: All of the above conditions may present with the clinical and laboratory findings described above. Aspiration of the joint and examination of the synovial fluid is required to rule out pyogenic arthritis. Ancillary laboratory testing for juvenile rheumatoid arthritis and acute rheumatic fever may be required.

Textbook: Page 1463 ANSWER: A, B, C, D, E.

38. Skeletal tuberculosis is:

A. Of historical interest only.
B. Increasing in association with patients with human immunodeficiency virus (HIV) infection.
C. Most frequently encountered at the thoracolumbar junction.
D. Seen in the absence of visceral tubercular infection.

DISCUSSION: Skeletal tuberculosis is still present and is occurring with increased frequency in patients with HIV infection. The thoracolumbar junction is most frequently affected. Skeletal tuberculosis is a sequel to pulmonary or gastrointestinal tuberculosis.

Textbook: Pages 1461–1462 ANSWER: B, C.

39. A radical margin in the resection of a musculoskeletal tumor removes:

A. The entire limb.
B. A 5-cm. margin of normal tissue around the neoplasm.
C. The anatomic compartment in which the tumor arises.
D. The joint adjacent to the neoplasm.
E. The reactive capsule around the tumor.

DISCUSSION: A radical resection defines removal of the anatomic compartment in which the tumor arises and does not necessarily mandate an amputation.

Textbook: Page 1464 ANSWER: C.

40. The appropriate surgical procedure for the treatment of an osteosarcoma is based on:

A. Staging information.
B. The age of the patient.
C. The response of the lesion to neoadjuvant chemotherapy.
D. The radiographic aggressiveness of the lesion.

DISCUSSION: The surgical treatment of an osteosarcoma is either amputation or wide excision with limb salvage. The decision to do a limb-salvage operation is based on the staging information and on the response of the lesion to chemotherapy. If staging studies indicate involvement of vital structures or if the response to neoadjuvant chemotherapy is inadequate, amputation may be selected rather than limb salvage. The age of the patient and the radiographic appearance of the lesion are not factors in this decision.

Textbook: Pages 1467–1468 ANSWER: A, C.

41. Which of the following statements about selection of an amputated part for replantation is/are correct?

A. A good choice for replantation is an amputated thumb at the level of the proximal phalanx of the dominant hand of a 35-year-old salesman.
B. The index finger should be replanted in an adult male if the amputation is at the base of the proximal phalanx.
C. In a 12-year-old child with an arm amputated above the elbow by an avulsion injury, replantation should be attempted.
D. In a 42-year-old male accountant with a complete amputation of the leg just below the knee, replantation should be attempted.
E. Replantation is advisable for a 20-year-old male with a complete amputation at the proximal forearm with 11 hours of warm ischemic time.

DISCUSSION: The thumb is a prime choice for replantation. If the patient is healthy replantation of the thumb is advisable at just about any level and any age. Amputations of fingers proximal to the flexor superficialis tendon insertion (middle phalanx) generally result in poor active digital motion, and in most adults isolated finger amputations at this level are not replanted. In general, in children replantation should be attempted at any level. Replantation of lower extremity amputations is seldom indicated in adults because of leg-length discrepancy, pain, and poor function. Prosthetic replacement usually results in a more functional gait. Replantation of a forearm amputated at the proximal forearm level is difficult because of the large amount of muscle mass and the multiple nerves entering the muscle. Additionally, over 6 hours of warm ischemia time at this level will most likely cause massive myonecrosis and replantation failure.

Textbook: Pages 1487–1488 ANSWER: A, C.

42. Which of the following statements about preservation of a completely amputated digit is/are correct?

A. The amputated digit should be wrapped in a sterile, dry cloth and kept at body temperature.
B. The amputated digit should be wrapped in a cloth moistened with saline or Ringer's lactate solution and kept at body temperature.
C. The amputated digit should be wrapped in a clean cloth and placed directly on ice.
D. The amputated digit should be placed in a plastic bag containing Ringer's lactate or saline solution, and the plastic bag placed on ice.
E. The amputated digit should be wrapped in a cloth or sponge moistened with Ringer's lactate or saline solution and placed in a plastic bag to rest on ice.

DISCUSSION: The amputated part must be kept cool (4° C or less) but not frozen. Cooling lowers the metabolic needs of the severed part, which allows replantation for up to 12 to 14 hours for major limb amputations and 24 to 36 hours for major digital amputations. The amputated part is preserved by one of the two following methods: (1) Place the amputated part in a plastic bag containing lactated Ringer's or saline solution and place the bag on ice or (2) wrap the amputated part in a cloth and place it in a plastic bag to be put on ice.

Textbook: Page 1487 ANSWER: D, E.

43. Which of the statements about major limb replantations (amputation proximal to the hand or foot) is/are correct?

A. Bone shortening is usually necessary.
B. If the amputation occurred more than 6 hours before arrival in the operating room some type of temporary vascular shunting is indicated.
C. Primary closure of all of the skin is generally recommended.

D. Myonecrosis is a common cause of failure of the replantation.
E. There are few indications for replantation of the lower extremity in adults.

DISCUSSION: Bone shortening of at least 2 cm. is critical in most major limb replantations, to allow thorough débridement of injured structures and approximation of normal tissue to normal tissue (e.g., nerve, vessel, and tendon repair). If the anticipated cold ischemic time for an amputated limb will exceed 6 hours before circulation can be re-established, a temporary silicone shunt should be applied. This is usually the setting, for rarely can the artery be reconnected within 6 hours of the amputation. Primary closure of all of the skin is rarely recommended. Because of the edema associated with reperfusion of the ischemic limb, tight skin closure can compromise the circulation. Skin grafts and/or delayed closure is indicated. Some degree of myonecrosis occurs in all major limb replantations. Thorough surgical excision of damaged muscle tissue diminishes the amount of necrosis. Excessive myonecrosis leads to infection and failure. There are few indications for replantation of lower extremities in adults. The amount of débridement and shortening that is necessary to obtain a viable lower extremity replantation results in excessive leg length discrepancy. Prosthetic replacement can result in a nearly normal gait, especially when the amputation is below the knee.

Textbook: Pages 1488–1489 ANSWER: A, B, D, E.

44. The most crucial elements of the flexor retinacular or pulley system needed for full digital flexion include which annular pulleys?

A. A_1.
B. A_2.
C. A_3.
D. A_4.
E. A_5.

DISCUSSION: The flexor retinacular system from the metacarpophalangeal joint to the distal interphalangeal joint maintains the flexor tendons against the digit during flexion, preventing bow stringing and allowing the digital tip to flex to the distal palmar crease. Division of the A_1, A_3, or A_5 pulleys minimally compromises this function; however, division of the A_2 or A_4 pulleys can significantly limit digital excursion.

Textbook: Page 1471 ANSWER: B, D.

45. Continuous passive mobilization following flexor tendon repair of Zone II injuries produces:

A. Increased total arc of digital range of motion.
B. Decreased incidence of poor results.
C. Increased incidence of postoperative tendon rupture.
D. Increased incidence of infection.

DISCUSSION: Continuous passive mobilization (CPM) causes a 16% improvement in range of digital motion compared to intermittent mobilization. The incidence of poor results is much lower (3% versus 26%) despite no postoperative ruptures or infections. Continuous passive mobilization appears to be a more effective yet safe means of improving postoperative function following flexor tendon injury.

Textbook: Pages 1474–1475 ANSWER: A, B.

46. Isolated flexor digitorum superficialis tendon function is determined by assessing:

A. Flexion of the metacarpophalangeal joint.
B. Flexion of the proximal interphalangeal joint with the adjacent digits held in extension.
C. Flexion of the distal interphalangeal joint.
D. Flexion of the proximal interphalangeal joint.

DISCUSSION: Metacarpophalangeal joint flexion is effected by intrinsic flexor digitorum profundus or flexor digitorum superficialis contraction and therefore cannot be utilized to assess isolated flexor digitorum superficialis integrity. The flexor digitorum superficialis tendon, by inserting on the middle phalanx, acts to flex the proximal interphalangeal joint. Since the flexor digitorum profundus tendon inserts distal to this level, it may also flex this joint. To negate this influence of the flexor digitorum profundus, the adjacent digits should be passively maintained in full extension to isolate flexor digitorum superficialis function in the digit. Distal interphalangeal flexion is the isolated function of the flexor digitorum profundus. The proximal interphalangeal joint may be flexed by the flexor digitorum profundus or flexor digitorum superficialis.

Textbook: Pages 1472–1473 ANSWER: B.

47. The zone of flexor tendon injury that carries the poorest prognosis following injury and repair is:

A. Zone I.
B. Zone II.
C. Zone III.
D. Zone IV.
E. Zone V.

DISCUSSION: Zone I extends from the distal margin of the flexor digitorum superficialis insertion to the flexor digitorum profundus insertion. Injury at this level involves only the profundus tendon. Zone II is defined as the proximal edge of the first annular pulley to the distal margin of the flexor digitorum superficialis insertion. At this level both the superficialis and profundus tendons are contained in a rigid fibroosseous canal. The smooth gliding required at the interfaces at this level may be compromised by adhesions following injury, thus making this the level with the poorest functional prognosis after injury. Injuries in Zones III, IV, and V, at the level of the palm, carpal canal, and distal forearm, respectively, may injure both or either of the flexor tendons to a digit. However, because of a less constrictive environment at the levels, adhesions that limit motion are less likely and the prognosis better than with Zone II injuries.

Textbook: Page 1471 ANSWER: B.

48. The contraindications to primary repair of a flexor tendon injury are:

A. Contaminated wound.
B. Severe soft tissue trauma.
C. Inexperienced surgeon.
D. Compromised general condition of the patient prohibiting prolonged anesthetic.

DISCUSSION: The prerequisites for primary repair (within 24 hours of injury) of a flexor tendon injury are (1) a clean wound or one that may be débrided to a clean status, (2) minimal soft tissue injury providing a relatively stable soft tissue environment, (3) a surgeon experienced in flexor tendon repair, (4) adequate anesthetic condition of the patient, and (5) appropriate supportive staff (operating room personnel). If all of these conditions are met, primary repair may be performed allowing accurate anatomic alignment and quicker rehabilitation. Delayed repair is indicated if one or more of these prerequisites are not met.

Textbook: Page 1472 ANSWER: A, B, C, D.

NOTES

NOTES

CHAPTER 19

GYNECOLOGY

1. Which of the following is/are correct regarding the embryology of the female reproductive system?

A. The external genitalia develop from the genital tubercle.
B. The wolffian system regresses.
C. The müllerian system fuses in the midline.
D. The ovaries are derived from the upper müllerian system.
E. The testicle regresses as the female duct system forms.

DISCUSSION: Knowledge of embryology is necessary for proper understanding of gynecology, particularly as it relates to problems such as congenital malformations, hermaphroditism, endocrine interrelationships, and generative neoplasms. The external genitalia develop from the genital tubercle. If there is no genetic material for testicle formation, then there is neither androgen nor müllerian inhibiting factor produced by a testicle. In this setting the wolffian duct regresses, and the müllerian system grows. The müllerian system then fuses in the midline to form the upper vagina, cervix, and uterus. Resorption of the midline septum must occur for the single intact structures normally seen. The ovary forms after migration of primordial germ cells to the genital ridge and their subsequent development into primordial follicles. The testicle is not present and does not regress as the female duct system forms in the normal female.

Textbook: Pages 1493–1494 ANSWER: A, B, C.

2. The vascularity of the female reproductive system includes:

A. The middle sacral veins, which empty into the middle colic vein.
B. The uterine arteries, which arise from the hypogastric arteries.
C. The uterine veins, which empty into the inferior epigastric veins.
D. The ovarian arteries, which arise from the aorta.
E. The ovarian veins, which empty into the vena cava.

DISCUSSION: The primary vasculature of the female reproductive system includes the ovarian artery and vein and the uterine artery and vein. The ovarian arteries both arise from the aorta, while the right ovarian vein empties into the vena cava and the left ovarian vein empties into the left renal vein. The uterine arteries are derived from the hypogastric arteries (internal iliac arteries), and the venous return from the uterine system is via the hypogastric veins, the common iliac veins, to the vena cava. Of particular concern is the close proximity of ureter and uterine artery and vein, which pass just above the ureter, approximately 2 to 3 cm. lateral to the uterine cervix. This makes the ureter vulnerable to injury if caution is not exercised in clamping and ligating the uterine vessels.

Textbook: Page 1496 ANSWER: B, D.

3. Which of the following statements describe important endocrine mechanisms in human ovulation?

A. Gonadotropin-releasing hormone (GnRH) release in the hypothalamus is controlled by the neuromodulators (opioids, prostaglandins, and catechol estrogen).
B. Pulsatile release of GnRH is important in causing the proper secretion of follicle-stimulating hormone (FSH) and luteinizing hormone (LH).
C. FSH and LH are necessary for normal ovulatory function.
D. Excessive amounts of androgen inhibit hypothalamic control of pituitary secretion.
E. Ovarian estrogen is produced principally by the ovarian stroma.

DISCUSSION: The ovulatory endocrine process in women is quite complex. Cells in the hypothalamus serve as the primary control center for the reproductive endocrine system. The system is dormant until late childhood, when activation begins; and neuromodulators activate the production of GnRH, which is transmitted by the hypophyseal portal system to the anterior lobe of the pituitary. There, GnRH causes the appropriate pulsatile release of FSH and LH necessary to cause normal ovulatory function. Excessive amounts of androgen inhibit hypothalamic control of pituitary secretion and are associated with disordered ovulatory kinetics. FSH and LH cause 17-beta estradiol production, primarily from the theca interna cells and the parafollicular apparatus. Estrogen is the feedback hormone on hypothalamic control of the ovulatory process, but it also stimulates growth of endometrium, myometrium, other tissues of müllerian origin, the vulva, the breast, and there is increasing evidence to suggest bone and blood vessel function.

Textbook: Pages 1497–1498 ANSWER: A, B, C, D.

4. Which of the following statements is/are correct as related to pathology of the vulva?

A. Vitiligo of vulvar skin is no different than the same lesion in other areas.
B. Whitened or thickened areas of the vulva should undergo Pap cytology study.
C. The primary therapy of vulvar cancer is surgical.
D. Vulvar cancer is spread by hematogenous dissemination.
E. Leukoplakia of the vulva is associated with an increased risk of vulvar cancer.

DISCUSSION: The vulva is subject to a variety of medical problems, including trauma, allergy, inflammatory conditions, infections, degenerative changes, and neoplasia. The vulva is rich in pigment, which increases in pregnancy. Vitiligo of the vulvar skin is no different from the same lesion in other sites, nor does it require treatment. On the other hand, leukoplakia or other degenerative diseases tend to be associated with hypertrophy, whitening, thickening, and even ulceration. These lesions should be subjected to vulvar biopsy, as genital cytology (Pap) is notoriously inaccurate. If cancer is detected, the primary therapy is surgical. Vulvar cancer spreads by lymphatic dissemination. Patients with leukoplakia of the vulva do have an increased risk of vulvar cancer if the area is not appropriately treated. Varicose veins of the vulva are often found and associated with varicosities of the lower extremities. A severe direct blow to the vulva may be complicated by subcutaneous hematoma formation, which may dissect widely beneath the fascia of the vulva and require surgical evacuation.

Textbook: Pages 1502–1505 ANSWER: A, C, E.

5. Which of the following statements about defects in support of female pelvic structures is/are correct?

A. Cystocele, rectocele, and enterocele are hernias.
B. Stress urinary incontinence is usually due to altered neurologic control of bladder function.
C. Culdoplasty should be considered only after hysterectomy by the abdominal route.
D. Urodynamic testing is indicated for women with urinary incontinence.
E. Uterine prolapse can only be treated by hysterectomy.

DISCUSSION: Defects in pelvic support are common problems for women. These are accentuated by vaginal childbearing, which sharply distends the pelvic supporting structures, exposing them to defects in support. Cystocele, rectocele, and enterocele are vaginal hernias. Stress urinary incontinence is usually due to loss of support of the urethrovesical angle, not to altered neurologic control. More commonly, this yields a neurogenic bladder, which is associated with overflow incontinence. In repairing pelvic defects, it is important to close the cul-de-sac to reduce the risk of subsequent enterocele. This should be done after abdominal or vaginal hysterectomy. For patients with urinary incontinence, careful examination and urodynamic testing are important parts of assessment. Increasingly, it is indicated in the assessment of all patients with urinary incontinence before attempts at therapy. Uterine prolapse can be treated by hysterectomy, but it may also be treated by the use of pessaries in patients who are not good operative risks. Usually surgical therapy of uterine prolapse or other hernias of the pelvic structures is not done until after childbearing is completed.

Textbook: Pages 1506–1507 ANSWER: A, D.

6. Which of the following statements regarding Papanicolaou genital cytology is/are true?

A. One should start Pap smears by age 18—or earlier if a woman becomes sexually active.
B. Exfoliated cells are obtained by gentle scraping of the cervix and aspiration, spread evenly on a glass slide, and immediately placed in fixative.
C. Cytologic studies should never be used as an indication for surgical or irradiation therapy.
D. Pap smears are quite reliable to diagnose or exclude neoplastic lesions of the cervix or endometrium.

DISCUSSION: Genital malignancies account for approximately 20% of neoplasms in women. Pap cytology provides an established method for screening for such changes, even before they are malignant or premalignant. Thus, early detection and therapy should be—and has been—associated with falling rates of reproductive malignancy. In the absence of symptoms (pain, abnormal bleeding) Pap smears should be initiated whenever a woman becomes sexually active or by age 18. Most authors advise yearly smears thereafter, although some suggest that after three consecutive, normal yearly smears they may be done less frequently. Proper technique for obtaining a Pap smear includes gentle scraping of the transitional zone of the cervix and aspirations of the pool of fluid in the posterior fornix. These materials are promptly spread thinly on a glass slide. *Immediate* placement in fixative is mandatory to avoid air drying. Cytologic studies are clues to abnormalities that must be sought further by biopsy. Only on histologic diagnosis should therapeutic surgical or irradiation therapy be initiated. Pap smears are quite reliable for cervical or vaginal neoplasms (90%) but very inaccurate for lesions higher in the reproductive tract. If frankly invasive cancer of the cervix is present, the false-negative rate is increased, probably as a result of increased secretions. Thus, any visible lesion of the cervix should be biopsied, even if cytology is benign.

Textbook: Pages 1500–1501 ANSWER: A, B, C.

7. Müllerian agenesis and androgen insensitivity are both associated with absence of the vagina, cervix, and uterus. Regarding these conditions, which of the following statements is/are correct?

A. Chromosome studies are indicated for all women with congenital absence of the vagina.

B. Urologic evaluation should be performed in all women with vaginal agenesis.
C. In patients with androgen insensitivity the gonads should be excised at puberty.
D. Patients with müllerian agenesis have normal ovaries *in situ.*

DISCUSSION: Congenital absence of the vagina, cervix, and uterus is a relatively unusual condition. It is often detected in the evaluation of primary amenorrhea in a young woman who has otherwise gone through a normal puberty. The two conditions associated with it are müllerian agenesis and androgen insensitivity. Leukocytic karyotyping is the primary test used to differentiate these conditions. In androgen insensitivity, the karyotype is 46,XY, whereas in müllerian agenesis a normal female karyotype (46,XX) is found. Buccal smears and serum testosterone levels are useful but not as accurate. Urologic evaluation (intravenous pyelography) is needed for patients with müllerian agenesis because up to 50% will be found to have abnormalities, some severe. Urologic anomalies are rarely found in patients with androgen insensitivity, and urologic testing is not mandatory. Most authors advise leaving the gonads *in situ* through puberty in patients with androgen insensitivity, then removing them in the late teens. Testicular neoplasms occur in about 25% of these women but only very rarely before the third decade of life. Patients with müllerian agenesis have normal ovaries *in situ*, and these do not need to be removed. In fact, these ovaries function quite normally in hormone production and ovulation. Such women may provide oocytes (through ultrasound-guided oocyte harvest) for *in vitro* fertilization and, with a surrogate who would carry the pregnancy, can become genetic mothers.

Textbook: Page 1502 ANSWER: A, D.

8. Which of the following statements is/are correct concerning vulvovaginal infections?

A. *Candida* vulvovaginitis is commonly seen after systemic antibiotic therapy.
B. Bacterial vaginosis is confirmed by finding "clue cells" on wet preparations.
C. The diagnosis of trichomoniasis is usually made by culture.
D. Gonococcal infections are usually associated with vaginal discharge and irritation.

DISCUSSION: Vulvovaginal infections are very common problems. Inflammation can occur from protozoan, fungal, bacterial, or viral infection and also from deficiencies of estrogen. *Candida albicans* is the most common vaginal infection and is associated with systemic antibiotic use, diabetes mellitus, and oral contraceptive use. Other causes of vulvovaginitis include bacterial vaginosis, a symbiotic infection between anaerobic bacteria and *Gardnerella* species. The diagnosis of bacterial vaginosis is confirmed by finding clue cells on wet preps of vaginal secretions. Trichomoniasis is caused by a protozoan, probably primarily transmitted sexually. The diagnosis of trichomoniasis is also based on wet prep. Gonococcal infections are rarely associated with vaginal discharge in adult women but may cause such problems if contracted by a child.

Textbook: Pages 1505–1506 ANSWER: A, B.

9. Which of the following statements about neoplasms of the vagina is/are correct?

A. Dysplasia of the vagina may be the source of abnormal Pap smears, even if the cervix is absent.
B. Intraepithelial carcinoma of the vagina is usually associated with abnormal bleeding, most often occurring post-contact.
C. Most vaginal carcinomas are adenocarcinomas.
D. The best treatment for vaginal carcinoma is usually irradiation.

DISCUSSION: Neoplastic lesions of the vagina are less common than similar lesions of the cervix or vulva but exhibit similar types of change. Lower genital tract neoplasia is often multicentric in origin, and neoplasia or carcinoma *in situ* may develop in any one or all of these structures. Dysplasia of the vagina may be the source of abnormal Pap smears, with or without the presence of the cervix or uterus. Dysplasia and intraepithelial carcinoma of the vagina cause no specific symptoms and are usually suspected from abnormalities of Pap smears. Most vaginal carcinomas are epidermoid (squamous) lesions. Rarely, melanocarcinoma, sarcoma, and mesonephric adenocarcinoma may be found. Adenocarcinomas are more commonly seen in women who were exposed to diethylstilbestrol (DES) while *in utero*. Treatment of vaginal carcinoma may be by surgery or irradiation, but most prefer irradiation. Exenterative surgery may be used for primary therapy or therapy for recurrence, but results of primary surgical therapy are not as good as those achieved with irradiation, and the operative and postoperative morbidity and mortality are significant.

Textbook: Page 1506 ANSWER: A, D.

10. Which of the following statements is/are correct regarding carcinoma of the cervix?

A. Carcinoma of the cervix is the second most common pelvic malignancy.
B. Invasive carcinoma of the cervix should be a preventable disease.
C. There are no gross lesions or symptoms of carcinoma *in situ* of the cervix.
D. Appropriate therapy for microinvasive carcinoma of the cervix is routine abdominal or vaginal hysterectomy with removal of the upper 2 to 3 cm. of the vagina.
E. More than half of patients who die from cervical carcinoma die because of ureteral obstruction.

DISCUSSION: Carcinoma of the cervix has now become the second most common gynecologic malignancy (endometrial carcinoma being first). This decline in frequency is due primarily to enhanced screening and the development of effective therapies for lesions of lesser severity and greater curability. Through widespread use of Pap cytologic screening, adequate evaluation, and various therapies (cryosurgery, laser ablation, conization, hysterectomy), invasive carcinomas of the cervix should become a preventable disease. There are no symptoms or gross lesions of carcinoma *in situ* of the cervix. It is detected only by Pap smears or found by biopsy. There has been considerable debate as to both the diagnosis and the treatment of microinvasive carcinoma of the cervix, a condition in which carcinoma *in situ* exists and there is less than 3 mm. of invasion from the basement membrane. Data showing lack of lymphatic metastasis have led to effective treatment of patients as if the lesions were only carcinoma *in situ*. Thus, hysterectomy with excision of the upper vagina is considered appropriate. The most common cause of patient death from carcinoma of the cervix is by direct extension to adjacent pelvic structures. More than 50% of patients who die with cervical cancer die of ureteral obstruction and uremia.

Textbook: Pages 1508–1511 ANSWER: A, B, C, D, E.

11. Which of the following statements is/are correct regarding pelvic infections (pelvic inflammatory disease or PID) in women?

A. Gonorrhea is by far the most common cause of primary pelvic infection.
B. Severe tenderness is associated with cervical manipulation in most patients with acute PID.
C. The absence of significant peritoneal signs and fever may allow outpatient treatment of acute PID.
D. "Test of cure" by repeat culture must be done after treatment of all gonococcal infections.
E. Infertility due to tubal damage and adhesive disease follows acute PID in approximately 5% of patients.

DISCUSSION: *Chlamydia* and *Neisseria gonorrhoeae* are, together, the most common causes of acute PID. Other causes include pelvic surgery and use of an intrauterine contraceptive device. *Chlamydia* may account for up to 40% of such cases. The signs and symptoms of acute pelvic infection are those of pelvic peritonitis. Fever and leukocytosis are less certain signs. Exquisite tenderness is usually present with cervical manipulation, and bilaterality of adnexal tenderness is an important diagnostic finding. The diagnosis usually rests upon cervical smear and culture. Laparoscopy may be needed to establish accurately the diagnosis, particularly to differentiate PID from appendicitis. Therapy of acute PID is based on the severity of peritonitis and fever. If significant peritonitis or fever is present, then hospitalization and intravenous antibiotic therapy is indicated. In a relatively asymptomatic patient treatment can be accomplished on an outpatient basis. In all patients treated for acute PID, a follow-up culture should be done approximately 1 week after treatment to provide a "test of cure." Each separate episode of acute PID causes an approximately 15% to 20% risk of secondary infertility. The incidence of ectopic pregnancy is increased approximately threefold in patients with a history of PID.

Textbook: Pages 1514–1515 ANSWER: B, C, D.

12. Which of the following statements is/are true of ectopic or intrauterine pregnancy?

A. The incidence of ectopic pregnancy has increased and is approximately 3 in 100 births.
B. In a normal pregnancy, before 12 weeks' gestation, human chorionic gonadotropin (hCG) levels double approximately every 48 hours.
C. Pelvic ultrasound will usually demonstrate an intrauterine pregnancy at hCG levels of 750 to 1000 mIU per ml.
D. Treatment of unruptured tubal ectopic pregnancy is usually salpingectomy.
E. In patients who have previously had an ectopic pregnancy the likelihood of another pregnancy being ectopic is approximately 10%.

DISCUSSION: An ectopic pregnancy is one in which the ovum implants outside the uterine cavity. The incidence of ectopic pregnancy has steadily increased and now accounts for approximately 3 in 100 births. This increase is likely due to increased rates of acute pelvic infections but probably also to enhanced diagnostic capabilities. The contemporary evaluation of possible ectopic pregnancy includes an integrated use of serial, quantified hCG levels and pelvic ultrasound. HCG levels usually double every 48 hours during the first 80 days of normal pregnancy. Less rapid increases are more likely seen in abnormal pregnancies, including ectopic gestations. Pelvic ultrasound is useful in the evaluation of ectopic pregnancy, not by demonstrating the actual ectopic pregnancy but in documenting an intrauterine pregnancy if one is present. Normal intrauterine pregnancy should be documentable by transvaginal ultrasound when serum hCG levels exceed 2000 mIU per ml. Treatment of unruptured tubal ectopic pregnancy is usually by linear salpingostomy (done by laparotomy or laparoscopy) rather than by salpingectomy, as was usually done in years past. In women who do (or may) desire to preserve fertility, all possible efforts should be made to leave at least the uterus and one ovary so future fertility might be allowed by the newer reproductive technologies. Tubal disease or damage is rarely unilateral. Thus, patients who have had one ectopic pregnancy have a threefold increased risk (10%) that another pregnancy will be ectopic.

Textbook: Pages 1517–1518 ANSWER: A, B, E.

NOTES

NOTES

CHAPTER 20

THE URINARY SYSTEM

1. The most ominous sign or symptom of urinary system disease is:

A. Urinary frequency.
B. Pyuria.
C. Pneumaturia.
D. Dysuria.
E. Hematuria.

DISCUSSION: While urinary frequency (voiding more than three to five times daily) or dysuria (painful voiding) may be a sign of malignant disease, they are more commonly associated with nonmalignant inflammatory disease, neurologic disease, or calculous disease of the urinary tract. Pyuria (pus in the urine) is most commonly associated with infection and not malignancy. Pneumaturia (air or gas in the urine) indicates a fistula between bowel and the urinary tract or infection by fermination in diabetic urine. Hematuria (blood in the urine) is most worrisome. While this may be produced by infection or by calculous disease, it is most commonly associated with malignant disease in the absence of associated signs or symptoms such as pyuria, frequency, and dysuria. Thus, of the ones mentioned, hematuria is the most ominous single sign or symptom.

Textbook: Pages 1526–1528 ANSWER: E.

2. A patient with acute urinary tract infection (UTI) usually presents with:

A. Chills and fever.
B. Flank pain.
C. Nausea and vomiting.
D. 5 to 10 white blood cells per high-power field (hpf) in the uncentrifuged urine specimen.
E. Painful urination.

DISCUSSION: Cystitis or infection of the bladder is the most common UTI. Lower UTI, or cystitis, is an infection in the bladder. Painful urination and frequency are the most common presenting complaints. Hematuria may occur, but is associated with painful urination and frequency. Flank pain, fever, chills, nausea, and vomiting usually occur only when the infection involves the kidney. An acute UTI is identified in unspun urine only when there are more than 10 leukocytes per hpf in the unspun urine. The normal urine may have as many as 10 WBC/per hpf without being infected.

Textbook: Page 1532 ANSWER: E.

3. Renal adenocarcinomas:

A. Are of transitional cell origin.
B. Usually are associated with anemia.
C. Are difficult to diagnose.
D. Are extremely radiosensitive.
E. Frequently are signaled by gross hematuria.

DISCUSSION: Renal adenocarcinomas arise from the renal tubular cells and not from the transitional cells that line the collecting system of the kidney. Although one fifth of all patients with renal cancer may present with anemia, the most common presenting symptom is hematuria, either gross or microscopic. Ultrasonography may confirm that a renal lesion is either cystic or solid but computed tomography (CT) is probably the most accurate imaging study for diagnosing the disease. Renal adenocarcinoma is little sensitive to current chemotherapeutic agents. Radiotherapy plays almost no role in the management of the primary tumor. Operation is the treatment of choice when the disease is confined to the kidney itself or when it has extended just outside the renal capsule. An operation has little effect once the disease is extended to adjacent structures or to regional lymph nodes.

Textbook: Pages 1536–1538 ANSWER: E.

4. Ureteral obstruction:

A. Is associated with hematuria.
B. Is associated with deterioration of renal function and rising blood urea nitrogen (BUN) and creatinine values.
C. Is commonly caused by a urinary tract calculus.
D. Usually requires open surgical relief of the obstruction.
E. Is usually associated with infection behind the obstruction.

DISCUSSION: Ureteral obstruction produces loss of renal function when there is only one renal unit and the ureter is obstructed or when obstruction is bilateral. Ureteral obstruction often is best identified by either intravenous pyelography (IVP) or retrograde pyelography, which allows one to identify the specific site of obstruction. Calculous disease is the most common cause of ureteral obstruction. Ureteral obstruction is not a surgical emergency that requires open surgical intervention, but it may be relieved by retrograde or antegrade passage of a double-J stent to bypass the obstruction, permitting orderly nonemergent identification of the cause of obstruction and selection of a treatment process.

Textbook: Pages 1541–1542 ANSWER: C.

5. Stress urinary incontinence:

A. Is principally a disease of young females.
B. Occurs only in males.
C. Is associated with urinary frequency and urgency.
D. May be corrected by surgically increasing the volume of the bladder.
E. Is a disease of aging produced by shortening of the urethra.

DISCUSSION: Stress urinary incontinence is seen principally in older females and is produced by pelvic floor relaxation with shortening of urethral length. The symptom of stress urinary incontinence is urinary leakage produced by an increase in intra-abdominal pressure, as with straining to lift or to laugh. Urgency and frequency are symptoms of urge incontinence, not stress incontinence. Stress incontinence classically is not seen either in males or in young females who have good pelvic floor support.

Textbook: Page 1547 ANSWER: E.

6. Which of the following is/are true of blunt renal trauma?

A. Blunt renal trauma and penetrating renal injuries are managed similarly.
B. Blunt renal trauma with urinary extravasation always requires surgical exploration.
C. Blunt renal trauma must be evaluated by contrast studies using either IVP or CT.
D. Blunt renal trauma requires exploration only when the patient exhibits hemodynamic instability.
E. Any kidney fractured by blunt renal trauma must be explored.

DISCUSSION: Blunt renal trauma should be explored. Only those who have gross hematuria need undergo contrast studies. Microscopic hematuria is no longer an indication for contrast evaluation. Patients who have blunt renal trauma need to undergo exploration only if they are hemodynamically unstable. Conservative management in the absence of hemodynamic instability is the current trend. All penetrating injuries should undergo exploration.

Textbook: Pages 1539–1540 ANSWER: D.

7. Carcinoma of the bladder:

A. Is primarily of squamous cell origin.
B. Is preferentially treated by radiation.
C. May be treated conservatively by use of intravesical agents even if it invades the bladder muscle.
D. May mimic an acute UTI with irritability and hematuria.
E. Is preferentially treated by partial cystectomy.

DISCUSSION: Carcinoma of the bladder is primarily of transitional cell origin, arising from the transitional epithelium that lines the bladder. It may be confused with an acute UTI by producing urgency, frequency, and hematuria. Bladder carcinoma may be treated conservatively using intravesical agents if the tumor is intraepithelial in origin and does not invade through the basement membrane. Neither radiation nor chemotherapy is the treatment of choice for disease that invades the muscle of the bladder. Partial cystectomy may be chosen only when the disease is focal and there are no mucosal changes in other parts of the bladder.

Textbook: Pages 1548–1550 ANSWER: D.

8. The *major* blood supply to the testes comes through the:

A. Hypogastric arteries.
B. Pudendal arteries.
C. External spermatic arteries.
D. Internal spermatic arteries.

DISCUSSION: Testes arise from portions of the wolffian bodies on the genital ridge close to the kidneys; therefore, the major blood vessels from the testes arises from the aorta just below the renal arteries and are termed the *internal spermatic arteries*. Secondary blood supply to the testes comes from the artery of the vas deferens, and a small branch from the epigastric artery termed the *external spermatic artery* forms during descent of the testes from the abdomen to the scrotum. The surgical importance of this phenomenon is that operations involving the region of the renal arteries may sacrifice the internal spermatic artery. If the two other arteries are intact, the testes will survive; however, if the patient has had a vasectomy and the artery of the vas has been sacrificed, there is a possibility of testicular atrophy, since the testicle will have to be totally dependent on the arterial supply derived from the small external spermatic artery.

Textbook: Page 1553 ANSWER: D.

9. Patients who have undergone operations for benign prostatic hypertrophy or hyperplasia:

A. Require routine rectal examinations to detect the development of carcinoma of the prostate.
B. Do not need routine prostate examinations.
C. Have a lesser incidence of carcinoma of the prostate.
D. Have a greater incidence of carcinoma of the prostate.

DISCUSSION: Patients who have undergone operations for benign prostatic hyperplasia or hypertrophy have had only the inner portion of the prostate removed, which consists of the periurethral glandular structures that give rise to hyperplasia and hypertrophy. The posterior segment of the prostate, which is compressed by the anterior (inner) portion, comprises the surgical capsule and is left behind. The posterior portion of the prostate gland is the most frequent site of origin of prostate cancer. There is no difference in the incidence of carcinoma of the prostate in patients with benign prostatic hypertrophy and those without benign prostatic hypertrophy or those who have and have not undergone operation for prostatic hypertrophy. Since prostate carcinoma can develop at any time in a patient's life, routine examinations and prostate-specific antigen assay are the most efficient methods of detecting this disease.

Textbook: Pages 1555, 1564–1566 ANSWER: A.

10. The male contribution to a couple's infertility is approximately:

A. 10%.
B. 25%.
C. 50%.
D. 75%.

DISCUSSION: In the United States of America it has been estimated that approximately 15% of couples have difficulty with conception. Adequate evaluation of the marital unit for infertility demands assessment of the male partner since infertile status may be attributed to the male as much as 50% of the time. A full evaluation of the male partner is important to avoid extended fruitless evaluation and management of the female partner when the male is infertile.

Textbook: Page 1556 ANSWER: C.

11. To maximize fertility potential, orchidopexy for cryptorchidism should be done before:

A. Age 15 years.
B. Age 12 years.
C. Marriage.
D. Age 2 years.

DISCUSSION: The testes are exquisitely sensitive to temperature; therefore there is progressive deterioration of testes that are not within the scrotum. Cryptorchid testes, whether they be in the inguinal canal, in an intra-abdominal position, or in an ectopic position, will undergo progressive spermatogenic failure, although adequate amounts of androgens may be produced and secreted. The timing of orchidopexy has been moved progressively backward, and now the recommendation is that orchidopexy should be accomplished before age 2 years, to maximize the possibility of production of spermatozoa of normal quantity and quality. In cases of unilateral cryptorchidism the matter of surgical exploration is less critical; however, to provide maximum potential for both testes, the earlier cryptorchidism is surgically corrected the better are the chances for normal spermatogenesis.

Textbook: Pages 1556, 1557 ANSWER: D.

12. Within the age group 10 to 35 years, the incidence of carcinoma of the testis in males with intra-abdominal testes is:

A. Equal to that in the general population.
B. Five times greater than that in the general population.
C. Ten times greater than that in the general population.
D. Twenty times greater than that in the general population.

DISCUSSION: The incidence of carcinoma of the testis is greater in patients who have cryptorchidism, whether corrected or not; because of this, routine self-examination by patients who have undergone operation for cryptorchidism is important. For patients who have uncorrected intra-abdominal testes it is estimated that the incidence of the development of carcinoma of the testis in the age group 10 to 35 years is approximately 20 times greater than that for the general population. If cryptorchidism is diagnosed after the age of 10 to 12 years, orchiectomy may be the preferred treatment, since such testes rarely exhibit normal function, despite adequate scrotal placement, and put the patient at great risk for an intra-abdominal neoplasm that will be difficult to diagnose.

Textbook: Page 1557 ANSWER: D.

13. The appropriate surgical treatment for suspected carcinoma of the testis is:

A. Transscrotal percutaneous biopsy.
B. Transscrotal open biopsy.
C. Repeated examinations.
D. Inguinal exploration, control of the spermatic cord, biopsy, and radical orchectomy if tumor is confirmed.

DISCUSSION: If, after physical examination, and even scrotal ultrasound, a tumor of the testicle is still suspected, the appropriate surgical treatment is high inguinal exploration with control of the cord, delivery of the testicle onto a protected field, biopsy if necessary, and then orchiectomy at the level of the internal ring if tumor is confirmed. Transscrotal manipulations, whether they be percutaneous or open, are to be condemned because of the possibility of tumor spillage with the ultimate necessity for hemiscrotectomy to control local recurrence. Certainly, repeated examinations over a very short period of time are appropriate, but no time should be lost if there is true suspicion of a testicular tumor. Before the high inguinal exploration it is helpful to obtain serum levels of the beta subunit of human chorionic gonadotropin and alpha-fetoprotein, which are important tumor markers. Surgical exploration should not be delayed until the actual laboratory values are determined, as they are important to the longitudinal course of the patient and not necessarily to the diagnosis.

Textbook: Pages 1558–1559 ANSWER: D.

14. If torsion of the testicle is suspected, surgical exploration:

A. Can be delayed 24 hours and limited to the affected side.
B. Can be delayed but should include the asymptomatic side.
C. Should be immediate and limited to the affected side.
D. Should be immediate and include the asymptomatic side.

DISCUSSION: Torsion of the testicle should be corrected as soon as possible after the diagnosis is entertained. Incomplete torsion can cause partial strangulation, the effects of which may be overcome if surgical intervention is accomplished within 12 hours, whereas severe torsion with complete compromise of the blood supply results in loss of the testis unless surgical intervention occurs within approximately 4 hours. The contralateral scrotum should also be explored at the time of the operation, since the primary anatomic defect—insufficient attachment of the testicle to the scrotal sidewall—most often is a bilateral phenomenon. If the contralateral scrotum is not explored, the patient runs a very high risk of undergoing torsion on the other side and the possible complication of loss of both testes.

Textbook: Pages 1558, 1559–1560 ANSWER: D.

15. Epididymitis, either unilateral or bilateral, in a prepubertal male:

A. Is a frequent diagnosis.
B. Can be dealt with on an outpatient basis.
C. Is a major scrotal problem in this age group.
D. Is a rare phenomenon.

DISCUSSION: Epididymitis can occur in prepubescent males, but it is a rare phenomenon and usually occurs only in patients with chronic UTI, obstructed urethra, or very high voiding pressure. The diagnosis of epididymitis in the prepubertal male should be reviewed with suspicion because one of the more common causes of the clinical situation that presents as epididymitis is torsion of the testicle. If there is any concern about the validity of the diagnosis, the patient should undergo scrotal exploration. Epididymitis will not be compromised by surgical exploration, but delay in surgical exploration leads to loss of the testicle if the problem is torsion.

Textbook: Page 1561 ANSWER: D.

16. Patients with prostatitis, especially acute suppurative prostatitis:

A. Should have residual urine measured by intermittent catheterization.
B. Should have bladder decompression by urethral catheter.
C. Should have repeated prostatic massage.
D. Should have no transurethral instrumentation if possible.

DISCUSSION: Acute suppurative prostatitis should be treated with vigorous antibiotic therapy with broad-spectrum agents initiated immediately and changed in response to results of culture and sensitivity studies. Urethral instrumentation and repeated prostate examination should not be done, if at all possible, since sepsis is not unusual after either diagnostic examination or urethral catheterization. If the patient does need to have the bladder decompressed, it is beneficial to use a suprapubic catheter rather than a urethral catheter.

Textbook: Page 1563 ANSWER: D.

17. Benign prostatic hypertrophy with bladder neck obstruction:

A. Is always accompanied by significant symptoms.
B. Is best diagnosed by endoscopy and urodynamic studies.
C. Is easily diagnosed by the symptoms of frequency, hesitancy, and nocturia.
D. Is always accompanied by residual urine volume greater than 100 ml.

DISCUSSION: Benign prostatic hypertrophy with bladder neck obstruction is difficult, in some patients, to diagnose as they are totally asymptomatic, even if they have residual urines of greater than 1000 ml. or renal compromise consisting of the syndrome of so-called "silent prostatism."

Textbook: Page 1564 ANSWER: B.

NOTES

NOTES

CHAPTER 21

VASCULAR SURGERY

1. A 55-year-old woman gives a history of tiredness, aching, and a feeling of heaviness in the left lower leg for the past 3 months. These symptoms are relieved by leg elevation. She is also awakened frequently by calf and foot cramping, which is relieved by leg elevation, walking, or massage. On physical examination there are superficial varicosities, nonpitting edema, and a slightly painful, 2 cm. diameter superficial ulcer 5 cm. above and behind the left medial malleolus. What is the most appropriate diagnosis?

A. Isolated symptomatic varicose veins.
B. Superficial lymphatic obstruction.
C. Deep venous insufficiency.
D. Arterial insufficiency.
E. Incompetent perforating veins.

DISCUSSION: The most common symptoms associated with venous insufficiency are aching, swelling, and night cramps of the involved leg, which often occur after periods of sitting or inactive standing. Leg elevation frequently provides relief of symptoms due to venous insufficiency, while it increases pain due to arterial insufficiency. Although edema can occur with varicose veins alone, usually it is associated with deep venous abnormalities and incompetent perforators. In such cases, ulcers usually are located above and posterior to the malleoli, reinforcing their relationship with perforator abnormalities. The ulcers associated with arterial insufficiency may occur anywhere on the lower leg, eventually penetrate the fascia, and are more painful than venous ulcers.

Textbook: Pages 1588–1589 ANSWER: C.

2. The best treatment plan for the patient described in the preceding question should include:

A. Varicose vein ligation and stripping as soon as possible.
B. Ulcer débridement, vein stripping, and skin grafting.
C. Ligation of the medial perforating veins.
D. Transposition of saphenous vein valve.
E. Leg elevation, external Unna boot support, and ambulation without standing.

DISCUSSION: Operative treatment of venous insufficiency is in most instances an adjunct after failure of aggressive conservative management. Leg elevation, active exercise, and elastic compression form the cornerstones of nonoperative management. The goals of compression are to relieve symptoms and reduce swelling. The indications for superficial vein ligation and stripping are moderate to severe symptoms without other signs of deep venous insufficiency. If ulceration persists despite appropriate conservative management, ligation of the underlying incompetent perforators helps ulcer recurrence, and split-thickness skin grafting provides immediate coverage and healing of the ulcer. The patient must, however, comply with a program of external stocking support and prevention of leg edema since the underlying venous pathophysiology remains and ulcers tend to recur.

Textbook: Pages 1588–1589 ANSWER: E.

3. In patients who develop a documented episode of deep venous thrombosis (DVT) the most significant long-term sequela is:

A. Claudication.
B. Recurrent foot infections.
C. Development of stasis ulcer.
D. Pulmonary embolization.
E. Diminished arterial perfusion.

DISCUSSION: The increased hydrostatic pressure from incompetent venous valves following DVT predisposes to erythrocyte extravasation, hemosiderin deposition, and brown pigmentation around the ankle. Although the edema that occurs with deep venous insufficiency can predispose to skin infections, these usually are located about the ankle and resolve with adequate short-term care. When patients with a history of DVT are followed beyond 10 years, as many as 80% ultimately develop venous stasis ulcers. While there may be recurrence of DVT in a minority of patients, the incidence of pulmonary embolization is no greater than with the initial episode. Even in a leg severely affected by venous stasis changes, the arterial circulation is unimpaired unless there is concomitant arterial obstructive disease.

Textbook: Page 1589 ANSWER: C.

4. A 28-year-old woman developed a painful thrombosis of a superficial varix in the left upper calf 2 days previously. After spending the 2 days in bed with her leg elevated, she felt better and the tenderness resolved; however, when out of bed she developed a twinge of right-sided chest pain when walking and a feeling of heaviness in the calf. Which treatment is most appropriate?

A. Check for leg swelling, tenderness, and Homan's sign, and obtain a Doppler ultrasound study.
B. Begin antibiotics for a probable secondary bacterial infection.
C. Order emergency venography, and if it is abnormal, begin heparin administration.
D. Begin ambulation and discontinue bed rest that probably caused muscle pain by hyperextension of the knee.
E. If there is no pain on dorsiflexion of the left foot reassure her, since a negative Homan's sign precludes the diagnosis of DVT.

DISCUSSION: Associated DVT may occur during treatment of superficial venous thrombosis, especially if the process is near the groin or popliteal fossa. Although a positive Homan's sign or calf, popliteal, or groin pain is suggestive of DVT, clinical examination alone may be incorrect in more than 50% of cases. Noninvasive tests, including Doppler ultrasonography, are accurate for diagnosing DVT in the thigh but are less dependable in the calf. Emergency venography performed on an outpatient basis remains the most accurate and cost-effective technique for diagnosing DVT of the calf veins. Because 85% of pulmonary emboli arise from the lower extremity, early diagnosis and aggressive treatment are important.

Textbook: Pages 1590–1591 ANSWER: C.

5. In a 55-year-old grocery store cashier with an 8-month history of leg edema increasing over the course of a work day, associated with moderate to severe lower leg bursting pain, the most appropriate investigative study or studies are:

A. Doppler duplex ultrasound.
B. Brodie-Trendelenburg test.
C. Ascending and descending phlebography.
D. Measurement of ambulatory and resting foot venous pressure.
E. Venous reflux plethysmography.

DISCUSSION: While the Brodie-Trendelenburg test was an early attempt to clinically evaluate valve competence and function, it is neither quantitative nor precise. The development of phlebography allowed anatomic delineation of normal and abnormal veins and, when used in combination with invasive measurement of venous pressures in the foot at rest and on ambulation, helped correlate the venous hypertensive state with postphlebitic changes. Noninvasive plethysmography to quantitate the degree of venous valvular incompetence was more easily accepted; however the combination of B-mode duplex ultrasound (to accurately locate the vein of interest) plus pulsed Doppler flow signal is now the "gold standard" for venous assessment.

Textbook: Pages 1584–1585 ANSWER: A.

6. Which of the following statements are *true* of pulmonary embolism?

A. Most cases occur postoperatively.
B. In the majority of patients pulmonary emboli are ultimately lysed *in situ* without the administration of pharmacologic agents.
C. The preferred therapy for most patients is intravenous heparin.
D. It is generally safe to give thrombolytic agents as early as 48 hours postoperatively.

DISCUSSION: Although many patients develop pulmonary embolism postoperatively, the majority of such lesions reported in most series do not follow operation. These patients develop thromboembolism as a complication of an underlying condition such as congestive heart failure, cerebrovascular accident, malignancy, chronic infection, and a variety of other debilitating diseases. Generally, postoperative patients comprise approximately one third of those with pulmonary embolism. Serial pulmonary scans following pulmonary embolism generally show gradual clearing of the emboli with re-establishment of perfusion in the occluded vessels. Depending on the magnitude of the embolism, most patients show the clearing at the end of a month to 6 weeks. The presence of persistent congestive heart failure, chronic infection, and atelectasis retard thrombolysis. This dissolution of emboli is generally agreed to be caused by naturally circulating thrombolysins. In fewer than 1% of cases the emboli persist and often increase with the passage of time, with the development of chronic pulmonary embolism leading to severe respiratory insufficiency, chronic cor pulmonale, pulmonary hypertension, right ventricular failure, and death. The majority of patients with pulmonary embolism are managed by continuous intravenous heparin. Thrombolytic agents are generally reserved for the management of extensive thromboembolism in patients with a stable cardiovascular system. Thrombolytic agents are generally withheld from postoperative patients until at least the fifth postoperative day, or preferably later. Earlier administration of these agents is apt to produce bleeding at the operative site. While it may occasionally be indicated to proceed earlier, it is generally best to wait until the thrombi in the vessels divided at the time of the surgical procedure have become organized.

Textbook: Pages 1594, 1601–1605 ANSWER: B, C.

7. Which of the following can cause a radioactive pulmonary perfusion scan to demonstrate an appearance similar to that of acute pulmonary embolism?

A. Atelectasis.
B. Pneumonitis.
C. Pleural fluid.
D. Emphysematous bullae.

DISCUSSION: It has been shown by routine radioactive pulmonary perfusion scans that atelectasis, pneumonia, pleural fluid, emphysematous bullae, and pulmonary embolism may reduce pulmonary arterial blood flow to the involved segment. For this reason, it is *imperative* simultaneously to obtain chest film to exclude any significant radiopacity, which is usually associated with any defect that causes diminished pulmonary vascular perfusion.

Textbook: Pages 1599–1600 ANSWER: A, B, C, D.

8. In an otherwise healthy male with previously normal pulmonary and cardiac function, how much of the pulmonary vascular bed must usually be occluded to produce an unstable cardiovascular state (shock)?

A. 10%.
B. 20%.
C. 40%.
D. More than 50%.

DISCUSSION: If the patient had normal cardiovascular and respiratory function before the onset of pulmonary embolism, experimental and clinical studies have documented the fact that more than 50% of the pulmonary circulation must be occluded to produce cardiovascular collapse or shock. This can be considered similar to ligation of the pulmonary artery during the course of pneumonectomy, as occlusion by this procedure is also tolerated well, without development of hemodynamic instability. While bronchoconstriction may reduce pulmonary function in the normally perfused lung after embolism, this effect is generally short lived, as demonstrated by pulmonary ventilation scans.

Textbook: Page 1597 ANSWER: D.

9. Lytic therapy in pulmonary embolism:

A. Should precede anticoagulation.
B. Can be considered for all patients.
C. Can be considered for hemodynamically unstable patients.
D. Is indicated for the majority of patients with documented pulmonary embolism.

DISCUSSION: Thrombolytic therapy in pulmonary embolism involves use of streptokinase or urokinase. This therapy is indicated for hemodynamic compromise from documented pulmonary embolism that has not responded to anticoagulation and inotropic support. Additionally, lytic therapy is contraindicated after neurosurgery or cranial trauma and in persons who have a history of internal bleeding or hemorrhagic cerebral infarction. The majority of patients with documented pulmonary embolism do not require lytic therapy.

Textbook: Pages 1603–1604 ANSWER: C.

10. The single most important indication for emergency pulmonary embolectomy is:

A. The likelihood of another episode of embolism.
B. The inability to determine whether the problem is acute pulmonary embolism or acute myocardial infarction.
C. The presence of persistent and intractable hypotension.
D. Pulmonary emphysema.

DISCUSSION: The likelihood of another episode of pulmonary embolism is not an indication for pulmonary embolectomy since recurrent embolism may also be managed nonoperatively in most cases. Myocardial infarction should definitely be ruled out before pulmonary embolectomy is considered. In the presence of intractable cardiopulmonary collapse the only measure apt to correct the condition is emergency pulmonary embolectomy employing extracorporeal circulation. In such instances emboli generally are massive, with more than 50% of the pulmonary arterial circuit being occluded. The presence of cardiac and/or respiratory insufficiency before the attack of embolism is important, as that is apt to mean that a smaller pulmonary embolism is present that can cause serious cardiovascular changes.

Textbook: Pages 1604–1606 ANSWER: C.

11. In prevention of the fat emboli syndrome the primary therapy can be accomplished by which of the following?

A. Systemic anticoagulation achieving a partial thromboplastin time greater than 50 seconds.
B. Intravenous administration of alcohol.
C. Prophylactic administration of methyl prednisolone.
D. Maintaining a serum albumin value greater than 3 gm. per 100 ml. in the days immediately following injury.

DISCUSSION: The mechanism producing fat emboli syndrome is primarily release of free fatty acids that produce a change in the capillary alveolar membrane. Albumin is the primary binder of fatty acids. With serum levels greater than 3 gm. per 100 ml., 99% of the circulating free fatty acid remains in the bound configuration. Alcohol, heparinization, and steroids have been shown to have no direct effect on fat emboli syndrome, and serious side effects are related to their use.

Textbook: Page 1616 ANSWER: D.

12. Significant tachypnea and hypoxia follow development of fat emboli syndrome, and the goal of ventilatory support should be:

A. Keeping the respiratory rate below 30.
B. Preventing respiratory alkalosis.
C. Reversing pulmonary shunting using positive end-expiratory pressure.
D. Maintaining an adequate total volume.

DISCUSSION: The primary defect is increased pulmonary shunting secondary to reduced functional residual capacity. Use of positive end-expiratory pressure reverses this and is the primary goal of therapy.

Textbook: Page 1616 ANSWER: C.

13. Which of the following statements about the role of the endothelium is/are correct?

A. Endothelial cells only mediate vasorelaxation.

B. Endothelial cell–derived nitric oxide (NO) is produced by a constitutive and an inducible NO synthase.
C. The anticoagulant properties of the endothelium reside in its barrier function.
D. A local renin-angiotensin system is found in the walls of arteries and veins.
E. There are no significant differences in the vasomotor characteristic of endothelial cells in the macro- and microcirculation.

DISCUSSION: Endothelial cells have the ability to mediate both contractile (prostanoids, oxygen free radicals, endothelins, angiotensins, and uncharacterized endothelium-derived constriction factors) and relaxant (prostanoids, nitric oxide and nitric oxide–containing compounds, hyperpolarization factor) responses. NO is synthesized from the conversion of L-arginine to citrulline by at least two categories of enzymes—constitutive nitric oxide synthases (cNOS, predominantly membrane bound) and inducible nitric oxide synthases (iNOS, predominantly cytosolic), both of which are calcium- and calmodulin dependent. Constitutive NOS is present in endothelial cells, and following cytokine stimulation endothelial cells also synthesize iNOS. In addition to its basic barrier function, the endothelium regulates intravascular coagulation by three other separate, but related, mechanisms: participation in procoagulant pathways, inhibition of procoagulant proteins, regulation of fibrinolysis and production of thromboregulating compounds. There is a local renin-angiotensin system in the vessel wall of both vein and arteries, and this system is considered important in the maintenance of blood pressure, the control of hypertension, and the response of the vessel wall to injury. In contrast to the macrocirculation, the microcirculation has distinctive vasomotor characteristics. Vessels of the microcirculation are the conduits that are responsible for the local delivery and transfer of cell substrates and metabolites. The endothelium regulates the microvasculature, reacting to the metabolic needs of tissue; it is essential in organ autoregulation and in the responses of these microvasculatures to changes in local blood flow. Reactive hyperemia appears to be dependent on the immediate production of endothelium-derived cyclooxygenase products, predominantly prostaglandin E_2 (PGE_2), as opposed to PGI_2, in the short term.

Textbook: Pages 1620–1623 ANSWER: B, D.

14. Which of the following statements on smooth muscle cells is/are correct?

A. Smooth muscle cells can undergo pheotypic changes in response to injury.
B. Platelet-derived growth factor (PDGF) requires a progression factor to initiate smooth muscle cell growth.
C. NO can be produced by smooth muscle cells.
D. Changes in the composition of the extracellular matrix modulate smooth muscle cell growth.
E. Smooth muscle cells are the principal cell involved in the development of intimal hyperplasia.

DISCUSSION: Smooth muscle cells are the principal cells found in the media of a vessel. They are embedded in a matrix of connective tissue elements and provide mechanical and structural support to the vessel. In addition to their vasoreactive characteristics, smooth muscle cells are capable of synthesizing and secreting elements of the extracellular matrix, particularly proteoglycans. The exact mechanisms whereby smooth muscle cell proliferation is initiated, controlled, reduced, and eventually suppressed are not fully understood. Quiescent vascular smooth muscle cells are well-differentiated cells characterized by an abundance of contractile proteins, predominantly smooth muscle cell actin and myosin but little rough endoplasmic reticulum. Once activated, smooth muscle cells lose their differentiated state, acquire abundant endoplasmic reticulum, and commence the synthesis of extracellular matrix. After cytokine stimulation, smooth muscle cells synthesize iNOS and produce nanomoles of NO for at least 24 hours. Smooth muscle cell proliferation depends on the presence of PDGF, basic fibroblast growth factor (bFGF), and insulin-like growth factor 1 (IGF-1). IGF-1 acts as a progression factor for PDGF in smooth muscle cells, and both *in vivo* and *in vitro* there is synergism between these two growth promoters. Smooth muscle cell growth in the wall can be modulated by various extracellular matrix substances such as collagen (type V), several glycoproteins, and the glycosoaminoglycans. Both NO and prostacyclin inhibit cell proliferation. Intimal hyperplasia is a structural lesion that develops in injured blood vessels after injury and is the result of smooth muscle cell migration into and proliferation within the intima of a blood vessel.

Textbook: Pages 1620–1623 ANSWER: A, B, C, D, E.

15. Which of the following statements correctly characterizes the healing of prosthetic arterial grafts in humans?

A. Complete healing occurs within 3 months of graft implantation.
B. Complete healing occurs within 1 year of graft implantation.
C. Prosthetic grafts do not heal completely in humans.
D. Polytetrafluoroethylene (PTFE) grafts heal completely whereas Dacron grafts do not.
E. Dacron grafts heal completely but PTFE grafts do not.

DISCUSSION: Prosthetic grafts of any kind do not heal completely in humans as they do in experimental animals. Some healing occurs in the perianastomotic regions, but the majority of the graft's luminal surface never develops a living neointima; rather, it remains covered with a compacted layer of fibrin.

Textbook: Page 1634 ANSWER: C.

16. Which of the following adversely influence the patency of lower extremity autogenous vein grafts?

A. Poor arterial outflow from the distal anastomosis of the graft.
B. Diabetes.
C. Small-caliber (less than 4 mm. in diameter) veins.
D. Use of reverse, rather than *in situ*, grafting technique.
E. Grafts performed for limb salvage indications rather than claudication.

DISCUSSION: Small-caliber veins perform poorly as arterial substitutes. The long-term patency of infrainguinal vein grafts is better when the indication for operation is claudication rather than limb salvage and is improved when there is a good outflow tract. Reverse vein and *in situ* bypass have equal patency rates at all levels. Surprisingly, the presence of diabetes has not been shown to negatively affect the patency of autogenous vein infrainguinal arterial bypass.

Textbook: Page 1630 ANSWER: A, C, E.

17. Arterial autografts are:

A. Limited by the length of available artery.
B. When available, always appear to function superiorly to venous autografts.
C. Are the graft of choice for pediatric renal artery grafting.
D. Are performed infrequently.
E. Are immune from the fibrointimal hyperplasia that frequently complicates venous autografts and prosthetic grafts.

DISCUSSION: Arterial autografts have limited but well-established clinical uses. They are the graft of choice for pediatric renal artery revascularizations, as they do not appear to be subject to the aneurysmal dilatation that complicates pediatric renal artery vein bypass. The internal mammary artery autograft provides superior patency for coronary artery bypass as compared with the saphenous vein and is thus a very common arterial autograft procedure. Radial artery autografts for coronary bypass are, however, rapidly narrowed by fibrointimal hyperplasia.

Textbook: Pages 1627–1628 ANSWER: A, C.

18. PTFE grafts:

A. Are a variant of a woven textile graft.
B. Provide patency superior to that with Dacron grafts for suprainguinal revascularization procedures.
C. Provide patency equal to that of autogenous saphenous vein for above-knee femoropopliteal bypass.
D. May be more resistant than Dacron grafts to pseudoaneurysm formation.
E. Are currently the prosthetic graft of choice for hemodialysis access.

DISCUSSION: PTFE grafts are manufactured from a unique polymer extrusion process and are not textile grafts. For most surgeons they are currently the prosthetic graft of choice for hemodialysis access. For suprainguinal bypass, PTFE and Dacron provide comparable patency, although PTFE grafts may be more resistant than Dacron grafts to pseudoaneurysm formation. PTFE at all levels in comparable patients is inferior to good-quality saphenous vein for infrainguinal bypass.

Textbook: Pages 1633–1634 ANSWER: D, E.

19. Which of the following statements about the evaluation of arterial substitutes are correct?

A. A graft is considered to have continued primary patency, even if it requires revision, as long as it has not actually thrombosed.
B. *Secondary patency* refers only to grafts whose patency has been restored following an episode of thrombosis.
C. Patency figures should be derived from life table calculations.
D. Primary patency is the best indicator of the natural history of an arterial substitute.
E. Secondary patency is the best indicator of the natural history of an arterial substitute.

DISCUSSION: Patency is the most important variable in the evaluation of the clinical effectiveness of an arterial substitute, and it should always be derived from life table calculations. Both primary and secondary graft patency are important. Primary patency is the best indicator of the natural history of a graft. A graft remains primarily patent as long as it has not thrombosed or had any graft- or anastomosis-directed procedures. Grafts are considered to be secondarily patent if patency has been restored after an episode of thrombosis or if, in order to maintain patency, operation on a patent graft is directed toward the graft itself or its anastomoses.

Textbook: Page 1627 ANSWER: C, D.

20. Which of the following statements about aneurysms of the sinus of Valsalva is/are true?

A. Aneurysms of the sinus of Valsalva are dilatations of the aortic sinuses that eventually rupture into a cardiac chamber, the pulmonary artery, or the pericardium.
B. The most common cause of an acquired sinus of Valsalva aneurysm is bacterial endocarditis.
C. Congenital aneurysms of the sinus of Valsalva usually cause symptoms long before they rupture.
D. The most common defect associated with congenital sinus of Valsalva aneurysms is aortic insufficiency.
E. The most common symptoms of sinus of Valsalva aneurysm rupture include symptoms caused by obstruction of the ventricular outflow tract, heart block, and embolization.

DISCUSSION: A sinus of Valsalva aneurysm is a dilatation of the aortic sinus that eventually ruptures into a cardiac chamber, the pulmonary artery, or the pericardium. The cause may be either congenital or acquired, and the most common cause of an acquired sinus of Valsalva aneurysm is bacterial endocarditis. The vast majority of sinus of Valsalva aneurysms are asymptomatic before they rupture, but if symptomatic they present as obstruction to either the left or right outflow tract, heart block, or embolization. When sinus of Valsalva aneurysms rupture, they present with symptoms of an acute left-to-right shunt and these include dyspnea, palpitations, and chest pain. Finally, associated defects occur commonly with congenital sinus of Valsalva aneurysms, the most common being ventricular septal defect followed by aortic insufficiency.

Textbook: Pages 1638–1639 ANSWER: A, B.

21. Which statements about treatment for sinus of Valsalva aneurysms are correct?

A. Close observation is appropriate for patients who have an asymptomatic sinus of Valsalva aneurysm without rupture.
B. Patients with sinus of Valsalva aneurysms that rupture should undergo operative repair because progressive heart failure may well lead to death.
C. All patients with suspected sinus of Valsalva aneurysm ruptures need to undergo cardiac catheterization prior to operation.
D. The best operative approach for closure of a ruptured sinus of Valsalva aneurysm is a dual approach through the aorta and the chamber of entry of the fistula.
E. When a sinus of Valsalva aneurysm ruptures into the pericardium, emergency operation is required.

DISCUSSION: When a found intact sinus of Valsalva aneurysm is asymptomatic, the patient should be followed closely for symptoms but does not usually require operative intervention without symptoms or rupture. A ruptured sinus of Valsalva aneurysm should be repaired by surgical intervention because the significant left-to-right shunt that occurs often leads to progressive heart failure and death. While it is true that cardiac catheterization was the gold standard, the accuracy of noninvasive transesophageal color-flow Doppler echocardiography has replaced it in some cases recently. Operative intervention is not emergent unless the aneurysm ruptures into the pericardial space. If this occurs, symptoms of cardiac tamponade are present and emergent operation is required. Finally, the best operative approach is a dual approach via the aorta and the chamber of entry of the fistula. The major advantage of this approach is that the fistula can be identified through the aorta into the chamber involved and closed securely from both sides. The aortic valve can be protected or replaced as necessary, and the ventricular septum can be inspected for a ventricular septal defect.

Textbook: Pages 1639–1641 ANSWER: A, B, D, E.

22. Transection of the thoracic aorta following trauma usually:

A. Is located just distal to the left subclavian artery.
B. Produces a false aneurysm.
C. Is fatal in 80% of cases.

DISCUSSION: Transection of the thoracic aorta may occur at multiple sites from the isthmus down into the abdominal aorta. Transection of the ascending aorta occurs but is uncommon. Those who survive the initial injury and do not rupture into the pleural space do so because the false aneurysm is supported by the adventitia and pleura. The majority of transections occur just distal to the left subclavian and the immediate mortality is about 80%.

Textbook: Pages 1643–1644 ANSWER: A, B, C.

23. Which of the following *confirms* the diagnosis of transection of the descending thoracic aorta?

A. Widened mediastinum.
B. Fractured first rib.
C. Left pleural effusion.
D. Positive aortogram.
E. All of the above.

DISCUSSION: The diagnosis of transected aorta should be suspected with severe injury especially if the patient is thrown from the vehicle. A widened mediastinum, fractured first rib, or a pleural effusion can each be seen with chest trauma that does not involve the thoracic aorta. The diagnosis is best made by the use of the aortogram even though the diagnosis can be made with CT, MRI, and occasionally echocardiography.

Textbook: Page 1644 ANSWER: D.

24. The following is/are true of a descending dissecting aortic aneurysm:

A. It originates distal to the subclavian artery.
B. It is usually found in hypertensive patients.
C. It may extend the entire length of the aorta.

DISCUSSION: Descending dissections are almost always seen in hypertensive patients. The diagnosis is made by locating the tear in the aorta distal to the left subclavian artery. Type III dissections may involve only the descending thoracic aorta but can extend the entire length of the aorta.

Textbook: Pages 1647–1648 ANSWER: A, B, C.

25. The optimal management of Type A or ascending aortic dissection includes:

A. Aortography.
B. Hemodynamic monitoring and frequent recording of blood pressure, urinary output, and neurologic status.
C. Emergency operation.

DISCUSSION: Type A dissections are Type I or Type II dissections that originate in the ascending aorta. These may be associated with aortic insufficiency or hypertension or hypotension depending upon whether or not there has been bleeding into the pericardial space and an element of tamponade and/or neurologic deficit has occurred. Aortography is the best method to establish this diagnosis. Patients with dissecting aortic aneurysms originating in the ascending aorta are considered as emergencies. The operation involves grafting of the ascending aorta to prevent rupture in the mediastinum or into the pericardium with correction of the aortic insufficiency while redirecting the blood into the true lumen.

Textbook: Pages 1651–1652 ANSWER: A, B, C.

26. Aneurysms of the ascending aorta may be caused by:

A. Type II aortic dissection.
B. Atherosclerosis.
C. Cystic medial necrosis.

DISCUSSION: Aneurysms of the ascending aorta are classically associated with Marfan's syndrome, cystic medial necrosis, and, in past years, syphilis. Today, aneurysm formation in the ascending aorta is secondary to the manifestations of degenerative disease occurring within the aorta and the aorta wall.

Textbook: Page 1647 ANSWER: A, B, C.

27. When complications occur after operating on a descending thoracic aorta, perhaps the most devastating is:

A. Recurrent nerve injury.
B. Bleeding with hemothorax.
C. Paraplegia.
D. Renal insufficiency.

DISCUSSION: Although the recurrent nerve can be stretched and hoarseness seen after operations in the area of the isthmus of the thoracic aorta and bleeding associated with aneurysm repair as well as renal insufficiency from the cross-clamping of the vessel above the renals, they are usually insignificant compared to the problem that occurs when paraplegia follows operation on the descending thoracic or thoracoabdominal aorta. Not only is there a loss of function in the legs, but bowel and bladder function are usually seriously affected. The psychological effects of paraplegia may also be devastating.

Textbook: Page 1657 ANSWER: C.

28. The most common risk associated with carotid artery aneurysm is:

A. Thrombosis of the aneurysm.
B. Embolization of mural thrombus.
C. Rupture of the aneurysm.
D. Compression of the hypopharynx.

DISCUSSION: Thrombosis of the aneurysm and internal carotid artery may occur through deposition of laminated clot within the aneurysm and kinking of the outflow tract of the internal carotid artery. However, this is a relatively uncommon clinical presentation for such an aneurysm. The majority of patients with carotid artery aneurysm present with transient ischemic attacks in the ipsilateral cerebral hemisphere secondary to embolization of laminated clot lining the aneurysm wall. If the aneurysm is left uncorrected, most patients ultimately suffer a stroke. Although rare, rupture of a carotid aneurysm is almost always fatal. Rupture usually occurs into the oral cavity or nasopharynx, and death occurs from *suffocation.* Aneurysms may present with symptoms of dysphagia secondary to pressure on neighboring cranial nerves and the lateral wall of the pharynx. Nevertheless, these presentations do not represent serious risks to the patient.

Textbook: Page 1658 ANSWER: B.

29. Risks associated with carotid artery aneurysms are treated most successfully by which of the following?

A. Proximal ligation.
B. Observation.
C. Resection and graft replacement.
D. Resection and reanastomosis.

DISCUSSION: Proximal ligation was the first method of surgical treatment and was employed during the nineteenth and early twentieth centuries, but a high incidence of stroke was associated with its use. Gradual occlusion over several days with a Crutchfield clamp can be used in the rare instance when resection and restoration of flow cannot be performed. Reports from the first part of this century indicate that observation of symptomatic carotid aneurysms yielded a high incidence of stroke and subsequent death. The preferred management of carotid aneurysms is resection and either reanastomosis of the internal and common carotid arteries or interposition graft replacement. Large aneurysms frequently require interposition grafting. Most aneurysms can be removed successfully, and flow can be re-established by reanastomosis. Currently, this is being achieved with a combined operative stroke and mortality rate of less than 2%.

Textbook: Pages 1659–1660 ANSWER: C, D.

30. Which of the following statements about carotid body tumors are true?

A. Cells from which carotid body tumors arise normally sense changes in systemic blood pressure.
B. Most carotid body tumors are malignant and usually metastasize to the ipsilateral cerebral hemisphere.
C. Carotid body tumors are extremely vascular.
D. Carotid body tumors most frequently present as a palpable, painless mass at the carotid bifurcation.

DISCUSSION: Cells of the carotid body function as receptors for changes in PO_2, PCO_2, and pH. Interestingly, carotid body tumors are more prevalent in persons living at high altitudes. Although carotid body tumor cells may have characteristics of malignancy, only about 5% of them metastasize. A carotid body tumor characteristically appears as a hypervascular oval mass situated at the carotid bifurcation and widening the angle between the origins of the internal and external carotid arteries. Although large or malignant carotid body tumors may cause dysfunction of the vagus and hypoglossal nerves and cause dysphagia from their mass effect on the hypopharynx, most tumors are recognized when they still have no associated symptoms and are only a painless mass over the area of the carotid bifurcation.

Textbook: Pages 1660–1661 ANSWER: C, D.

31. Treatment of carotid body tumors most frequently consists of:

A. Radical neck dissection, including the extracranial carotid artery.
B. Radiation therapy.
C. Resection of the common, internal, and external carotid arteries with interposition grafting.
D. Subadventitial dissection of the carotid bifurcation and simple excision of the tumor.

DISCUSSION: Malignant carotid body tumors are uncommon. They are treated either by limited resection of the structures involved with the tumor or by radiation therapy. Although radiation therapy has been demonstrated to shrink some tumors, it should be used only for the rare tumor that is unresectable. Most tumors are benign and can be separated from the wall of the carotid artery without resection of the bifurcation. Such resection is possible because the tumor is located in a plane outside the media. Therefore, upon creation of a subadventitial plane, one can separate the tumor from the carotid artery bifurcation without entering the vessel.

Textbook: Page 1661 ANSWER: C, D.

32. The cause of subclavian arterial aneurysms is most often:

A. Sepsis.
B. A congenital defect.
C. Atherosclerosis.
D. Fibromuscular dysplasia.

DISCUSSION: The most common cause of subclavian aneurysms is atherosclerosis followed by trauma. The thoracic outlet syndrome may cause dilatation of the distal subclavian artery secondary to compression with poststenotic dilatation. Mural thrombi are quite common in these aneurysms and may cause embolism in an arm, a serious complication.

Textbook: Page 1662 ANSWER: C.

33. Of the visceral aneurysms, which is the most common?

A. Celiac.
B. Superior mesenteric.
C. Hepatic.
D. Splenic.

DISCUSSION: Splenic aneurysms are the most common visceral type. They are usually caused by medial degeneration of the arterial wall, although fibromuscular dysplasia can be a cause.

Textbook: Page 1662 ANSWER: D.

34. Aneurysms of the renal artery are most common:

A. At its origin from the aorta.
B. In the main renal artery or the bifurcation into the primary branches.
C. Within the kidney.

DISCUSSION: The majority of renal aneurysms are located either in the main renal artery or at the point of bifurcation into the branches. The appropriate treatment is resection of the aneurysm with restoration of continuity of the artery whenever possible, often with the use of a graft.

Textbook: Pages 1664–1665 ANSWER: B.

35. An aortic abdominal aneurysm was first successfully resected by:

A. Matas.
B. Linton.
C. Dubost.
D. None of the above.

DISCUSSION: Charles Dubost was the first to successfully correct an aortic abdominal aneurysm by resecting the entire aneurysm and replacing it with an aortic homograft. In his paper he presented preoperative as well as postoperative arteriograms demonstrating correction of both the aortic aneurysm and severe stenosis of the left iliac artery.

Textbook: Page 1665 ANSWER: C.

36. Evaluation of the *natural history* of abdominal aortic aneurysms in patients who are followed without any surgical procedure indicates that:

A. Approximately 20% are alive at the end of 5 years.
B. Seventy-five per cent of patients succumb by the end of the first year.
C. Aortic rupture is quite common in this group, occurring in more than half by the second year.
D. None of the above.

DISCUSSION: In the classic study of Estes in 1951, during an era before surgical correction, the survival at 5 years of patients with aortic abdominal aneurysms was 20%.

Textbook: Page 1665 ANSWER: A.

37. The appropriate treatment in most situations of an aortic abdominal graft that has become infected is:

A. Intravenous antibiotics and observation for future complications.
B. Catheter drainage at the site of infection.
C. Replacement of the infected graft with another prosthetic graft.
D. Excision of the entire graft and insertion of axillobifemoral grafts.

DISCUSSION: Many forms of management have been tried and occasionally recommended. The most appropriate treatment for most patients with an infected graft is removal of the entire graft, closure of the iliac or femoral arteries distal to the insertion of the graft, and placement of axillobifemoral grafts.

Textbook: Page 1671 ANSWER: D.

38. In a patient with an abdominal aortic aneurysm and a history of several previous abdominal procedures for release of dense peritoneal adhesions causing episodes of intestinal obstruction, consideration should be given to which one of the following at operation?

A. Cardiopulmonary bypass.
B. An incision from the xiphoid process to the symphysis pubis.
C. Incision in the left flank with a retroperitoneal approach.
D. An axillobifemoral graft.

DISCUSSION: A retroperitoneal approach has been recommended, particularly for patients who have had previous abdominal procedures when peritoneal adhesions might represent a serious technical problem. In these circumstances, the retroperitoneal approach can be quite satisfactory, especially in the management of small aneurysms and those located in the *midportion* of the abdominal aorta between the renal arteries and aortic bifurcation. However, prolonged postoperative incision pain may be a complication in some patients with this incision.

Textbook: Pages 1668–1669 ANSWER: C.

39. After emergency correction of an aortic abdominal aneurysm, the two most common causes of mortality are:

A. Acute renal insufficiency.
B. Severe hemorrhage from dehiscence of the suture line postoperatively.
C. Myocardial infarction.
D. Infection of the graft.

DISCUSSION: Although all these complications may follow correction of an aortic abdominal aneurysm, the most common ones are fatal complications from myocardial infarction and acute renal insufficiency.

Textbook: Page 1672 ANSWER: A, C.

40. The incidence of inflammatory aortic abdominal aneurysms with dense periaortic adhesions and possible involvement of adjacent structures such as the duodenum, renal vein, and ureter is approximately:

A. 2%.
B. 10%.
C. 25%.

DISCUSSION: Increased attention is being given to inflammatory aortic abdominal aneurysms. These are characterized by aneurysms surrounded by dense periaortic inflammation and at times involvement of surrounding structures such as the duodenum, renal vein, and ureter. This problem occurs in some 7% to 10% of patients undergoing aneurysmectomy.

Textbook: Page 1665 ANSWER: B.

41. Which of the following statements about true femoral artery aneurysms is/are correct?

A. All three layers of the blood vessel wall are involved in true aneurysms.
B. There is a very high association with aortoiliac and popliteal aneurysms.
C. Femoral artery aneurysms occur bilaterally in about 10% of cases.
D. Type I femoral artery aneurysms involve the orifice of the deep femoral artery.
E. The most common complication of femoral aneurysms is rupture.

DISCUSSION: By definition, a true aneurysm involves the intima, media, and adventitia. Femoral aneurysms are very often associated with other aneurysms, ranging from 70% to 95% in most reports. They are most commonly associated with aortoiliac or popliteal aneurysms. Approximately 50% of femoral aneurysms are bilateral. Type I femoral aneurysms are limited to the common femoral artery; type II aneurysms involve the orifice of the deep femoral artery. Rupture of femoral artery aneurysms is rare. The most common complications are due to thrombosis, embolism, or local compression.

Textbook: Page 1673 ANSWER: A, B.

42. Which of the following statements about false aneurysms of the femoral artery is/are correct?

A. The incidence of iatrogenic false aneurysms has increased in recent years.
B. Arteriography is the most useful study for diagnosis of iatrogenic femoral aneurysms.
C. Ultrasound-guided compression of iatrogenic false aneurysms is usually successful in achieving thrombosis.
D. Femoral anastomotic aneurysms usually involve the proximal anastomosis of a prosthetic infrainguinal bypass.
E. Rupture is the most common complication associated with femoral anastomotic aneurysms.

DISCUSSION: With the introduction of invasive percutaneous procedures such as angioplasty, valvuloplasty, atherectomy and coronary stenting, the incidence of iatrogenic false aneurysms has risen to about 0.6% to 1.0% in recent years. Color-flow duplex ultrasound is the best test for diagnosis of these aneurysms, owing to its ability accurately to delineate the anatomy. Additionally, compression of these false aneurysms using ultrasound guidance is very effective in achieving thrombosis. Femoral anastomotic aneurysms are most commonly seen after aortofemoral bypass grafting and only rarely are associated with infrainguinal procedures. Thromboembolic complications are the most common complication of these lesions.

Textbook: Pages 1673–1674 ANSWER: A, C.

43. Which of the following statements about popliteal artery aneurysms is/are correct?

A. They are the most common site of peripheral artery aneurysms.

B. For a patient with an abdominal aortic aneurysm the risk of a popliteal aneurysm is approximately 50%.
C. For a patient with a popliteal artery aneurysm the risk of a contralateral popliteal aneurysm is approximately 50%.
D. Popliteal artery aneurysms most commonly present with local symptoms secondary to compression of the adjacent vein or nerve.
E. Arteriography is the most accurate test for the diagnosis of popliteal artery aneurysm.

DISCUSSION: Although rare, popliteal artery aneurysms are the most common site of peripheral artery aneurysms. While the incidence of associated aneurysms in patients with popliteal aneurysms is high, the opposite is not true. The likelihood of a patient with an abdominal aortic aneurysm having a popliteal artery aneurysm is less than 10%. About 50% of popliteal aneurysms are bilateral. The most common presenting symptom in patients with popliteal aneurysms is leg ischemia, secondary to either thrombosis or embolism. Local symptoms due to the aneurysm are relatively rare. Ultrasonography is the best test for diagnosis of a popliteal aneurysm. Arteriography should be reserved for patients undergoing operative repair.
Textbook: Pages 1675–1676 ANSWER: A, C.

44. Which of the following statements about management of popliteal artery aneurysms is/are correct?

A. All symptomatic aneurysms should be treated with surgery.
B. The most common operation is excision of the aneurysm with arterial reconstruction.
C. Thrombolytic therapy may be useful when there is thrombosis of the aneurysm and the distal runoff vessels.
D. The results for surgery for asymptomatic aneurysms are better than those for symptomatic ones.
E. The long-term results with prosthetic grafts are equivalent to those of autogenous vein grafts.

DISCUSSION: It is generally felt that all symptomatic popliteal aneurysms should be treated with surgery. Treatment of asymptomatic aneurysms is more controversial; some advocate repair of all of these as well. A reasonable approach is to consider surgery for asymptomatic aneurysms larger than 2 cm. Aneurysm ligation with bypass is the most commonly performed operation for popliteal aneurysm, excision being reserved for aneurysms that cause local compressive symptoms. Thrombolytic therapy, given either before or during operation, is useful in clearing the tibial and pedal vessels in cases of acute thrombosis. The patency and limb salvage rates are better for asymptomatic lesions than for symptomatic ones. Autogenous vein is superior to prosthetic material and is the conduit of choice for ligation and bypass of popliteal aneurysms.
Textbook: Pages 1676–1677 ANSWER: A, C, D.

45. Which of the following statements about thrombo-obliterative disease of the aorta and its branches are correct?

A. The most common cause of obstructive disease is thrombi.
B. Atherosclerosis is the most common pathologic cause of arterial obstruction.
C. Lesions occur with greater frequency at the origin of vessels from the aorta.
D. Obstructive lesions are preferentially managed by endarterectomy.

DISCUSSION: Thrombo-obliterative disease of the aorta and its branches is primarily due to atherosclerosis. The lesions occur most frequently at the origin of blood vessels and are usually localized and short. Surgical management consists primarily of bypass grafts since endarterectomy is often followed by later reocclusion with reappearance of symptoms.
Textbook: Pages 1678–1679 ANSWER: B, C.

46. Which of the following statements about Takayasu's disease is/are correct?

A. Atherosclerosis is restricted to the ascending aorta and innominate artery.
B. It primarily affects patients of Asian descent.
C. It is a nonspecific arteritis affecting the thoracic and abdominal aorta and its major branches.
D. The disorder is also characterized by systemic symptoms, including fever, malaise, arthritis, and pericardial pain.
E. Surgical bypass of the involved vessel should be undertaken in nearly all patients, since the results are excellent.

DISCUSSION: While it may affect others, Takayasu's disease occurs primarily in those of Asian descent and usually attacks young females. It is basically a nonspecific arteritis involving all layers of the arterial wall with proliferation of connective tissue and degeneration of elastic fibers. Clinical manifestations include fever, malaise, arthritis, and pericardial pain. Some believe that it may be an autoimmune disease, and steroids have been effective in some patients. Late manifestations include ischemia of both cerebral and upper extremity circuits. While surgical management is occasionally successful, it usually is not recommended except for patients with disabling symptoms.
Textbook: Pages 1679–1681 ANSWER: B, C, D.

47. A 65-year-old man complains of having had slurred speech and no motor function or sensation of his right hand for 15 minutes. A left carotid bruit is heard in the neck. Which of the following diagnostic studies should be done?

A. Carotid duplex scan.
B. Electroencephalography (EEG).
C. Carotid arteriography.
D. Computed tomography (CT) of the brain.

DISCUSSION: Although a carotid duplex scan provides valuable information on the presence of significant carotid artery disease at its bifurcation, it cannot be used as the final test of the circulation to the brain in this particular case. Carotid duplex scanning has its greatest value in the assessment of asymptomatic patients who have cervical bruits. In that circumstance, it can provide information on which the decision for further workup can be based. When symptoms suggest a transient ischemic attack, no noninvasive study provides a complete evaluation and arteriography is mandatory. EEG is a valuable test for evaluating patients when seizure activity is suspected. In this patient, an EEG would be valuable only if all other diagnostic studies had been unrevealing. An arteriogram is mandatory in this patient to adequately evaluate the entire extracranial and intracranial cerebral circulation. If a duplex scan had been performed and had revealed no disease, an arteriogram would still be necessary to exclude brachiocephalic trunk disease as a source of emboli. Likewise, intracranial narrowing would also be missed by such a noninvasive study. For these reasons, duplex scanning might be considered redundant and inadequate in these circumstances. CT of the head would be imperative in the evaluation of this patient. Its primary role is to exclude cerebral infarction, even in the presence of transient symptoms. It also distinguishes an ischemic cerebral event from an intracranial hemorrhage and rules out other potential causes of the symptoms, such as a brain tumor, other space-occupying intracranial lesions, and arteriovenous malformation.

Textbook: Pages 1683–1684 ANSWER: C, D.

48. Carotid artery occlusive disease most often produces transient ischemic attacks or stroke by which of the following mechanisms?

A. Reduction of flow to the affected area of the brain through stenotic or occluded vessels.
B. Embolization of atheromatous debris and/or clot with occlusion of intracranial branches of the carotid artery.
C. Thrombosis and propagation of the clot into the intracranial branches.
D. All of the above are equally common.

DISCUSSION: The collateral network to the brain is extensive. Collateral flow to an area supplied by a carotid artery is provided by the contralateral carotid artery and vertebrobasilar system around the circle of Willis, by the external carotid artery branches around the eye, and by direct intracerebral connections between the anterior cerebral arteries. For these reasons, low-flow cerebral symptoms are extremely rare, even when carotid lesions are present bilaterally. Approximately 70% of all cerebral symptoms produced by carotid artery occlusive disease are embolic in origin. The surface of an atherosclerotic lesion at the carotid bifurcation is thrombogenic and acts as a nidus for the accumulation of platelet-rich thrombi. Similarly, the interior of the plaque can degenerate and rupture into the lumen, embolizing its contents into the distal bed of the carotid circulation. The final event in the progression of an atherosclerotic carotid lesion is total thrombosis. Because there are no extracranial branches of the internal carotid artery, the thrombus propagates distally. If the propagation of the clot stops at the first major intracranial branch (the ophthalmic artery) and does not disturb collateral flow through it, no cerebral ischemic event may occur. When propagation continues into the intracranial branches, a massive stroke may occur. This mechanism accounts for a minority of strokes.

Textbook: Pages 1682–1683 ANSWER: B.

49. The majority of patients with "subclavian steal" syndrome have which of the following conditions?

A. Reversed flow in the involved vertebral artery.
B. Disabling neurologic symptoms.
C. Upper extremity claudication.
D. Decreased systolic blood pressure in the ipsilateral arm.

DISCUSSION: Subclavian steal syndrome results from occlusion of a subclavian artery, rarely the innominate, with decreased systolic pressure distal to this obstruction. This causes blood to flow up the contralateral vertebral area and across the basilar artery (from which more blood is "stolen") as it courses down (in a retrograde manner) the ipsilateral vertebral artery to help supply that subclavian artery. Most patients with this phenomenon are asymptomatic, although limb weakness and paresthesias or symptoms of vertebral basilar insufficiency may occur. Strokes do not occur in patients with subclavian disease alone. Most affected patients, however, have associated atherosclerotic disease of other extracranial arteries, particularly the carotid vessels, which may contribute to symptoms of cerebral ischemia.

Textbook: Pages 1685–1686 ANSWER: A, D.

50. Which of the following treatments is/are appropriate for symptomatic subclavian steal syndrome?

A. Subclavian endarterectomy.
B. Carotid-subclavian bypass.
C. Subclavian-carotid transposition.
D. Intra-arterial streptokinase.

DISCUSSION: Because most patients with the abnormal flow phenomena demonstrated in subclavian steal syndrome are asymptomatic, surgical treatment is not necessary. Furthermore, some patients with subclavian steal have symptoms caused by other extracranial arterial disease and benefit from therapy directed at carotid disease. For patients whose symptoms are attributed to the subclavian steal phenomenon, a variety of surgical procedures have been proposed. Relief of symptoms has been obtained in 70% to 80% of these patients. Currently, both carotid-subclavian bypass and subclavian-carotid transposition are considered acceptable.

Textbook: Pages 1687–1688 ANSWER: B, C.

51. Which statements about thrombo-obliterative disease of the terminal abdominal aorta (Leriche syndrome) are true?

A. It is characterized by a combination of atherosclerotic and thrombotic occlusion of the terminal aorta.
B. It is characterized by acute thrombosis of the terminal aorta.
C. It requires emergency revascularization when the diagnosis is made.
D. It is often associated with distal obstructive lesions.
E. Patients often show signs of ischemia in the legs, and males may have difficulty maintaining a stable erection.
F. The preferred surgical procedure is bypass with a prosthetic graft.

DISCUSSION: Leriche syndrome usually affects males 35 to 60 years of age. It is caused by a combination of thrombosis superimposed on atherosclerosis. The symptoms are usually those of ischemia of the legs, including weariness or claudication, atrophic changes, and the inability to maintain a stable erection owing to inadequate arterial flow to the penis. Distal sites of segmental occlusion are not uncommon. This disorder is often tolerated well for 5—and even 10—years, but ultimately serious symptoms of ischemia require operation. The procedure of choice is a bypass with a prosthetic graft from the aorta to the iliac or femoral arteries bilaterally.

Textbook: Pages 1689–1690 ANSWER: A, D, E, F.

52. Following surgical correction of Leriche syndrome, which of the following are true?

A. Gangrene is usually prevented, but symptoms of claudication persist.
B. The symptoms of claudication are usually improved.
C. Sexual function is improved in some patients.
D. Patients who continue to smoke following surgical correction have a higher incidence of reocclusion.
E. Prevention of damage to the sympathetic and parasympathetic nerves in the periaortic region reduces the postoperative incidence of retrograde ejaculation.

DISCUSSION: Following corrective operation, patients with a history of claudication as well as ischemic manifestations are usually considerably improved. Those who have one or more patent internal iliac (hypogastric) arteries are more likely to have improved sexual function. It is important that patients cease smoking following bypass grafts since there is objective evidence that thrombosis of grafts is appreciably increased by continuance of smoking. Minimal dissection in the region of the abdominal aorta is important in minimizing damage to the sympathetic and parasympathetic nerves, since injury is related to the incidence of postoperative retrograde ejaculation.

Textbook: Pages 1690–1691 ANSWER: B, C, D, E.

53. In a patient who has chronic, complete occlusion of a common iliac artery, which of the following are true?

A. The primary symptom is claudication of the calf muscles.
B. Symptoms are usually claudication of the thigh and calf.
C. The decision as to whether or not to operate can be based on clinical examination findings.
D. Collateral iliac arterial vessels are prevalent.
E. Balloon angioplasty is appropriate in some patients.

DISCUSSION: Occlusion of the common iliac artery is usually associated with claudication of the thigh and calf. Arteriography should be done to establish the diagnosis and to assess the peripheral arterial system. Arteriography is also quite helpful in deciding whether or not balloon angioplasty is indicated, since it can be used successfully in some patients. Collateral vessels are usually apparent on the arteriogram. Bilateral involvement of the iliac vessels is quite common, and if symptoms are not present at the outset they may develop later. The preferred surgical management is bypass grafts from the aorta to the patent distal circulation.

Textbook: Page 1691 ANSWER: B, D, E.

54. Which of the following does not describe intermittent claudication?

A. Is elicited by reproducible amount of exercise.
B. Abates promptly with rest.
C. Is often worse at night.
D. May be an indication for bypass surgery.

DISCUSSION: Intermittent claudication characteristically is elicited by a relatively reproducible amount of exercise, and it is promptly relieved by cessation of that exercise. Furthermore, it is usually felt in a defined muscle group such as the calf muscles. Rest pain, indicating impending limb loss, is felt in the toes and forefoot as opposed to a muscle group, and this pain often begins at night. Claudication, when sufficiently disabling, may be an indication for revascularization, particularly if it interferes with gaining a livelihood.

Textbook: Page 1692 ANSWER: C.

55. In terms of long-term graft patency, the best results in the femoral tibial bypass position have been achieved with:

A. A modified human umbilical cord graft.
B. Polytetrafluoroethylene (PTFE [Gore-Tex]).
C. Saphenous vein allograft.
D. Segments of greater and lesser saphenous and cephalic veins spliced together.

DISCUSSION: Particularly for distal bypass grafting, the autogenous saphenous vein is the graft material of choice. When this is not available intact, several segments of this vein, as well as lesser saphenous and upper extremity veins, can be used for creating a graft of sufficient length. When the distal anastomosis is below the popliteal artery autogenous tissue grafts are clearly superior to synthetic ones.

Textbook: Pages 1696–1697 ANSWER: D.

56. Which of the following statements about femoral popliteal bypass grafting is/are true?

A. Long-term graft surveillance by duplex scanning has no effect on graft patency rates.
B. Graft failure and amputation occur in half the patients within 5 years.
C. If grafting is successful, long-term mortality is improved.
D. Patency rates of 80% to 90% at 1 year currently are expected.

DISCUSSION: Graft surveillance and repair of acquired defects in the vein before graft thrombosis improve long-term patency rates. Patients who require lower extremity bypass for limb salvage have poor 5-year survival because of concomitant coronary and cerebrovascular disease. Current graft patency rates approach 90% at 1 year.

Textbook: Page 1698 ANSWER: D.

57. Which of the following statements about percutaneous renal artery transluminal angioplasty (PRTA) are true?

A. Patients with renovascular hypertension are usually cured after successful PRTA.
B. Patients with renovascular hypertension due to atherosclerosis are more likely to benefit from PRTA than those in whom it is due to fibromuscular dysplasia.
C. PRTA of ostial atherosclerotic lesions is more successful than PRTA of nonostial lesions.
D. PRTA is associated with a higher morbidity and mortality than angioplasty for peripheral vascular disease.

DISCUSSION: The results of treatment for renovascular hypertension depend on the nature of the obstructing lesion and its anatomic location. Treatment of obstruction due to fibromuscular dysplasia is technically successful in 90% of patients and helps to control hypertension in almost 85%. However, fewer than 60% are cured. The results of treating atherosclerotic causes are substantially worse. Approximately 60% of patients show improvement in blood pressure control, but fewer than 25% are cured. The results of treating nonostial atherosclerotic lesions are better than those for ostial lesions. Unfortunately, the majority of patients with renovascular hypertension have ostial atherosclerotic lesions as the obstructing lesion. The complication rate associated with PRTA is substantially higher than that for angioplasty of vascular disease of the lower extremities, averaging almost 20% in patients with atherosclerotic lesions. Renal insufficiency is more likely. The mortality averages 1%, but higher rates are reported.

Textbook: Pages 1706–1708 ANSWER: D.

58. True statements about percutaneous transluminal angioplasty (PTA) of peripheral vascular lesions include which of the following?

A. PTA of iliac lesions is more often successful than PTA of femoral artery lesions.
B. PTA of iliac occlusions produces results similar to PTA of iliac artery stenoses.
C. PTA of infrapopliteal occlusive disease is associated with an increased rate of vasospasm, which can cause thrombosis.
D. A short, singular arterial stenosis is the optimal situation for a successful angioplasty.

DISCUSSION: Clinical results using PTA to treat occlusive vascular disease of the lower extremities depend on the morphologic nature of the obstruction as well as the anatomic location. PTA of iliac lesions is technically successful in approximately 90% of patients with 3-year patency rates of approximately 80%. PTA of superficial femoral artery lesions is technically successful in 75% to 85% of patients with 3-year patency rates of approximately 60% to 70%. PTA of infrapopliteal vessels is associated with increased risk of vasospasm, which can cause thrombosis. Improvements in the technique and pharmacologic treatment of vasospasm have reduced the risk of vessel thrombosis to less than 10%. Although some series have reported PTA of infrapopliteal lesions in patients with claudication, most authors recommend treating only patients with threatened limbs. Ideal patients for PTA are those with stenotic lesions less than 5 cm. long; the best results occur in the shortest lesions. Although total occlusions and multiple stenoses have been treated successfully, there are fewer technical successes, and long-term patency rates are substantially lower than in the treatment of stenotic lesions.

Textbook: Pages 1703–1705 ANSWER: A, C, D.

59. Advantages of PTA, as compared with surgical revascularization, include which of the following?

A. Decreased initial cost, shorter convalescence, and earlier return to full activity.
B. Because PTA is performed under local anesthesia, it is applicable to a greater number of patients with peripheral vascular disease.
C. PTA is more durable and requires fewer subsequent procedures.
D. Repeat PTA is well-tolerated, morbidity is equivalent to that for the initial procedure, and success rates are comparable to those expected with the initial procedure.

DISCUSSION: The primary advantages of PTA over surgical revascularization are the lower initial cost of the procedure, decreased hospital stay, earlier return to full activity, lower morbidity, and the ability to repeat the procedure without markedly increasing patient morbidity or compromising clinical results. The procedure can be performed in patients who would have a high operative risk related to coexisting medical conditions; however, angioplasty is not applicable to the majority of patients with vascular occlusive disease because of the presence of long stenoses, occlusion, or multiple lesions in the vascular system. Restenosis and progression of disease in the vascular system also limit the long-term results of PTA and are the cause of a greater need for subsequent procedures.

Textbook: Pages 1700, 1701–1702 ANSWER: A, D.

60. Which of the following statements are true?

A. All arterial injuries are associated with absence of a palpable pulse.
B. Preoperative arteriography is required to diagnose an arterial injury.
C. The presence of Doppler signals indicates that an arterial injury has not occurred.
D. Patients with critical limb ischemia have paralysis and paresthesias.
E. In all patients with multiple trauma, arterial injuries should be repaired before other injuries are addressed.

DISCUSSION: Although arteriography may be required to diagnose partially severed or damaged arteries with persistent flow, it is not required for the diagnosis of most injuries. In a patient who is not in shock, a diminished pulse on physical examination indicates an arterial injury; however, patients with only partial severance or intimal injury may maintain axial flow through the injury and distal pulses will be palpable. In a patient who has adequate collateral flow, Doppler signals may be heard even in the presence of complete occlusion of an axial artery. These patients may have audible flow, but their Doppler-derived pressure will be decreased. Patients who do not have adequate collateral flow present with critical ischemia manifested by paralysis and paresthesias, the latter in a stocking or glove distribution. Patients who have neither paralysis nor paresthesia do not have immediately limb-threatening injuries and, for them, arterial reconstruction can be deferred until more acute life- and limb-threatening lesions have been treated.

Textbook: Pages 1714–1716 ANSWER: D.

61. A patient presents with a gunshot wound of the mid-neck. Although drunk, he exhibits no lateralizing neurologic signs. After control of his airway is achieved, he is taken directly to the operating room for control of hemorrhage. The common carotid artery has a 2-cm. destroyed segment. There is also a major esophageal injury. The best treatment for this carotid injury is:

A. Vein graft replacement of the common carotid artery.
B. Ligation of the common carotid artery.
C. Ligation of the common carotid artery proximally with a subclavian carotid bypass.
D. Ligation of the common carotid artery with sympathectomy.
E. Prosthetic graft replacement of the common carotid artery.

DISCUSSION: The treatment of carotid artery injury in a patient without neurologic deficit consists of reconstruction of the carotid. This patient had no neurologic deficit preoperatively and should have a good result. Autogenous material is preferred over prosthetic material. Ligation without reconstruction may be tolerated in the common carotid artery but is not recommended. Subclavian carotid bypass has no advantage over reconstruction unless it can be performed in a clean operative field. Cervical sympathectomy is not performed in these circumstances. Although the presence of an esophageal wound means that there is a potential for infection, it should not deter reconstruction with autogenous material. This potential for infection, however, should alert the physician to the possible development of false aneurysm in the postoperative period. If an infected false aneurysm develops, alternative methods of carotid reconstruction must be utilized.

Textbook: Pages 1717–1718 ANSWER: A.

62. Which of the following statements about iatrogenic arterial injuries are true?

A. Femoral artery pseudoaneurysms occurring after arteriography require urgent operative intervention.
B. Symptomatic axillary sheath hematomas require urgent operative intervention.
C. Arterial occlusions after catheterization occur more commonly in the femoral artery than in the brachial artery.
D. The Allen test identifies patients with an incomplete palmar arch.

DISCUSSION: Small pseudoaneurysms after arterial puncture often close spontaneously. Duplex-guided compression may be used to cause thrombosis of the pseudoaneurysm. Surgery is usually reserved for large or expanding pseudoaneurysms that are not successfully occluded by duplex-guided compression. On the other hand, axillary sheath hematomas can cause permanent nerve injury and require urgent surgical decompression. Occlusions after catheterization are more common in smaller arteries such as the brachial artery, but ischemic signs and symptoms are more likely with larger vessel occlusions. The Allen test should be performed before all radial artery cannulations to show that there is an adequate palmar arch.

Textbook: Page 1718 ANSWER: B, D.

63. A 35-year-old man involved in a motor vehicle accident presents with a knee dislocation that is easily reduced. Radiography of the knee shows no fracture. Which of the following statements about his treatment are true?

A. If he has normal pulses he can be discharged.
B. If he has normal pulses he requires either close observation or arteriography.
C. If he has absent distal pulses and severe ischemia he should undergo arteriography in the radiology suite.

D. A popliteal vein injury is best treated with ligation.
E. A popliteal artery injury should be repaired with the ipsilateral saphenous vein if available.

DISCUSSION: Knee dislocations commonly cause popliteal vessel injury. Early after injury, flow may be sustained in the injured popliteal artery; therefore, these injuries require close observation or arteriography. When an occluded popliteal artery is evident clinically, immediate repair is indicated and arteriography is unnecessary. Repair should ideally utilize the contralateral saphenous vein, to maintain optimal venous return in the injured leg. Injured popliteal veins should be repaired if at all possible. Ligation may jeopardize the arterial repair and increase the likelihood of chronic venous insufficiency and the risk of pulmonary embolism.

Textbook: Page 1721 ANSWER: B.

64. A 24-year-old man is involved in an industrial accident in which he sustains a crushed pelvis. Diagnostic peritoneal lavage is positive. At exploration, a large pelvic hematoma is found. What is the best treatment?

A. Explore all the major arteries and veins of the pelvis and surgically control the bleeding if possible.
B. Do not explore the pelvic hematoma. Close the abdomen and apply a MAST suit.
C. Do not explore the pelvic hematoma. Apply a pelvic fixator and send the patient to radiology for possible embolization of bleeding pelvic vessels.
D. Use sustained hypotensive anesthesia to try to control bleeding.
E. Open the pelvic hematoma and apply laparotomy pads with topical hemostatic agents.

DISCUSSION: Pelvic hematomas are not usually the result of common or external iliac artery disruption. Therefore, unless the hematoma is rapidly expanding in the area of one of the major iliac arteries, it is not opened. Instead, the pelvic fracture is fixed externally and arteriography is performed. Usually, bleeding is from smaller arteries as they exit through the fracture site. These are best controlled with embolization. The other options are poor surgical choices that have little chance of success.

Textbook: Pages 1712, 1721–1722 ANSWER: C.

65. Which of the following statements about acute arterial occlusion today is/are *not* true?

A. Most arterial emboli originate in the heart as a result of underlying cardiac disease.
B. It can be treated under local anesthesia.
C. It is usually due to atherosclerotic disease.
D. Surgical treatment can usually be avoided if the lesion is diagnosed early.

DISCUSSION: The majority of arterial emboli originate in the heart as a result of atherosclerotic disease manifested by myocardial infarction, atrial fibrillation, congestive heart failure, or ventricular aneurysm. The incidence of embolization from rheumatic mitral stenosis has decreased significantly. Elderly and debilitated patients who are poor risks for general anesthesia can be treated with the balloon embolectomy catheter technique, which can be performed under local anesthesia via groin incisions. Atherosclerotic disease in the peripheral vessels can cause thrombosis at the site of atheroma. Acute arterial occlusion represents an emergency that is best treated promptly via heparinization and balloon catheter embolectomy.

Textbook: Pages 1723–1725, 1726 ANSWER: D.

66. Which of the following statements about lytic agents is/are true?

A. They were first introduced well after the advent of balloon embolectomy.
B. Streptokinase is nonantigenic.
C. Systemic use is the most effective means of delivery.
D. The interval to reperfusion limits their utility in the treatment of advanced ischemia.

DISCUSSION: The balloon catheter technique for embolectomy and thromboembolectomy was introduced in 1963. Lytic agents were undergoing clinical investigation at that time. Streptokinase, derived from streptococci, is antigenic. Urokinase is a naturally occurring enzyme and is not antigenic. Lytic agents have yet to play a major role in the treatment of advanced ischemia in the periphery because of delayed reperfusion, cost, risk of complications, the danger of increased tissue loss.

Textbook: Pages 1729–1730 ANSWER: D.

67. Which of the following is not an indication for postoperative heparinization?

A. Suspected venous thrombosis.
B. Risk of embolism following acute myocardial infarction.
C. Advanced ischemia secondary to acute embolic occlusion.
D. Dissolution of residual thrombus after balloon thromboembolectomy.

DISCUSSION: Conditions that would cause undesirable consequences from rethrombosis (e.g., venous thrombosis, additional embolization from the cardiac source, pre-existing ischemia) are indications for postoperative heparinization. Heparin prevents additional clotting; it is not a thrombolytic agent.

Textbook: Page 1729 ANSWER: D.

68. Which of the following is/are not true of the embolectomy catheter technique?

A. The balloon should be inflated by the same person who withdraws the catheter.

B. Distal exploration should be carried out in all major branches of the affected extremity.
C. The balloon is designed to dilate as it traverses areas of luminal narrowing.
D. Removal of adherent thrombus requires alternate catheter-based therapy in addition to balloon exploration.

DISCUSSION: The embolectomy balloon should be adjusted in diameter as the catheter is withdrawn to accommodate changes in luminal diameter and to effect appropriate traction. To do so, the operator must simultaneously control the withdrawal and the balloon inflation. The propensity of clot to propagate distally and proximally requires nearby branches to be explored. When it is technically feasible, major branches should be explored. The embolectomy balloon is made of a distensible elastomer that conforms to the intra-arterial surface to maintain wall contact. Dilatation balloons, in contrast, are made of a nondistensible material that can effect dilating force on the arterial narrowing. An increase in the incidence of adherent thrombus from chronic atherosclerotic disease and failed synthetic grafts has promoted the development of more aggressive catheter-based systems. Graft thrombectomy and adherent clot catheters are specifically designed to remove adherent thrombus left behind after balloon exploration.

Textbook: Pages 1726–1728 ANSWER: C.

69. Which of the following is the least reliable indicator of successful thrombectomy?

A. Vigorous back-bleeding after removal of thrombotic material.
B. Arteriographically demonstrated patency of all runoff vessels.
C. Normal distal pulses.
D. Return of normal skin color and temperature.

DISCUSSION: The significant incidence of discontinuous thrombus makes the presence of vigorous back-bleeding an unreliable indicator of distal patency. Proximal material can be cleared, precipitating back-bleeding from all side branches yet still leaving the main vessel occluded more distally. Arteriography, normal distal pulses, and the return of normal skin color and temperature are the best indicators of distal patency, and thus of successful reperfusion. It must be borne in mind that the primary goal of most thromboembolectomy procedures is to return the limb to its preocclusive state. Optimal distal perfusion may require additional therapy for the patient with chronic atherosclerotic disease.

Textbook: Pages 1727–1728 ANSWER: A.

70. Which of the following statements about arteriovenous fistula are correct?

A. The local features characteristic of an arteriovenous communication are demonstrated by the presence of a thrill and bruit with aneurysmal dilatation.
B. An arteriovenous fistula is best managed by ligation of the feeding vessels.
C. The most common type of arteriovenous fistula is iatrogenic, created for vascular access.
D. Branum's or Nicoladoni's sign is increased heart rate when the fistula is compressed.

DISCUSSION: Local features characteristic of an arteriovenous fistula include a thrill and bruit at the site of the fistula associated with aneurysmal dilatation. Simple ligation of feeding vessels often leads to vascular insufficiency of the peripheral vascular bed secondary to drainage of the flow via collateral circulation. Repair of the artery and vein is considered the optimal therapy. If this is not possible, ligation of the feeding artery and vein proximally and distally can be performed if sufficient collateral circulation has developed, which generally takes months or more after the fistula develops. Branum's or Nicoladoni's sign is a decrease in the heart rate following compression of the fistula.

Textbook: Pages 1731–1734 ANSWER: A, C.

71. Of the following statements about congenital arteriovenous malformations, which are correct?

A. Patients with complex congenital arteriovenous malformations should as early as possible undergo ligation of feeding vessels.
B. Embolizing large arteriovenous malformations has not been demonstrated to be beneficial.
C. The most common complications of a large arteriovenous fistula are symptoms of congestive heart failure, pain, ulceration, and cosmetic deformity.
D. Most congenital arteriovenous malformations are easily managed with simple excision.

DISCUSSION: Complex congenital arteriovenous malformations are often one of the greatest challenges a surgeon may encounter. Management includes accurate diagnosis and determination of the extent of the lesion. The site of communication should be localized by arteriography; however, computed tomography (CT), magnetic resonance imaging (MRI), and duplex Doppler imaging may prove useful in the diagnosis of arteriovenous communications. Ideal surgical management includes closure of the fistula with restoration of arterial and venous continuity. Complex arteriovenous malformations require a multidisciplinary approach, including intra-arterial embolization in conjunction with surgical therapy. Indications for surgery include secondary ischemic complications and congestive heart failure, pain, nonhealing ulcers, and a cosmetic deformity. Ligation of feeding vessels is effective only temporarily, making further treatment, especially embolization, difficult or impossible. Preoperative embolization may allow surgical resection and reduce operative blood loss.

Textbook: Page 1735 ANSWER: A, B, C.

72. Thrombosis occurs frequently in thromboangiitis obliterans (Buerger's disease) in which of the following vessels?

A. Superficial femoral artery.
B. Radial or ulnar artery.
C. Digital arteries.
D. Superficial veins.

DISCUSSION: Thromboangiitis obliterans is characterized by thrombosis and inflammation of small and medium-sized peripheral arteries and veins, and by migratory superficial phlebitis. Unlike atherosclerosis, it often involves the upper extremity. Thromboangiitis obliterans rarely involves large vessels such as the brachial or femoral arteries.

Textbook: Pages 1738–1739 ANSWER: B, C, D.

73. Which of the following statements about thromboangiitis obliterans (Buerger's disease) are true?

A. The disease affects only young men.
B. The disease is more common in Asia and the Middle East than in the United States.
C. Life expectancy is limited.
D. The usual cause is smoking.

DISCUSSION: Thromboangiitis obliterans was originally described in young men, who still constitute the overwhelming majority of patients. In recent years, however, several cases have been reported in women, perhaps a reflection of the marked increase in the number of female smokers. For reasons unknown, there is marked geographic variation in the prevalence of thromboangiitis obliterans. The number of cases in the United States has decreased markedly since World War II, but the incidence is much higher in other countries, particularly in the Far East. Although thromboangiitis obliterans often results in peripheral gangrene and may necessitate amputation, long-term life expectancy differs little from that for the general population, unlike that of atherosclerosis. Although rare instances of thromboangiitis obliterans have been reported in nonsmokers, the most common cause is cigarette addiction, which usually starts at an early age. Prolonged remissions often follow cessation of smoking.

Textbook: Page 1738 ANSWER: B, D.

74. A 52-year-old man presents with sudden onset of profound cyanosis of the second and third digits of the right hand with gangrene of the tip of the second digit. The remaining digits and the other hand are not affected. Which of the following statements are true?

A. This is characteristic of vasospastic Raynaud's syndrome.
B. Evaluation should include arteriography.
C. A coagulation abnormality may be the cause of this problem.
D. Thoracic sympathectomy is the first-line treatment.

DISCUSSION: Gangrene is indicative of occlusive disease and not of vasospastic disease. The other factor that makes this unlikely to be vasospasm is the involvement of only two fingers. Because of the possibility of a surgically correctable upstream vascular lesion such as a subclavian aneurysm, patients presenting with embolic-type lesions should have arteriography. Thus this patient, presenting with ischemia of sudden onset in just two digits, should undergo arteriography. Coagulation abnormalities such as antithrombin-III, protein C, or protein S deficiency, or the presence of antiphospholipid antibodies or the lupus anticoagulant, may cause digital gangrene. Conservative therapy—local wound care and débridement—leads to healing in most patients. Sympathectomy should be reserved for patients who fail to heal after months of conservative therapy.

Textbook: Pages 1741–1742 ANSWER: B, C.

75. A 21-year-old woman presents with digital color changes in response to cold stimulation. Physical examination and laboratory data, including an autoimmune disease screen, are normal. She should be advised that:

A. Her condition is characteristic of vasospastic Raynaud's syndrome and, while she may be at a slightly higher risk for developing a connective tissue disease in the future, there is no evidence of one currently.
B. Her problem with her fingers will get progressively worse and she will eventually lose fingers.
C. She has scleroderma, which will manifest itself at a later date.
D. Her problem is "all in her head."

DISCUSSION: This presentation is classic for vasospastic Raynaud's syndrome. While these patients are probably at a slightly higher risk for developing a connective tissue disorder in the future, this risk is low. These patients do not invariably progress to tissue loss. This patient has no evidence of scleroderma at the present, and there is no reason to predict that she will develop it. Even though her physical and laboratory examinations are negative, her history is positive for Raynaud's syndrome.

Textbook: Pages 1742–1744 ANSWER: A.

76. Obstructive Raynaud's syndrome can be differentiated from vasospastic Raynaud's syndrome by the:

A. Ice water test.
B. Digital hypothermic challenge test.
C. Antinuclear antibody levels.
D. Digital blood pressure measurement.

DISCUSSION: Patients with obstructive Raynaud's syndrome have fixed palmar and digital arterial lesions with a decrease in digital blood pressure at rest. In contrast, patients with vasospastic Raynaud's syndrome have normal digital arteries at rest and normal digital blood pressure. Therefore the only test that differentiates the two conditions is measurement of digital blood pressure. The ice water and digital hypothermic challenge tests both test for the presence of Raynaud's syndrome, but do not differentiate the spastic from the obstructive type. The presence or absence of antinuclear antibodies does not determine whether obstruction is present, although it is true that many patients with obstructive Raynaud's syndrome will have a positive test.

Textbook: Pages 1740–1741 ANSWER: D.

77. Which of the following statements about upper extremity arterial insufficiency is/are true?

A. Symptomatic ischemia is more common in the upper extremity than in the lower extremity.
B. Vascular injuries from blunt trauma are more common in the upper extremity arteries than in the lower extremity ones.
C. Arteriovenous fistulas frequently follow blunt trauma.
D. The inflammatory process of arteries obstructed by an arteritis should be controlled before a bypass graft is inserted.

DISCUSSION: The larger muscle mass and heavier work loads of the lower extremities may lead to the development of ischemic symptoms in them more often than in the upper extremities. Blunt trauma occurs more often in the lower extremities. Arteriovenous fistulas more frequently follow penetrating trauma than blunt trauma. If the arteritis is not controlled before a bypass graft is placed, the inflammatory process may contribute to early occlusion of the graft.

Textbook: Pages 1747–1748 ANSWER: D.

78. Which of the following statements about upper extremity edema is/are true?

A. Lymphedema is more common than venous edema.
B. Signs and symptoms of venous obstruction include edema, distention of superficial veins, tightness, aching, cyanosis, and pain.
C. Distal venous obstructions are more likely than proximal venous obstructions to cause symptoms in the upper extremity.
D. All patients with symptomatic upper extremity venous thrombosis should receive fibrinolytic therapy.

DISCUSSION: Venous edema is much more common than lymphedema. Any of the signs and symptoms listed may be seen in patients with venous obstruction. The proximal venous obstructions in the axillary, subclavian, and innominate veins are more likely to cause symptoms in the upper extremities than is obstruction of the distal veins. The treatment for symptomatic upper extremity venous thrombosis varies according to the cause of the thrombosis.

Textbook: Pages 1748–1749 ANSWER: B.

79. Which of the following statements about chronic mesenteric ischemia due to atherosclerosis is/are correct?

A. Postprandial pain in these patients is due to gastric hyperacidity and in most cases is relieved with H_2 blockers.
B. Men are more often affected than women.
C. Mesenteric endarterectomy is the surgical treatment of choice, since long-term patency rates are superior to mesenteric bypass.
D. Arteriography is no longer necessary in these cases since noninvasive diagnosis can be established using duplex ultrasound scanning.
E. Surgical treatment is indicated to prevent intestinal infarction in symptomatic patients.

DISCUSSION: The precise cause of postprandial pain in patients with chronic mesenteric ischemia is unknown. Hyperacidity has been observed in some patients with this disease, and gastric pH may be reduced after successful revascularization. No medical therapy, including H_2 blockers, has provided symptomatic relief. Unlike most syndromes of ischemia due to atherosclerosis (coronary, cerebrovascular, peripheral vascular), chronic mesenteric ischemia occurs more frequently in women. The long-term success rates for mesenteric bypass and mesenteric endarterectomy are equivalent; either technique is acceptable. While duplex scanning is a useful noninvasive screening technique in these cases, arteriography is required for definitive diagnosis and to plan revascularization. While prospective, natural history studies have not been done, an increased risk of intestinal infarction is undeniable in these patients. When this occurs, patients rarely survive. Elective surgical revascularization is indicated in symptomatic patients with severe mesenteric arterial occlusive disease.

Textbook: Pages 1756–1758 ANSWER: E.

80. In patients with acute mesenteric ischemia due to mesenteric embolism, which of the following statements is/are correct?

A. Patients often have a history of postprandial pain and weight loss.
B. The use of digitalis may be a predisposing factor to the acute event.
C. Thrombolytic therapy may be attempted in patients without signs of bowel infarction or gastrointestinal bleeding.
D. Arteriography usually reveals the embolus lodged at the orifice of the superior mesenteric artery.
E. At the time of exploration, the proximal jejunum is often viable and ischemia is most severe in the more distal small bowel and colon.

DISCUSSION: Patients who suffer mesenteric embolism usually have otherwise normal mesenteric arterial anatomy, and ischemic symptoms are acute and profound. A history of chronic gastrointestinal symptoms is most often seen in patients with mesenteric thrombosis. Although cardiac arrhythmias like atrial fibrillation (which predispose to mesenteric emboli) may be treated with digitalis, this has no causative role in mesenteric embolism. Digitalis use has been associated with the development of "nonocclusive" mesenteric ischemia. Thrombolytic therapy with streptokinase or urokinase has been used successfully to treat mesenteric emboli; however, patients with any signs of local or generalized peritonitis should have immediate surgical exploration. Mesenteric emboli usually lodge distally in the main superior mesenteric artery beyond the first jejunal branches and the origin of the middle colic artery. The orifice of the superior mesenteric artery and the proximal branches are normal, which explains the "jejunal sparing" often observed at the time of surgical exploration, even when arteriography has not been performed.

Textbook: Pages 1752–1755 ANSWER: C, E.

81. Which of the following statements about angiotensin II is correct?

A. It is a decapeptide.
B. It is an enzyme found in high concentration in the pulmonary circulation.
C. It is a direct vasoconstrictor and stimulates aldosterone production.
D. It is a vasoconstrictor and inhibits aldosterone secretion.

DISCUSSION: Angiotensin II is an octapeptide cleaved from angiotensin I by angiotensin-converting enzyme. A direct vasoconstrictor, it also stimulates the adrenal cortical production of aldosterone.

Textbook: Pages 1759–1760 ANSWER: C.

82. Which of the following statements about atherosclerotic obstruction of the renal arteries is true?

A. Lesions are usually short.
B. These lesions are usually found in the distal renal arteries, particularly just beyond branch points.
C. Ostial lesions are best treated with balloon angioplasty.
D. Lesions of this type are the second most common cause of renal artery stenosis.

DISCUSSION: Atherosclerotic renal artery lesions are usually short and found in the proximal renal arteries. Ostial lesions in particular do not respond well to balloon angioplasty, and such lesions are responsible for more than two thirds of renal artery obstructions.

Textbook: Pages 1760–1761 ANSWER: A.

83. Which of the following statements about the treatment of renal artery stenosis is/are true?

A. Though a significant cause of hypertension, renal artery stenosis seldom results in loss of renal function.
B. In patients with medically controlled renovascular hypertension there is no need to consider revascularization.
C. Balloon angioplasty is more effective in patients with atherosclerotic disease as compared with those with fibromuscular disease.
D. In patients with severe atherosclerosis of the aorta, bypass from the splenic or hepatic arteries should be considered.

DISCUSSION: In a significant percentage of patients with renovascular hypertension there is loss of renal mass, which may progress to end-stage renal insufficiency. Ostial lesions respond poorly to balloon angioplasty. If the aorta is severely diseased bypass can be effective using either the hepatic or the splenic artery to supply blood to the kidney.

Textbook: Pages 1764–1765 ANSWER: D.

84. Which of the following statements about venous trauma is/are current?

A. All injured veins can be ligated without any immediate or long-term complications.
B. Attempted repair of injured veins is associated with increased incidence of thrombophlebitis.
C. Attempted repair of injured veins is associated with a high incidence of fatal pulmonary embolism.
D. Careful consideration should be made to repair the injured popliteal vein.
E. Anatomy of the venous system is more variable than anatomy of the arterial system.

DISCUSSION: Many patients treated by ligation of injured veins suffer no immediate or long-term sequelae. Unfortunately, there are patients who are difficult to identify initially who may have either acute venous hypertension or later suffer chronic venous insufficiency following ligation of large-caliber veins in the lower extremities. The popliteal vein is particularly important to repair if at all possible following injury, as are many of the larger-caliber central veins. Both civilian and military reports have documented that there is not an increased incidence of thrombophlebitis and/or pulmonary embolism associated with attempted repair of injured veins. In contrast to the arterial system, there are many more variations in venous anatomy. This complicates the evaluation of patients with injured veins with examples of a possible bifid popliteal vein and one to five channels comprising the superficial femoral vein.

Textbook: Pages 1768–1770 ANSWER: D, E.

85. All but one of the following statements is true. Which is *not* true?

A. Successful clinical repair of injured veins had been effected by the turn of the twentieth century.
B. Initial large experience in managing injured veins came from the battlefields of twentieth-century wars.
C. More than 50% of repaired injured veins thrombose.
D. Phlebography is useful in evaluating variable venous anatomy.
E. Repeated phlebography following attempted venous repair is useful in determining the success rate.

DISCUSSION: Murphy advocated venous repair as early as 1897, after others, including Schede (1882), noted success. Extensive experience in managing large numbers of venous injuries has resulted from major armed conflicts of the twentieth century. Phlebography is particularly valuable for determining venous anatomy and the success or failure of attempted venous repair, and repeated phlebography over the first 72 hours has proven particularly informative. There is a high degree of success in performing lateral suture of lacerations of large-caliber veins as demonstrated by follow-up phlebography.

Textbook: Pages 1767–1768, 1770 ANSWER: C.

86. Which of the following statements about injured veins is/are correct?

A. In contrast to the arterial system, it is more difficult to evaluate the patient for suspected venous trauma.
B. There is no simple method similar to palpating distal pulses following arterial repair to evaluate the status of attempted venous repair.
C. Recanalization of initial thrombosis of attempted venous repair is more common than in the arterial system.
D. Doppler ultrasound—and more recently color-flow duplex—have been increasingly helpful in evaluating integrity of the venous system.
E. Prevention of venous stasis is important in the immediate postoperative period after attempted venous repair.

DISCUSSION: There are significant differences between the arterial system and the lower-pressure venous system. Presence or absence of distal pulses associated with possible arterial injuries provides a simple mechanism for evaluating patients with potential injury, while there is no simple method of evaluating patients for potential venous injury. Doppler ultrasound—and more recently color-flow duplex—have been increasingly helpful in evaluating the integrity of the venous system. If thrombosis of an attempted venous repair occurs, there is a high probability that recanalization of the thrombus will occur. This is in contrast to the arterial system, where recanalization of thrombosis of an attempted arterial repair is a rare occurrence. Venous stasis must be prevented in the immediate postoperative period following attempted venous repair to reduce the possibility of thrombosis.

Textbook: Pages 1767–1768, 1770–1771 ANSWER: A, B, C, D, E.

NOTES

NOTES

CHAPTER 22

CHEST SURGERY

1. The bronchial circulation:

A. Is the blood supply to the conducting airways.
B. Drains into a peribronchial venous network that may expand considerably with conditions such as bronchiectasis and chronic obstructive pulmonary disease.
C. Is an especially important consideration in pulmonary transplantation.
D. All of the above.

DISCUSSION: The bronchial circulation is the primary blood supply for the conducting airways, pulmonary vessels, lymphoid tissue, and squamous cell carcinomas. In conditions such as mitral stenosis, bronchiectasis, or chronic obstructive pulmonary disease, the rich peribronchial venous network that drains the bronchial circulation may expand considerably, creating significant left-to-right shunts. Whenever the pulmonary artery circulation is obstructed, there is a tendency for bronchial circulation to increase; thus, the bronchial circulation is an important consideration during lung transplantation as well as in the surgical treatment of cyanotic congenital heart disease and chronic pulmonary embolism.

Textbook: Pages 1781–1783 ANSWER: D.

2. Clearance of mucus produced in the tracheobronchial tree in chronic bronchitis secondary to smoking may:

A. Be hampered by the fact that the amount of mucus is increased by the number of mucus-producing cells at the expense of ciliated cells.
B. Be slowed if patients have decreased lung volume and are therefore unable to generate a vigorous cough that would cause an inflammatory process.
C. Cause a decrease in diffusion capacity and associated hypoxemia.
D. All of the above.

DISCUSSION: Chronic bronchitis may have an acute component, and in these patients therapy with antibiotics and bronchodilators may improve the flow rate as measured by pulmonary function tests within 3 or 4 days of the cessation of smoking and treatment of the acute condition. However, the chronic bronchitic will continue to produce large amounts of mucus, most evident in the morning, even after the acute process has been resolved. Clearance of these secretions is hampered by the inability to cough, perhaps secondary to the pain of thoracotomy or abdominal surgery or by a decrease in the number of ciliary cells that help move mucus up the tracheobronchial tree. This causes plugging of small airways and atelectasis, which may progress to pneumonia. For this reason, cessation of smoking for 3 to 5 days before surgery is very beneficial in preventing pulmonary complications during the postoperative period.

Textbook: Pages 1778–1779 ANSWER: A.

3. The pulmonary circulation:

A. Is the only vascular system in which the veins do not have the same course as the arteries.
B. Has a direct connection of vein to adjacent lung tissue by connective tissue fibers, making the diameter of the tissue fibers dependent upon lung volume.
C. Supplies the metabolic needs of the alveoli.
D. All of the above.

DISCUSSION: Pulmonary artery circulation transports oxygenated blood to the alveoli level where gas exchange occurs, and it is here that the matching of ventilation and perfusion is so important during the postoperative period. The loss of lung volume that generally occurs after all surgical procedures does not return to baseline for 5 to 7 days and may play an important role in the ventilation-perfusion ratio. Improving or returning lung volume to normal is performed by manipulating functional residual capacity (FRC) and preventing atelectasis, which in turn maintains circulation to the alveolus and optimizes the ventilation-perfusion ratio.

Textbook: Pages 1780–1783 ANSWER: C.

4. Which of the following screening tests are important for preoperative evaluation of pulmonary function?

A. History and physical examination.
B. Room air arterial blood gases.
C. Chest film.
D. Vital capacity and forced expiratory volume in 1 second (FEV_1).
E. Cardiopulmonary exercise testing.

DISCUSSION: The most important clues to impairment of respiratory function are found in the history and physical examination. A negative history and physical examination in combination with a relatively normal room air arterial blood gas and normal chest film are sufficient to screen patients to support the clinical impression that there is minimal pulmonary disease. Patients with symptoms, positive physical findings, and/or abnormalities in the arterial blood gases or chest film can be screened most effectively with an additional evaluation of the vital capacity and FEV_1. More elaborate tests such as cardiopulmonary exercise testing are reserved for patients with obvious and marked impairment of pulmonary function who are being evaluated for the feasibility of surgical intervention.

Textbook: Pages 1787–1788 ANSWER: A, B, C, D, E.

5. Carbon monoxide diffusion capacity (DL_{CO}) has been shown to correlate with:

A. The thickness of the alveolar lining membrane.
B. The permeability of the erythrocyte to carbon dioxide.
C. Pulmonary emboli.
D. Total alveolar-capillary capacity.

DISCUSSION: The single-breath DL_{CO} is a screening test that has been shown to be decreased in all of the above examples. It is an estimate of the total capacity of the functional alveolar microarchitecture and has been demonstrated to be an independent measure of physiologic capability apart from the FEV_1 and forced ventilatory capacity.

Textbook: Pages 1790–1791 ANSWER: A, B, C, D.

6. The closing volume is:

A. The volume remaining in the lung at the end of expiration below which alveolar collapse begins to occur, resulting in physiologic shunting.
B. Higher in young persons.
C. Not changed during surgery.
D. Relative to the oxygen content of mixed venous blood.

DISCUSSION: The closing volume is conceptually the remaining lung volume at the end of expiration below which alveolar collapse begins to occur, causing intrapulmonary right-to-left shunting and thus desaturation of blood in the left atrium. In a normal young person this closing volume is well below the functional residual capacity (FRC); thus, such physiologic shunting does not occur until there is a decrease in the elastic properties of the lung. Although FRC gradually increases with age, so does the effective closing volume. Eventually some alveoli are being underventilated (at end-expiration), allowing physiologic right-to-left shunting to occur. Closing volume is unchanged, but FRC decreases during surgery (i.e., shunting occurs). Closing volume has no direct relationship to the oxygen content of the mixed venous blood.

Textbook: Page 1799 ANSWER: A, C.

7. The effect of high positive end-expiratory pressures (PEEP) on cardiac output is:

A. None.
B. Increased cardiac output.
C. Decreased cardiac output because of increased afterload to the left ventricle.
D. Decreased cardiac output because of decreased effective preload to the left ventricle.

DISCUSSION: Higher levels of PEEP can be associated with decreases in cardiac output as a consequence of an effective decrease in the preload to the left ventricle owing to impaired left ventricular filling.

Textbook: Page 1796 ANSWER: D.

8. Weaning patients from maximum ventilator support usually involves:

A. Weaning PEEP first, tidal volume second, and the fraction of inspired oxygen (FIO_2) third.
B. Weaning FIO_2 first, ventilator rate second, and PEEP third.
C. Weaning FIO_2 first, PEEP second, and tidal volume third.
D. Weaning FIO_2 first, PEEP second, and ventilator rate third.

DISCUSSION: When the inspired oxygen concentration is greater than 60% for more than 24 to 28 hours, the risk of oxygen toxicity increases. PEEP is usually weaned to physiologic levels (i.e., 5 to 7 cm. H_2O) before weaning either rate or tidal volumes. Generally, the optimal tidal volume to achieve alveolar recruitment is selected and usually is not decreased unless peak airway pressures increase. If decreases in ventilatory rate are not tolerated, airway pressure support can be added.

Textbook: Page 1796 ANSWER: D.

9. Which of the following statements about bronchoscopy is false?

A. The morbidity and mortality are approximately 0.2% and 0.08%, respectively.
B. The most common complications of bronchoscopy are related to premedication of patients.
C. Adjunctive cancer therapy such as laser treatment and brachytherapy may be administered via this route.
D. A chronic cough and unilateral wheezing are accepted indications for bronchoscopy.
E. Early postoperative bronchoscopy for atelectasis is contraindicated following pulmonary resection.

DISCUSSION: The stated complication rates are true and reported from a comprehensive review of over 24,000 patients. Although the most common complications are related to the premedication, significant hemorrhage, pneumothorax, bronchospasm, and dysrhythmias have been reported. In addition to laser and brachytherapy, phototherapy and immunotherapy have been given by bronchoscopy. Unilateral wheezing may represent a bronchial foreign body, and a chronic cough could signify myriad pulmonary disorders. Accordingly, both are amenable to diagnostic bronchoscopy. Most thoracic surgeons favor early

bronchoscopy for lobar atelectasis following pulmonary surgery.
Textbook: Pages 1802–1804 ANSWER: E.

10. Flexible bronchoscopy is preferred over rigid bronchoscopy for all of the following except:

A. Patients with cervical spine injuries requiring intubation.
B. The evaluation of a smoke inhalation injury.
C. Transcarinal needle aspiration of an enlarged subcarinal lymph node.
D. The removal of a bronchus intermedius foreign body from an infant.
E. A cost-effective evaluation of mild hemoptysis.

DISCUSSION: Neither patients with significant cervical spine disease or injuries nor those with large aortic arch aneurysms should undergo rigid bronchoscopy, given the greater risk of complications. Even if severe, smoke inhalation injury can be assessed adequately by flexible bronchoscopy. Transbronchial needle aspiration of lesions that on computed tomography (CT) look suspicious is safe and quite easily performed with fluoroscopic guidance. Hemoptysis as a presenting symptom should be evaluated by flexible bronchoscopy. In contrast, for massive hemoptysis an airway should be secured for ventilation with a rigid bronchoscope. Similarly, an airway needs to be maintained while removing endobronchial foreign bodies from infants or children. Since adequate port sites for instrumentation are also needed, the rigid bronchoscope is preferred in this setting.
Textbook: Page 1803 ANSWER: D.

11. Which of the following approaches is/are currently acceptable for the management of spontaneous pneumothorax?

A. Chest tube replacement alone for the patient with a first episode.
B. Operation on presentation for any patient with a first episode.
C. Video-assisted thoracic surgery (VATS) bleb excision and pleurodesis for recurrent pneumothorax on the same side.
D. Thoracotomy with bleb excision and pleurodesis for unilateral recurrent pneumothorax.
E. Operation after a first episode in an airline pilot.

DISCUSSION: Primary spontaneous pneumothorax typically occurs in young patients with congenital blebs at the apices of the lungs. Rupture of these blebs causes pneumothorax, which recurs in about 30% of patients. Standard care on initial presentation is chest tube placement alone. Operation traditionally has been performed during the initial episode only if there is prolonged air leakage (longer than 7 days); in patients with bilateral pneumothorax; those who live in an area where prompt medical care, if needed, is not available; and those frequently exposed to extremes of pressure (e.g., airline pilots). Both VATS and thoracotomy approaches to excision of blebs and pleurodesis have been shown to be effective. The availability of the apparently safer VATS approach has led some to favor earlier operation.
Textbook: Page 1809 ANSWER: A, C, D, E.

12. For which patient(s) with a pulmonary infiltrate of uncertain cause would you favor VATS over open wedge excision?

A. An AIDS patient with a diffuse infiltrate who is ambulatory but requires supplemental oxygen. Bronchoalveolar lavage is negative.
B. A 64-year-old previously healthy man with increasing shortness of breath, a diffuse infiltrate, and restrictive lung disease as shown by pulmonary function studies.
C. A 74-year-old diabetic woman with a rapidly progressing process throughout the right lung who is ventilator- and pressor-dependent.
D. A 44-year-old man with fever, left-sided infiltrate, and shortness of breath.
E. A 79-year-old man on a ventilator for right lower and middle lobe pneumonia which has been culture negative.

DISCUSSION: Lung biopsy by VATS or minithoracotomy is often indicated in the work-up of a pulmonary infiltrate that has not been successfully diagnosed by less invasive studies. This procedure probably is not indicated for cancer patients with acute pneumonitis, as broad-spectrum antibiotics frequently are successful treatments. For those who do require the procedure, the choice between VATS and thoracotomy is determined by the severity of illness. In those who are critically ill and ventilator dependent, changing the tube to an endobronchial tube for thoracoscopy may be risky, and in these cases an anterior thoracotomy with single-lumen ventilation is indicated. These patients, who are frequently heavily sedated and are likely to remain so for some time postoperatively, are unlikely to benefit from the greatest advantage of VATS, the reduction of postoperative pain. It is, then, the ambulatory patient with a chronic interstitial process who benefits the most from the VATS approach.
Textbook: Pages 1807–1808 ANSWER: A, B, D.

13. Which of the following statements about the cause and prevention of postintubation tracheal stenosis are correct?

A. Postintubation airway stenosis can largely be avoided by providing assisted ventilation via endotracheal tube rather than tracheostomy tube.
B. Postintubation tracheal stenosis at the cuff level results, more or less equally, from low blood pressure, advanced age, steroids, high intracuff pressure, sensitivity to tube materials, gas sterilization elution products, and systemic disease.
C. In women and smaller men large endotracheal tubes can produce lesions of the glottis and subglottis that can progress to stenosis.

D. Stomal stenosis is due principally to cicatricial closure of large stomas resulting from removal of a disk or segment of tracheal wall during tracheostomy.
E. A large-volume tracheostomy tube cuff such as that now used on most available tubes can become a high-pressure cuff if filled beyond its resting maximal volume.

DISCUSSION: Use of an endotracheal tube, of course, avoids a stoma and related complications. Cuff lesions, however, are incurred from cuffs on endotracheal tubes, cricothyroidostomy tubes, and tracheostomy tubes. A cuff is the common factor. Endotracheal tubes, on the other hand, cause erosion at the level of the glottis and subglottis, in particular. Although many factors may play some role in the origin of airway stenosis, the principal factor is pressure necrosis of the mucosa, submucosa, and ultimately of the cartilage, with subsequent cicatrization. Large endotracheal tubes do, indeed, cause necrosis and airway injury at narrow areas in the upper airway, at glottic and cricoid levels. Such injuries lead to posterior commissure stenosis, arytenoid fixation, vocal cord erosion and granulomas, anterior commissure stricture, and subglottic circumferential stenosis. While excision of a large amount of tracheal wall can lead inevitably to healing by contraction with narrowing of the tracheal circumference, the most usual cause of stomal stenosis is erosion of the stoma by pressure from the tracheostomy tube. This in turn may relate to leverage by equipment. Additional factors appear to be subsidiary. A large volume, low pressure tracheostomy tube cuff, such as those currently available, if properly constructed, will seal the trachea before it is necessary to stretch the cuff by adding an increasing volume of air. If the cuff is stretched beyond that resting volume, which usually occludes the normal trachea, high pressures will develop because the plastic material from which all of these cuffs are now made is not very extensible. Therefore, the pressure-volume curve rises sharply once the limit of unstretched volume is passed. A low-pressure cuff then becomes a high-pressure cuff.

Textbook: Pages 1816–1819 ANSWER: C, E.

14. Which of the following statements about the treatment of postintubation airway stenosis are correct?

A. Emergency management of airway obstruction due to stenosis at the level of a prior tracheal stoma is best accomplished by establishing a new tracheostomy in normal tracheal tissue just below the scar of the old stoma.
B. Radial lasering and dilatation usually leads to permanent resolution of postintubation tracheal stenosis.
C. Splinting of a cervical trachea with a silicone T-tube for 6 to 8 months generally leads to permanent resolution of stricture.
D. Postintubation tracheal stenosis that extends into the subglottic larynx is treated by resection of a cylindrical sleeve of stenotic airway and end-to-end reconstruction.
E. Acquired tracheoesophageal fistula due to intubation injury is corrected by surgical closure of the fistula concurrent with resection and reconstruction of the damaged trachea.

DISCUSSION: Emergency management of postintubation tracheal stenosis is accomplished by dilatation under general anesthesia using rigid bronchoscopes and dilators. Tracheostomy is employed only when the patient requires a prolonged or a permanent airway before or instead of resection and reconstruction. If a new tracheostomy is needed it is preferable to place it through the area of existing stenosis—in this case the site of prior tracheostomy—rather than to injure normal trachea that will be needed for resection and reconstruction. If the stenosis is below the sternal notch, a long tracheostomy tube is inserted at the usual position (second and third rings) but extends past the now dilated stenotic lesion.

Lasering almost never results in a permanently satisfactory airway; the exception is the very limited lesion described as a thin, weblike stenosis. Such lesions are rare. Unfortunately, laser is widely used and often compounds existing damage by concurrent placement of a tracheostomy tube below the lesion in the normal trachea. T-tubes are very useful for temporizing when repair is not possible or must be delayed. It almost never leads to resolution of a stricture unless it is an extremely limited one. Soon after removal of the T-tube the stricture reasserts itself.

If the lesion involves the subglottic larynx, complex repair is required to preserve the recurrent laryngeal nerve's anatomy and function. The posterior cricoid plate is salvaged and resurfaced with a flap of membranous tracheal wall; the anterior subglottic larynx is reconstructed with a "prow" of distal tracheal cartilage and mucosa.

A tracheoesophageal fistula is managed (*after* weaning from a respirator) by layered closure of the esophagus, interposition of a flap of well-vascularized tissue (such as a pedicled strap muscle), and resection and reconstruction of the damaged trachea. Since the fistula results from the pressure of a cuff, often against an esophageal feeding tube, there is circumferential damage to the trachea at the level of the fistula. Resection and reconstruction are therefore necessary, in addition to closure of the fistula, for successful treatment of this complex lesion.

Textbook: Page 1818 ANSWER: E.

15. Which of the following statements are true?

A. Pyogenic lung abscess occurs most frequently in the lower lobe of the left lung.
B. Anaerobic bacteria are commonly present in pyogenic lung abscess.
C. Operation is usually required to eradicate a pyogenic lung abscess.
D. Penicillin is the treatment of choice for lung abscess.

DISCUSSION: Pyogenic lung abscess is the result of aspiration of debris from the oropharynx. Since most patients are unconscious and supine when this occurs, the aspirated material usually finds its way into the most dependent bronchi. These are the superior division of the right lower lobe and the posterior segment of the right upper lobe. The organisms most commonly responsible for pyogenic lung abscess are the same anaerobic bacteria found in the mouths of patients with poor oral hygiene. In addition to anaerobic organisms alpha- and beta-hemolytic streptococci, staphylococci, nonhemolytic streptococci, and *Escherichia coli* may be present. Gram-negative rods and staphylococci are particularly common in hospital-acquired infections. These organisms are almost always penicillin sensitive. Surgical therapy is rarely necessary to eradicate a pyogenic lung abscess. Penicillin, alone or in combination with metronidazole, is the drug of choice. Metronidazole alone probably lacks sufficient activity against anaerobic and microaerophilic streptococci. Clindamycin is also effective against most anaerobic bacteria present in pyogenic lung abscesses.

Textbook: Pages 1821–1822 ANSWER: B, D.

16. Amphotericin B is effective for the following lung infections:

A. Histoplasmosis.
B. North American blastomycosis.
C. Aspergillosis.
D. Mucormycosis.
E. Sporotrichosis.

DISCUSSION: Amphotericin B is effective against most fungal infections, including histoplasmosis and North American blastomycosis. Aspergillosis is caused by the fungus *Aspergillus fumigatus,* an organism that is resistant to treatment with iodides, nystatin, hydroxystilbamidine, and amphotericin B. The treatment for this fungal infection is a surgical procedure, if the patient's condition permits. Surgical excision and amphotericin B usually are necessary to treat mucormycosis. Itraconazole is the drug of choice for sporotrichosis. Itraconazole, ketoconazole, and fluconazole should be considered as primary or secondary drugs when treating systemic fungal infections.

Textbook: Page 1824 ANSWER: A, B, D.

17. The following statements are true.

A. A distinguishing roentgenographic appearance of lung abscess, the air-fluid level can be seen only on roentgenograms obtained in the upright or lateral decubitus position.
B. The fungus ball characteristic of aspergillosis can be seen roentgenographically in either the upright or recumbent position.
C. Actinomycosis and nocardiosis are both fungal diseases of the lung that respond to treatment with the newer azole antifungal agents.
D. The commonest fungal lung infection in the United States is due to *Histoplasma capsulatum.*

DISCUSSION: An air-fluid level distinguishes a lung abscess. While this can be seen easily in an upright or lateral decubitus roentgenogram, it cannot be seen when the patient is recumbent. The fungus ball characteristic of aspergillosis is identified by its crescent-shaped shadow on a roentgenogram. When the patient changes from an upright to recumbent position, the fungus ball may also change position in the cavity in the lung. Both actinomycosis and nocardiosis are bacterial infections and do not respond to antimycotic treatment. *Actinomyces israelli* is treated with penicillin and *Nocardia asteroides* is sensitive to trimethoprim-sulfamethoxazole. The most common fungal infection in North America is histoplasmosis. More than 30 million people have been infected, most of whom are asymptomatic.

Textbook: Pages 1821–1827 ANSWER: A, B, D.

18. *Pneumocystis* pneumonia is an opportunistic infection caused by *Pneumocystis carinii.* Which of the following statements are true?

A. *P. carinii* is a fungus.
B. *Pneumocystis* pneumonia is the most common opportunistic infection in patients with AIDS.
C. The diagnosis of *Pneumocystis* pneumonia depends on the demonstration of *P. carinii* organisms in lung tissue.
D. There is no effective treatment for *Pneumocystis* pneumonia.

DISCUSSION: *P. carinii* is a protozoan that stains with silver methenamine and resembles a fungus. It responds to antiprotozoal drugs. *Pneumocystis* pneumonia occurs in 80% of AIDS patients. The diagnosis is made by demonstrating the organisms in lung tissue by transbronchoscopic lung or brush biopsy, percutaneous needle biopsy, or open lung biopsy. Both trimethoprin-sulfamethoxazole and pentamidine isethionate are effective against *P. carinii.*

Textbook: Pages 1828–1829 ANSWER: B, C.

19. Which of the following statements are true?

A. The pleural space does not extend into the neck.
B. Positive intrapleural pressures as high as 40 cm. H_2O and negative pressures as low as −40 cm. H_2O are possible.
C. The pleural cavities cannot absorb more than 500 ml. of fluid per day.
D. All pleural effusions are of clinical significance and should be investigated.

DISCUSSION: The pleural spaces extend into the neck as well as retrosternally and into the costophrenic sinuses. This should be kept in mind when performing procedures such as subclavian and jugular puncture, to avoid pneumothorax. Markedly elevated intrapleural pressures are obtained with the Valsalva maneuver, and extreme negative pressures can be produced with forced inspiratory effort against a closed glottis. Because of the many microvilli present on the mesothelial cells that line the pleural cavity, a liter or more of fluid is easily secreted or absorbed within a 24-hour period. Most pleural effusions are caused by infection, tumor, or congestive heart failure and should be investigated to determine the proper course of management.

Textbook: Pages 1830–1831 ANSWER: B, D.

20. Which of the following statements are true?

A. Chylothorax, or chyle in the pleural cavity, usually is not a serious condition.
B. Chyle is easily identified by its milky appearance, which looks like no other kind of pleural effusion.
C. The commonest causes of chylothorax are trauma and tumor.
D. The thoracic duct can be ligated with impunity.

DISCUSSION: Chylothorax is most often the result of trauma; however, spontaneous chylothorax is also a manifestation of tumor and should be investigated to identify occult malignancies. Chyle in the thorax is characteristically milky white but can be mistaken for the pseudochylothorax of rheumatoid disease or tuberculosis. If necessary, a diagnosis can be confirmed by lymphangiography. This also facilitates ligation of the thoracic duct, should this become necessary to control the loss of chyle.

Textbook: Page 1835 ANSWER: C, D.

21. Which of these statements about pleural tumors is/are true?

A. The commonest type of pleural tumor is primary pleural mesothelioma.
B. Exposure to asbestos dust is causally related to the development of malignant mesothelioma.
C. Localized benign mesotheliomas are asymptomatic.
D. Complete pleurectomy for malignant mesothelioma usually results in cure.

DISCUSSION: Pleural involvement by metastatic disease is much more common than primary pleural tumors. Patients with localized benign pleural mesotheliomas may have symptoms of arthralgia, clubbing of the fingers, or fever, which usually disappear after excisional surgery. The evidence relating industrial exposure to asbestosis and malignant pleural mesothelioma is quite strong. Excisional surgery for malignant mesothelioma is usually only palliative. Most patients succumb within 1 to 2 years of the diagnosis, regardless of the kind of treatment they receive.

Textbook: Page 1837 ANSWER: B.

22. Which of the following correctly describe a patient with spontaneous pneumothorax?

A. The patient is almost always elderly and debilitated.
B. An unsuspected primary or metastatic lung tumor may be present.
C. The administration of supplemental oxygen is of little benefit to the patient.
D. The patient should always be treated with an intercostal tube and closed pleural drainage.
E. Video-assisted thoracic surgery (VATS) should be considered for persistent air leak in patients with secondary spontaneous pneumothorax.

DISCUSSION: A patient with spontaneous pneumothorax may be old and debilitated, but the typical patient is an otherwise healthy young adult, usually one who smokes. An incidental, unsuspected lung cancer is discovered on rare occasions when operation is performed to control a persistent air leak. Perhaps smoking is a common factor. Absorption of air from the pleural space can be facilitated by the administration of supplemental oxygen. Increasing the oxygen tension lowers the partial pressure of nitrogen (P_{N_2}) of the capillary blood and increases the partial pressure difference between the pleural space and the pulmonary capillary. If the pneumothorax results in less than 20% collapse of the lung an asymptomatic patient can be safely observed; however, a larger or persistent pneumothorax is best treated with an intercostal tube thoracostomy. Patients with bullous emphysema may require stapling of bullae and pleurectomy, which can be done by open thoracotomy or thoracoscopically (VATS).

Textbook: Pages 1833–1834 ANSWER: B, E.

23. Which of the following statements about spontaneous pneumothorax (PSP) is/are correct?

A. The risk of recurrence after resolution of the first episode of PSP or secondary spontaneous pneumothorax (SSP) is 35% to 45%.
B. Patients with PSP are typically tall, thin, young adult males with a history of smoking.
C. Secondary spontaneous pneumothorax is associated with family history in 10% of cases.
D. For bleb resection and pleurodesis thoracoscopic thoracotomy and open thoracotomy provide similar cure rates for patients with primary spontaneous pneumothorax.
E. Causes of secondary pneumothorax include trauma and iatrogenic needle puncture.

DISCUSSION: Patients with PSP are usually 20- to 40-year-old males with a common long-chested body habitus. The majority of PSP patients have a history of tobacco use and 10% have a family history of PSP. The majority of cases of SSP are due to advanced emphysema in a population of patients aged 50 to 70 years. Additional causes of SSP include tuberculosis, cystic fibrosis, *P. carinii* infection, lung cancer, and lung abscess. For patients with PSP bleb resection and pleurodesis performed thoracoscopically provides cure rates similar to those of open thoracotomy. Because of the nature of underlying pulmonary diseases, open thoracotomy appears to provide better results for patients with SSP.

Textbook: Pages 1833–1834 ANSWER: A, B, D.

24. Which of the following are relative contraindications for surgical management of emphysema?

A. Rapidly progressive dyspnea.
B. Bullae occupying less than one third of a hemithorax on plain chest radiography.
C. Elevated room air PCO_2.
D. "Pink puffer" patients.
E. FEV_1 less than 35% of predicted value.

DISCUSSION: Relative contraindications to operation for bullous emphysema include patients with carbon dioxide retention, FEV_1 less than 35% of predicted value, small bullae that occupy less than one third of a hemithorax, and "blue bloaters," who are prone to the sequelae of chronic bronchitis. Patients who have primarily emphysema ("pink puffers") and rapidly progressive dyspnea are usually good candidates for operation.

Textbook: Pages 1840–1841 ANSWER: B, C, E.

25. Which of the following treatments would be appropriate therapy for symptoms that persist on medical therapy and bronchiectasis involving, in order of decreasing severity, the left lower lobe, the right middle lobe, and the left upper lobe?

A. Left pneumonectomy.
B. Wedge resection of the left lower lobe.
C. Left lower lobectomy.
D. Simultaneous left lower lobectomy and right middle lobectomy.

DISCUSSION: Pneumonectomy is seldom indicated today for bronchiectasis. Anatomic resection of involved segments with either segmentectomy or lobectomy is preferred to nonanatomic wedge resection. Bilateral pulmonary resections should generally be done as staged procedures, the most symptomatic side being resected first. Then, the contralateral side is resected only if symptoms persist during a prolonged course of medical therapy.

Textbook: Pages 1845–1846 ANSWER: C.

26. Which of the following would not be acceptable sequences of preoperative studies in a patient being prepared for lingulectomy for bronchiectasis?

A. CT alone.
B. CT, bronchoscopy, bronchography.
C. Bronchoscopy alone.
D. Bronchoscopy, bronchography.

DISCUSSION: Bronchoscopy alone is generally not diagnostic for bronchiectasis. Thin-section, high-resolution CT can diagnose bronchiectasis and define the airway anatomy sufficiently for resection. Bronchography is performed less frequently today but can be very useful in diagnosing bronchiectasis and defining airway anatomy for pulmonary resection.

Textbook: Pages 1845–1846 ANSWER: C.

27. Which of the following statements about pulmonary mycobacterial infection is/are correct?

A. Worldwide, tuberculosis no longer represents a significant public health problem.
B. *Mycobacterium tuberculosis* is responsible for the majority of cases of pulmonary mycobacterial disease.
C. *Mycobacterium kansasii* pulmonary infection almost always requires surgical treatment.
D. Atypical mycobacteria are never primary pulmonary pathogens in humans.
E. *Mycobacterium avium-intracellulare* is generally resistant to most antimycobacterial drugs *in vitro*.

DISCUSSION: Tuberculosis remains the leading infectious killer in the world today. *M. tuberculosis* is responsible for the vast majority of pulmonary mycobacterial disease. *M. kansasii* infection responds to multiple drug chemotherapy and relatively infrequently requires surgical treatment. Atypical mycobacteria can be primary pulmonary pathogens in humans. *M. avium-intracellulare* is usually resistant *in vitro* to most antituberculosis drugs.

Textbook: Pages 1847–1848 ANSWER: B, E.

28. Which of the following chemotherapeutic regimens are currently recommended for the treatment of pulmonary infection caused by *M. tuberculosis?*

A. Isoniazid, rifampin, pyrazinamide, and streptomycin for 24 months.
B. Isoniazid for 9 months with ethambutol for the first 3 months.
C. Isoniazid and rifampin for 6 months with pyrazinamide added for the first two months.
D. Isoniazid alternating with rifampin at 3-month intervals for 12 months.
E. Isoniazid and rifampin for 9 months.

DISCUSSION: Treatment of tuberculosis with a single drug leads to rapid emergence of drug-resistant organisms. Any treatment regimen that employs only one drug for a period of time encourages the development of drug-resistant tuberculosis. Currently, the American Thoracic Society recommends either (1) a 6-month regimen consisting of isoniazid, rifampin, and pyrazinamide for 2 months followed by isoniazid and rifampin for 4 months or, alternatively, (2) a 9-month course of isoniazid and rifampin. Prolonged courses of treatment beyond 9 to 12 months no longer are considered necessary.

Textbook: Pages 1850–1851 ANSWER: C, E.

29. Which of the following are appropriate indications for pulmonary resection for mycobacterial disease?

A. Localized pulmonary disease caused by *M. avium-intracellulare.*
B. Advanced lobar tuberculous pneumonia with massive hilar lymphadenopathy and bronchial obstruction in a young child.
C. Localized pulmonary disease due to multiple drug–resistant *M. tuberculosis.*
D. An asymptomatic tuberculous cavity greater than 12 cm. in diameter.

E. Massive hemoptysis from a right upper lobe cavity occurring during an appropriate course of chemotherapy for pulmonary tuberculosis in a sputum-negative patient.

DISCUSSION: Modern antimycobacterial chemotherapy is very effective. Surgical treatment of pulmonary mycobacterial disease is rarely necessary; however, pulmonary disease caused by *M. avium-intracellulare* or multiple drug–resistant *M. tuberculosis* is not likely to respond to chemotherapy and should be resected if the disease is localized. Chemotherapy for tuberculosis is almost invariably curative in children, regardless of the extent of disease. The size of a tuberculous cavity is not an indication for resection. Massive hemoptysis from a cavitary lesion is life threatening and is an indication for pulmonary resection.
Textbook: Pages 1851–1853 ANSWER: A, C, E.

30. Which statements about squamous papillomatosis of the trachea is/are correct?

A. It is the most common type of benign tracheal tumor in adults.
B. It is the most common type of benign tracheal tumor in children.
C. Most are treated with segmental tracheal resection.
D. There is no risk of malignant degeneration.
E. It is associated with a herpesvirus.

DISCUSSION: Squamous papillomatosis is the most common benign tracheal and bronchial tumor in adults. Up to 50% of untreated lesions may degenerate into squamous cell carcinoma. The lesion is associated with human papillomavirus types 6 and 11, and therefore, interferon therapy is under investigation. Most patients can be treated successfully by repeated bronchoscopic fulguration, laser ablation, or cryotherapy.
Textbook: Page 1854 ANSWER: A.

31. Which of the following statements about pulmonary hamartomas is/are true?

A. Hamartomas are benign chondromas.
B. Most are located in the conducting airways.
C. Wedge resection is curative.
D. A lobectomy is necessary to obtain draining hilar lymph nodes.
E. Hemoptysis is common.

DISCUSSION: Pulmonary hamartomas are benign masses consisting of cartilage, lymph tissue, fat, and epithelial elements. Eighty per cent are located in the lung periphery and are treated by a small wedge resection, usually with a thoracoscope. Most are asymptomatic, and there is no risk of malignant degeneration.
Textbook: Page 1858 ANSWER: C.

32. Which of the following statements about typical carcinoid tumors are true?

A. They make up the majority of bronchial adenomas.
B. They frequently have lymph node metastases.
C. The carcinoid syndrome is observed in 33%.
D. Overall survival at 5 years is 90%.
E. Overall survival at 5 years is 50%.

DISCUSSION: Eighty-five per cent of bronchial adenomas are carcinoid tumors. Typical carcinoid tumors have few mitotic figures and infrequent lymph node metastases (fewer than 10%). Only 10% to 15% of patients present with the carcinoid syndrome (flushing, wheezing, diarrhea). Survival after resection is more than 90% at 5 years but decreases to approximately 50% for atypical histology.
Textbook: Pages 1860–1861 ANSWER: A, D.

33. Which is/are true of adenoid cystic carcinoma?

A. It is a common type of salivary gland tumor.
B. Another name is cylindroma.
C. Most patients are completely resected for cure.
D. Different histological types have different prognoses.
E. Tissue invasion is rare.

DISCUSSION: Adenoid cystic carcinomas (cylindromas) are commonly observed salivary gland tumors that can occur in the conducting airways. The undifferentiated solid type is associated with distant metastases, of which the cribriform and tubular types are associated with perineural and submucosal invasion. Most patients (60%) can be resected for cure.
Textbook: Pages 1861–1863 ANSWER: A, B, C, D.

34. A solitary pulmonary nodule is discovered in an asymptomatic 55-year-old smoker with no evidence of extrathoracic dissemination. The most appropriate management would be to:

A. Obtain serial chest films every 3 months to determine the growth potential of the nodule.
B. Perform transthoracic needle aspiration (TTNA) before considering pulmonary resection to confirm malignancy.
C. Conduct an extensive systematic evaluation to exclude the possibility that the nodule represents a metastatic lesion.
D. Proceed with pulmonary resection after ascertaining that the patient would tolerate removal of the requisite amount of lung.
E. Obtain baseline serum levels of carcinoembryonic antigen and p53.

DISCUSSION: A patient with a solitary pulmonary nodule—a single spherical lesion within the lung—represents an important and challenging diagnostic problem in thoracic oncology. A solitary pulmonary nodule is assumed to be primary lung cancer until proved otherwise; the differential diagnosis includes metastatic carcinoma, granuloma, and benign pulmonary tumors. In most cases, solitary pulmonary nodules should be resected after thorough investigation to establish that systemic dissemination has not already occurred. CT of the chest, liver, and adrenals is performed to confirm the location of the tumor, to evaluate the mediastinum, and to assess the abdomen for systemic disease. If there is no evidence of metastases on CT, the patient should undergo bronchoscopy, which may establish the histologic diagnosis and determine resectability if an endobronchial lesion exists.

Pulmonary function studies are obtained preoperatively to assess the potential for pulmonary resection. A thorough review of systems is undertaken to rule out medical contraindications to thoracotomy. TTNA is not performed routinely and should be reserved for patients with marginal pulmonary function, for whom thoracotomy would be performed only after verification of a malignant histologic diagnosis.

Textbook: Pages 1868–1869, 1871 ANSWER: D.

35. After thoracotomy, pulmonary resection, and mediastinal lymph node dissection, a patient is determined to have a squamous cell carcinoma 2 cm. in diameter, located 1 cm. from the carina along the right mainstem bronchus. Three peribronchial lymph nodes are positive for cancer, and all other lymph node stations are negative. The correct stage, according to the TNM system, is:

A. T1N0M0 Stage I.
B. T1N1M0 Stage II.
C. T2N1M0 Stage II.
D. T3N1M0 Stage IIIa.
E. T2N3M0 Stage IIIb.

DISCUSSION: The TNM staging system for carcinoma of the lung provides a consistent, reproducible description of the anatomic extent of disease at the time of diagnosis. In the TNM system, T represents the primary tumor and numerical suffixes describe increasing size or involvement; N represents regional lymph nodes with suffixes to describe levels of involvement; and M designates the presence or absence of distant metastases.

TUMOR (T)

TX Occult carcinoma (malignant cells in sputum or bronchial washings but tumor not visualized by imaging studies or bronchoscopy)
T1 Tumor 3 cm. or less in greatest diameter, surrounded by lung or visceral pleura, but not proximal to a lobar bronchus
T2 Tumor larger than 3 cm. in diameter, or with involvement of main bronchus at least 2 cm. distal to carina, or with visceral pleural invasion, or with associated atelectasis or obstructive pneumonitis extending to the hilar region but not involving the entire lung
T3 Tumor invading chest wall, diaphragm, mediastinal pleura, or parietal pericardium; or tumor in main bronchus within 2 cm. of, but not invading, carina; or atelectasis of obstructive pneumonitis of the entire lung
T4 Tumor invading mediastinum, heart, great vessels, trachea, esophagus, vertebral body, or carina; or ipsilateral malignant pleural effusion

NODES (N)

N0 No regional lymph node metastases
N1 Metastases to ipsilateral peribronchial or hilar nodes
N2 Metastases to ipsilateral mediastinal or subcarinal nodes
N3 Metastases to contralateral mediastinal or hilar, or to any scalene or supraclavicular nodes

DISTANT METASTASES (M)

M0 No distant metastases
M1 Distant metastases

The TNM subsets are subsequently grouped in a series of stages of disease to identify groups of patients with similar prognosis and therapy.

STAGE	T	N	M
Occult	TX	N0	M0
Stage I	T1-2	N0	M0
Stage II	T1-2	N1	M0
Stage IIIa	T3	N0-1	M0
	T1-3	N2	M0
Stage IIIb	T4	N0-2	M0
	T1-4	N3	M0
Stage IV	Any T	Any N	M1

Textbook: Page 1869 ANSWER: C.

36. After complete resection of Stage I non-small cell lung cancer (NSCLC), the role of adjuvant therapy is best summarized thus as:

A. Postoperative radiation therapy improves disease-free survival.
B. Postoperative radiation therapy improves overall survival.
C. Postoperative chemotherapy improves disease-free survival.
D. Postoperative chemotherapy improves overall survival.
E. Adjuvant therapy is not indicated after complete resection of Stage I NSCLC.

DISCUSSION: Prospective randomized trials conducted by the Lung Cancer Study Group demonstrate that postoperative chemotherapy may be responsible for significantly longer disease-free survival in patients with Stage III (and perhaps Stage II) NSCLC. The efficacy of postoperative chemotherapy and radiotherapy in patients with extensive lymph node involvement or positive surgical margins in reducing systemic recurrences and prolonging disease-free survival has also been demonstrated. Adjuvant therapy is not associated with improved overall survival and has not been shown to be beneficial in patients with Stage I NSCLC.

Radiation therapy is an effective adjuvant treatment in many patients with carcinoma of the lung. Adjuvant radiotherapy, applied to patients with completely resected Stage II or Stage III (but not Stage I) NSCLC, has been shown to decrease local recurrence but has no significant effect on survival. However, postoperative irradiation may provide a survival advantage in patients who have resection and are found to have metastases to hilar or mediastinal lymph nodes. Thus, the purpose of adjuvant radiotherapy is prevention of local tumor recurrence, especially when lymph node sampling of the mediastinum at thoracotomy is incomplete.

Textbook: Pages 1873–1874 ANSWER: E.

37. Compared to segmentectomy or wedge resection, lobectomy for NSCLC is associated with:

A. Similar operative morbidity but higher operative mortality.
B. Similar operative mortality but higher operative morbidity.
C. More severe postoperative pulmonary dysfunction.
D. Lower incidence of locoregional recurrence.
E. Equivalent locoregional recurrence.

DISCUSSION: The risk of recurrence after surgical resection according to the magnitude of the resection has been analyzed by the Lung Cancer Study Group. In a prospective, randomized trial involving more than 400 patients with T1N0 lung cancer, lobectomy was compared to segmentectomy and wedge resection. There was no significant difference in morbidity and mortality among the procedures. Furthermore, no difference was observed in postoperative pulmonary function between patients who underwent lobectomy and those who underwent lesser procedures. The rate of locoregional recurrence was significantly lower in patients who underwent lobectomy (5%) as compared with those who underwent either segmentectomy or wedge resection (15%). In another study, segmentectomy was compared to lobectomy in patients with Stage I lung cancer. In this study, the rate of locoregional recurrence was lower in patients who underwent lobectomy (5%), as compared with those who underwent segmentectomy (23%). Furthermore, there was a survival advantage in the patients undergoing lobectomy for T2 disease.

Textbook: Pages 1871–1872 ANSWER: D.

38. In contrast to NSCLC, small cell lung cancer (SCLC) is characterized by:

A. Greater response rate to chemotherapy.
B. Inability to achieve surgical cure.
C. Less frequent association with paraneoplastic syndromes at the time of diagnosis.
D. Lower likelihood of metastases present at the time of diagnosis.
E. Slower growth.

DISCUSSION: For the purposes of staging, estimating prognosis, and selecting therapy, lung cancer is divided into two categories: NSCLC and SCLC. SCLC is characterized by more rapid growth, higher prevalence of metastases at the time of diagnosis, and greater responsiveness to chemotherapy and radiation therapy. After ascertaining the histological diagnosis of SCLC, staging is performed, including thorough neurological examination and CT evaluation of the chest, abdomen, and brain. For most patients with limited-stage disease, treatment is initiated with six cycles of combination chemotherapy. Radiotherapy to the chest is usually employed after three initial cycles of chemotherapy and is continued for 4 weeks. Among patients with limited-stage disease, thoracotomy for pulmonary resection is recommended for the subset of patients with stage I SCLC.

Textbook: Pages 1874–1875 ANSWER: A.

39. Which of the following statements about the diagnosis and staging of mesothelioma is/are correct?

A. Fluid obtained by thoracentesis is usually adequate for accurate diagnosis.
B. Open biopsy or thoracoscopy should be performed to obtain tissue for diagnosis.
C. Immunohistochemistry should be performed in all cases of suspected mesothelioma.
D. Chest CT and/or magnetic resonance imaging (MRI) are useful in the staging of mesothelioma.
E. Head CT and bone scans are useful in the staging of mesothelioma.

DISCUSSION: Approximately 90% of patients with mesothelioma develop pleural effusion, but cytologic specimens from pleural fluid are inaccurate for the diagnosis of mesothelioma, and open or thoracoscopic biopsy is required. Accurate diagnosis of mesothelioma is difficult: the epithelial variant must be differentiated from adenocarcinoma, whereas the sarcomatous form often resembles benign sarcomas. Immunohistochemistry using a panel of antibodies, and sometimes electron microscopy, is required for all cases. Relentless local spread is typical, and chest CT or MRI is essential to evaluate potential local extension into the chest wall, pericardium, mediastinum, or diaphragm. Metastatic disease is less common and occurs late (if at all) in the disease course, so head CT and bone scans are indicated only if clinical findings are suspicious for metastasis.

Textbook: Pages 1877–1880 ANSWER: B, C, D.

40. Which of the following statements about therapy for malignant pleural mesothelioma is/are correct?

A. The role of surgery is confined to biopsy for diagnosis and pleurodesis for palliation of effusion.
B. Extrapleural pneumonectomy involves resection *en bloc* of the lung, visceral and parietal pleura, pericardium, and diaphragm.
C. If a lesion is unresectable by extrapleural pneumonectomy, pleurectomy/decortication is contraindicated.
D. Neither surgery, chemotherapy, nor radiation therapy as a single therapy improves survival.
E. Multimodality therapy, combining surgery, chemotherapy, and radiation therapy may improve survival in select patients.

DISCUSSION: In debilitated patients, palliation by pleurodesis is indicated; however, cytoreductive techniques, including pleurectomy/decortication, and extrapleural pneumonectomy, are indicated for patients who can tolerate surgery. For Stage I disease, extrapleural pneumonectomy is offered. If the patient cannot tolerate pulmonary resection or if the lesion is unresectable by extrapleural pneumonectomy, pleurectomy/decortication is appropriate. Both cytoreductive procedures, when used in a multimodality setting, may improve survival in selected patients. They also improve quality of life by relieving or delaying two severe symptoms of mesothelioma: dyspnea secondary to lung restriction by the tumor and pain from tumor invasion. No single modality (surgery, chemotherapy, or radiation therapy) improves survival.

Textbook: Pages 1880–1882 ANSWER: B, D, E.

41. All of the following may be acceptable operative approaches to management of the thoracic outlet syndrome except:

A. Scalenectomy.
B. Excision of a cervical rib.
C. Thoracoplasty.
D. First rib resection.
E. Division of anomalous fibromuscular bands.

DISCUSSION: Supraclavicular decompression of the thoracic outlet is the preferred operative approach for the thoracic outlet syndrome. This procedure consists of extensive anterior scalenectomy, middle scalenectomy, removal of a cervical rib (if present), and, on occasion, first rib resection. Transaxillary first rib resection has been widely used as well but is associated with a greater risk for complications. Numerous fibromuscular anomalies have been described in association with the thoracic outlet syndrome. Thoracoplasty has no role in the management of this disorder.

Textbook: Pages 1886–1887 ANSWER: C.

42. Initial conservative (nonsurgical) management of the thoracic outlet syndrome may include all of the following except:

A. Weight reduction.
B. Improvement of posture.
C. Exercises to strengthen the muscles of the shoulder girdle.
D. Pentoxifylline.
E. Avoiding hyperabduction.

DISCUSSION: The initial management of the thoracic outlet syndrome is nonoperative. A trial of weight reduction, shoulder girdle strengthening exercises, improvement of posture, and avoidance of hyperabduction should be recommended for 4 months or longer. These measures are successful in 50% to 70% of patients, particularly in young to middle-aged females with poor posture. Pentoxifylline is a hemorrheologic agent used in selected patients with peripheral arterial insufficiency and has no known benefit in the thoracic outlet syndrome.

Textbook: Page 1886 ANSWER: D.

43. Which of the following statements about pectus excavatum are correct?

A. It is the most common congenital malformation of the chest wall.
B. The most frequent presenting complaint is the cosmetic deformity.
C. The manubrium and first and second costal cartilages typically are involved in the deformity.
D. It may be associated with cardiac defects and other skeletal defects such as scoliosis.
E. Restrictive alterations in chest wall mechanics and abnormalities in pulmonary function tests have been documented.

DISCUSSION: Congenital deformities of the chest wall represent a spectrum of deformities ranging from minor cosmetic defects to gross deformities incompatible with life. Pectus excavatum, or funnel chest, is the most common of the congenital deformities of the chest wall, accounting for 90% of such defects. It is characterized by a concave, posteriorly displaced sternum due to overgrowth of the costal cartilages. Most commonly the defect begins at the junction of the manubrium and the body of the sternum and becomes progressively deeper toward the xiphoid. The manubrium and the first and second costal cartilages typically are normal. The defects have both physiologic and psychologic consequences and are often associated with other abnormalities, including congenital heart disease, Marfan's syndrome, and other skeletal defects, including scoliosis. Patients most often present because of the cosmetic defect but frequently are found to have other symptoms, including impaired cardiopulmonary function and scoliosis. Pulmonary complaints include dyspnea and respiratory tract infections. Restrictive alterations in chest wall mechanics and abnormalities in pulmonary function tests, including decreased vital capacity, decreased total lung capacity, decreased maximal ventilatory volume, and decreased maximal breathing capacity, have been documented.

Textbook: Pages 1888–1890 ANSWER: A, B, D, E.

44. Surgical correction of pectus excavatum is characterized by which of the following?

A. Significant cosmetic improvement initially but a high incidence of recurrence of the defect on late follow-up.
B. An increase in exercise tolerance and respiratory reserve postoperatively.
C. Improvement in FEV_1, vital capacity, and total lung capacity.
D. Improvement in maximal ventilatory volume, total progressive exercise time, and maximal exercise capacity.
E. Prevention of the development of "thoracogenic scoliosis."

DISCUSSION: Because of the significant cosmetic and psychological improvement, subjective increase in exercise tolerance, documented improvement in cardiac and respiratory status, and prevention of the development of scoliosis following surgical intervention in these patients, surgical correction should be considered for all patients with moderate to severe deformity. Cosmetic results of surgical correction are excellent, and recurrence is uncommon. Objective improvement in cardiac function has been documented postoperatively, owing to relief of the sternal compression. Postoperatively, worsening of the FEV_1, vital capacity, and total lung capacity have been noted, whereas a significant improvement in maximal ventilatory volume, total progressive exercise time, and maximal oxygen consumption has also been documented. Following surgical correction there is a consistent increase in maximal exercise capacity at every level of workload, a lower heart rate at every workload, and an increase in exercise duration.

Textbook: Pages 1892–1893 ANSWER: B, D, E.

45. Which of the following statements about the diagnosis of chest wall tumors is/are correct?

A. Pain is a common presenting symptom.
B. Firmness and fixation to underlying bone and muscle are important to note in the physical examination as aids to diagnosis.
C. In general, chest wall tumors are slow growing and produce symptoms late in their course.
D. CT is the most useful imaging study for making the diagnosis and for planning surgical resection of chest wall tumors.
E. Angiography should be performed routinely.

DISCUSSION: Seventy-five per cent of patients present with a slow-growing, painless chest wall mass. A firm mass that is fixed to an underlying rib is more likely to be of bony or cartilaginous origin. Conversely, soft, mobile tumors are more likely to be of soft tissue origin. CT defines depth of invasion and extent of tumor and is the most useful imaging modality. Angiography should be employed selectively, primarily for very large and vascular tumors.

Textbook: Pages 1896–1897 ANSWER: B, C, D.

46. Which of the following statements about chest wall resection and reconstruction is/are correct?

A. Most tumors of soft tissue and bone require 4-cm. margins to be adequately resected.
B. At least one normal rib above and below the primary tumor should be included in the resection.
C. Techniques of chest wall reconstruction are directed at the prevention of paradoxical chest wall movement with respiration.
D. Soft tissue defects are most conveniently addressed by stretching the existing skin over the defect under tension.
E. Chest wall defects that are covered by the scapula require no special reconstructive procedures, even if the defects are quite large.

DISCUSSION: Margins of resection of chest wall tumors should be at least 3 cm. of skin, 4 cm. of muscle, and 6 cm. of bone. Old biopsy sites should be included in the specimen. A normal rib above and below the specimen should also be included. Prevention of paradoxical chest wall movement is the primary goal of chest wall reconstruction. Large soft tissue defects are best managed by myocutaneous pedicle flaps. In general, defects larger than 5 cm. require reconstruction. Defects covered by the scapula require no reconstruction.

Textbook: Pages 1897–1898 ANSWER: A, B, C, E.

47. Prolonged extracorporeal membrane oxygenation (ECMO):

A. Is highly successful in the treatment of severe respiratory failure in newborn infants.
B. Is contraindicated in adult respiratory distress syndrome (ARDS).
C. Causes hemolysis and renal failure.
D. Requires total systemic heparinization (activated clotting time longer than 500 seconds).
E. Is identical to heart/lung bypass for cardiac surgery.

DISCUSSION: The survival rate of newborn infants who are moribund from respiratory failure with ECMO is 80% to 90%. ECMO is also indicated in ARDS with a survival rate from 40% to 50%. Hemolysis and renal failure are rare complications. ECMO requires low-dose partial heparinization, with clotting times in the range of 200 seconds. Several modifications in the conventional heart/lung machine permit the extension of ECMO from hours to days.

Textbook: Page 1899 ANSWER: A.

48. Indications for ECMO include:

A. Newborn infants with pulmonary hypoplasia secondary to congenital diaphragmatic hernia.
B. Meconium aspiration syndrome in full-term babies (at least 35 weeks).
C. Children with pulmonary infection after bone marrow transplantation.
D. Adults with acute viral pneumonia.
E. Adults requiring mechanical ventilation and 100% oxygen for 2 weeks or longer.

DISCUSSION: At present ECMO is not used for infants smaller than 1500 gm. because of a high risk of intracranial bleeding. ECMO is very successful in the treatment of respiratory failure in full-term newborn infants. Immunosuppression is a relative contraindication to ECMO. ECMO is indicated in adults with acute, potentially reversible respiratory failure, but mechanical ventilation and high oxygen concentration for more than 10 days are contraindications.

Textbook: Page 1899 ANSWER: B, D.

49. Venovenous ECMO:

A. Avoids major arterial access.
B. Provides cardiac and pulmonary support.
C. Can be accomplished via cannulation at

separate venous sites or at a single venous site using a double-lumen catheter.

D. Provides greater venous drainage than venoarterial ECMO.

E. Maintains the normal pulsatile blood flow to the systemic circulation.

DISCUSSION: Venovenous ECMO has become the access technique of choice for patients with respiratory failure without significant requirement for cardiac (hemodynamic) support. In neonates, a double-lumen cannula allows ECMO to be performed through a single incision over the right internal jugular vein. It can also be performed by separate cannulation of the femoral and jugular veins. In either configuration, venovenous ECMO avoids cannulation of any major arteries and maintains the normal pulsatile circulation through the heart and lungs. Venous drainage is no different with venovenous ECMO.

Textbook: Pages 1899–1900 ANSWER: A, C, E.

50. As compared with venovenous ECMO, venoarterial ECMO:

A. Requires cannulation of a major artery and vein.
B. Provides both cardiac and respiratory support.
C. Can be performed with less anticoagulation.
D. Usually maintains a normal pulse pressure.

DISCUSSION: Venoarterial ECMO can provide total cardiorespiratory support via cannulation of a major vein and artery (usually the right internal jugular vein and common carotid artery in neonates). With most roller and vortex pumps, the arterial inflow from the ECMO circuit is nonpulsatile, and therefore pulse pressure is often reduced or absent. Venoarterial ECMO requires the same degree of anticoagulation as venovenous techniques.

Textbook: Pages 1899–1900 ANSWER: A, B.

51. A 24-year-old male has new onset of chest pain. Chest films demonstrate a large anterosuperior mass. Appropriate evaluation should include:

A. CT of the chest.
B. Measurement of serum alpha-fetoprotein and beta–human chorionic gonadotropin.
C. A barium swallow.
D. A myelogram.

DISCUSSION: Elevated levels of serum alpha-fetoprotein and beta–human chorionic gonadotropin are indicative of a malignant nonseminomatous germ cell tumor. Optimal therapy for such a tumor is based on a *cis*-platinum-containing chemotherapeutic regimen. After normalization of serum markers, resection of residual disease is performed. Extensive surgical procedures prior to chemotherapy are not warranted. Confirmation of the diagnosis can usually be obtained using needle biopsy techniques. In some institutions patients are treated based on elevated serum markers alone. CT imaging is useful to evaluate tumor invasiveness, airway compression, vascular involvement, and the likelihood of resectability. Barium swallow may be helpful in the evaluation of enteric cysts. Myelography may be useful in patients with posterior mediastinal masses to evaluate for spinal column involvement.

Textbook: Pages 1911–1914, 1920–1921 ANSWER: A, B.

52. Systemic syndromes frequently associated with mediastinal tumors include:

A. Myasthenia gravis.
B. Hypercalcemia.
C. Malignant hypertension.
D. Carcinoid syndrome.

DISCUSSION: Myasthenia gravis occurs in 10% to 50% of patients with thymoma. The incidence with which myasthenia gravis occurs in patients with a thymoma increases with the age of the patient. In males over 50 and females over 60 years of age, the incidence appears to be greater than 80%. Hyperparathyroidism due to a mediastinal parathyroid adenoma is a cause of hypercalcemia. Although parathyroid glands may occur in the mediastinum in 10% of the patients, they are usually accessible through a cervical incision. A sternotomy is required infrequently, even in those patients with a mediastinal parathyroid gland. Most often the adenomas are found embedded in or near the superior pole of the thymus. Mediastinal paraganglioma may produce significant catecholamines, predominantly norepinephrine. Catecholamine production causes a classic group of symptoms associated with pheochromocytomas, including periodic sustained hypertension often accompanied by orthostatic hypotension, and hypermetabolism manifested by weight loss, hyperhydrosis, palpitation, and headaches. Mediastinal carcinoid tumors have been more frequently associated with Cushing's syndrome because of the production of adrenocorticotrophic hormones. These tumors uncommonly cause the carcinoid syndrome.

Textbook: Pages 1918–1920 ANSWER: A, B, C.

53. A 36-year-old female developed dyspnea on exertion that has progressed over 3 months. Chest film reveals a left anterior mediastinal mass with evidence of elevated left hemidiaphragm. CT indicates probable invasion of the pericardium. Paratracheal or subcarinal adenopathy is not identified. Appropriate intervention in this patient would include:

A. A median sternotomy with radical resection of the tumor, sacrificing the left phrenic nerve and excising the involved pericardium.
B. A mediastinoscopy with biopsy.
C. A left anterolateral thoracotomy or median sternotomy with generous biopsy of the tumor.
D. Observation with repeat chest radiography in 3 months.

DISCUSSION: The differential diagnosis of an invasive anterosuperior mediastinal mass includes thymoma, lymphoma, germ cell tumor, undifferentiated carcinoma, and carcinoid tumors. These tumors often have a very similar histologic appearance, which may cause an inaccurate diagnosis based on light microscopy alone. Use of electron microscopy and immunohistochemistry may be necessary to correctly determine the specific histologic diagnosis. Frozen section should be used to determine adequacy of tissue biopsy. Histologic diagnosis based on frozen section examination in many of these tumors may be erroneous. Although radical resection of tumor is indicated for thymoma, chemotherapy and radiotherapy are the modalities used for the treatment of patients with lymphomas and germ cell tumors. Exact determination of tumor histology by permanent section should precede radical resectional therapy. Generous tissue biopsy is necessary for the precise subtyping of lymphomas. Mediastinoscopy is useful in patients with paratracheal and pericarinal masses or adenopathy, particularly when right-sided. Observation of a patient with invasive mediastinal mass is not warranted.

Textbook: Pages 1911–1912 ANSWER: C.

54. An 18-year-old male presents with a history of increasing shortness of breath that worsens in the recumbent position. On physical examination, the neck veins are noted to be distended, with facial plethora that is accentuated by lying the patient down. A 2.5-cm. left supraclavicular lymph node is palpable. Chest film reveals an extensive right anterosuperior mediastinal mass. Appropriate intervention may include:

A. An urgent biopsy of the mediastinal mass under general anesthesia with subsequent initiation of therapy.
B. CT.
C. Pulmonary function testing in the sitting and supine positions.
D. A biopsy of the right supraclavicular lymph node under general anesthesia.
E. A biopsy of the supraclavicular lymph node under local anesthesia.

DISCUSSION: Although most patients with a mediastinal mass may undergo surgical procedures under general anesthesia with a minimal risk, patients with a large anterior, superior, or middle mediastinal mass, particularly those with posture-related dyspnea and superior vena caval syndrome, have an increased risk of developing severe respiratory complications during general anesthesia. Useful techniques for identifying less symptomatic patients who have significant airway compression include CT imaging and pulmonary function tests. A reduction of the tracheal diameter by more than 35% on a CT scan and reduction of peak expiratory flow during pulmonary function testing are sensitive indicators of functional airway compression. In patients with airway compression and superior vena caval obstruction, the risk of general anesthesia is significant. Attempts to obtain a histologic diagnosis should be limited to needle biopsies or open procedures performed under local anesthesia. In situations in which histologic diagnosis cannot be obtained using these methods, therapy may be initiated with radiation, corticosteroids, and chemotherapy. However, a histologic diagnosis may not be obtainable in as many as 40% of these patients after initiation of treatment. Some proceed with biopsy of the mediastinal mass under general anesthesia. However, alterations in anesthetic management include: (1) induction of anesthesia in a semi-Fowler's or upright position, (2) availability of rigid bronchoscopy to allow reestablishment of an adequate airway, (3) use of a long endotracheal tube to allow advancement of the tube beyond the site of obstruction, (4) avoidance of muscle relaxants and the use of spontaneous ventilation when possible, (5) lower extremity intravenous cannulation, and (6) standby cardiopulmonary bypass.

Textbook: Pages 1910–1914 ANSWER: B, C, E.

55. A 42-year-old male who is scheduled to undergo elective knee surgery has a preoperative chest film that demonstrates a 5-cm. posterior mediastinal mass. The patient denies any neurologic symptoms and physical examination fails to elucidate any neurologic deficit. CT confirms the presence of a 5-cm. mediastinal mass in the left costovertebral gutter with minimal enlargement of the seventh thoracic foramen. Appropriate intervention includes:

A. Resection of the posterior mediastinal mass using a standard posterolateral incision.
B. A CT with myelography or magnetic resonance (MR) imaging.
C. Two-stage removal of the tumor, performing the resection of the thoracic component first with subsequent removal of the spinal column component at a later date.
D. One-stage removal of the dumb-bell tumor, excising the intraspinal component prior to resection of the thoracic component.

DISCUSSION: Approximately 10% of neurogenic tumors extend into the spinal column and are termed dumb-bell tumors because of the characteristic shape. Although 60% of patients with such tumors have neurologic symptoms related to spinal cord compression, the significant proportion of patients without symptoms underscores the importance of evaluating all patients with a posterior mediastinal mass for possible intraspinal extension. CT, MR imaging, and vertebral tomography may demonstrate an enlargement of the foramen, erosion of bone, or intervertebral widening, which are indicative of a dumb-bell tumor. If these findings are present, CT with myelography or MR imaging is indicated to evaluate the presence and extent of the intraspinal component. A one-stage removal of the tumor is recommended, with excision of the intraspinal component prior to resection of the thoracic component to minimize the risk of spinal column hematoma.

Textbook: Pages 1914–1918 ANSWER: B, D.

56. True statements regarding patients with a mediastinal mass include:

A. Asymptomatic patients have a benign mass in over 75% of cases.
B. Symptomatic patients are more likely to have a malignant lesion than a benign lesion.
C. In a patient with a chest film demonstrating a mediastinal mass, a Tru-cut needle biopsy is a safe procedure.
D. Seminomas usually produce alpha-fetoprotein.

DISCUSSION: Seventy-six per cent of the asymptomatic patients with a mediastinal mass seen in one series over a recent 20-year period had a *benign* leison. In contrast, 62% of the symptomatic patients had a malignant neoplasm during this period. A number of intrathoracic and extrathoracic lesions may have an appearance similar to a primary mediastinal mass on routine chest films, as do a large number of cardiovascular lesions. Although angiography was used in the past for this differentiation, CT with contrast and MRI now distinguish a primary mediastinal mass from a cardiovascular lesion. Tru-cut needle biopsy of a cardiovascular lesion may be associated with significant hemorrhagic complications. Seminomas rarely produce beta–human chorionic gonadotropin and never produce alpha-fetoprotein. In contrast, over 90% of the nonseminomas secrete one or both of these hormones.

Textbook: Pages 1910–1911 ANSWER: A, B.

57. Which of the following would be the least appropriate in the management of acute suppurative mediastinitis?

A. Wide débridement.
B. Irrigation under pressure.
C. Topical antibacterials.
D. Long-term systemic antibacterials.
E. Closure with muscle flaps.

DISCUSSION: Acute suppurative mediastinitis is a classic wound problem and forms a paradigm for principles of management. Wide débridement is perhaps the most important step in correcting this type of invasive wound sepsis. Drainage requires removal of tissue with vascular compromise. Tissue that is infected and can serve as an ongoing nidus for infection, particularly cartilage, must be removed. Irrigation is effective only when the irrigation fluid reaches into and flushes out débris and bacteria. The irrigation is insufficient if only dilutional and not also mechanically effective. Since infected tissue tends to become isolated from the systemic circulation the direct application of antibacterials reaches avascular areas. Some, such as silver sulfadiazine, penetrate avascular tissue better than, for instance, ointments or povidone iodine, and such an agent should be chosen. Wide débridement and the washing of debris with pressure irrigation make the wound then available to topical applications, which are often best packed into these deep, irregular cavities. Long-term systemic antibacterials serve no purpose and lead to potential resistant bacterial overgrowth. Although systemic antibacterials provide a measure of protection up to the margin where vascularized and nonvascularized tissues meet, topical agents are better in the actual infected site. Once closed, these wounds rapidly become sterilized. Even the infection at the bone level is far different from traditional osteomyelitis, and long-term systemic therapy is unnecessary. Muscle flaps are a great advance in closure technique, since they provide bulky protection, obliterate dead space, and help vascularize the wound.

Textbook: Pages 1907–1908 ANSWER: D.

58. Each of the following is appropriate for managing acute suppurative mediastinitis except:

A. Alloplastic material and skin flaps.
B. Rectus abdominis muscle flaps.
C. Omentum.
D. Pectoralis major muscle flaps.
E. Rigid internal fixation.

DISCUSSION: Alloplastic materials may be nonreactive in the laboratory and biologically acceptable in other areas (artificial hips, breast prostheses). Their introduction into a contaminated wound, however, would more likely promote rather than reduce infection. Various meshes and other types of "protection" devices are not necessary. Skin flaps alone do not obliterate dead space and have not been shown either to reduce or resist infection. The rectus abdominis muscle is a superb source of readily available tissue that can be rotated into very large cavities. The nature of the muscle allows it to be "dressed into" irregular cavities. It has an excellent, easily movable skin territory overlying it, which can also be transferred if locally available skin is wanting. The omentum has the great ability to fit into the many irregularities of some defects. For appropriately selected cases it is excellent. The pectoralis major muscle flaps are the usual initial choice since they are in the operative field. When the musculotendinous insertion is released their mobility is often sufficient. Additionally, it avoids the need for abdominal incisions. The latissimus dorsi muscle as a flap is dependable and includes sternal defects in the scope of its arc of rotation. It requires rotating the patient on the operating table and thus is less readily available than the other flaps.

Textbook: Pages 1907–1908 ANSWER: A.

59. Clinical features suggestive of myasthenia gravis include all of the following except:

A. Proximal muscle weakness.
B. Diplopia.
C. Sensory deficits of the extremities.
D. Dysphagia.

DISCUSSION: Weakness of proximal weight-bearing muscle groups is the hallmark of the clinical diagnosis of myasthenia gravis. The weakness or fatigue occurs with repetitive activity and improves with rest. The majority of patients (90%) experience ocular muscle involvement, manifested as diplopia or ptosis most easily demonstrated with sustained upward gaze. Cranial nerve involvement is uncommon but can be present, with symptoms of dysphagia, nasal regurgitation, and aspiration. Since myasthenia gravis is a disorder of neuromuscular transmission at the motor end plate, deep tendon reflexes and sensory examination are normal.

Textbook: Page 1934 ANSWER: C.

60. The diagnosis of myasthenia gravis can be confirmed most reliably using:

A. Anti–acetylcholine receptor antibody titers.
B. The Tensilon test.
C. Electromyography (EMG).
D. Single-fiber EMG.
E. Physical examination.

DISCUSSION: Although findings from a careful history and physical examination are suggestive of the diagnosis of myasthenia gravis, specific diagnostic testing is required to confirm the diagnosis. Elevated anti–acetylcholine receptor antibodies are present in 85% to 90% of patients with generalized myasthenia but are often negative in patients with early or ocular myasthenia gravis. The Tensilon test is also positive in approximately 90% of patients with generalized myasthenia gravis, but both false-negative and false-positive results occur, especially in patients with mild or early disease. Standard EMG studies are helpful if positive, but their overall sensitivity may be as low as 35%. The specialized technique of single-fiber EMG is the most reliable diagnostic test, being abnormal in 90% of patients with mild disease and in virtually 100% in patients with severe generalized myasthenia gravis.

Textbook: Page 1935 ANSWER: D.

61. All of the following statements are true about the pathogenesis of myasthenia gravis except:

A. The number of functional acetylcholine receptors at the motor end plate is reduced.
B. An autoimmune mechanism involving antibodies to the acetylcholine receptor has been proposed.
C. Complement system involvement has been demonstrated.
D. A nonspecific "thymitis" may initiate the autoimmune response.
E. Clinical improvement following thymectomy is correlated with decreased acetylcholine receptor antibody titers.

DISCUSSION: Myasthenia gravis is generally regarded as an autoimmune disorder due to antibodies directed toward the acetylcholine receptor. A variety of autoimmune mechanisms have been proposed; the ultimate result is a reduction in the number of functional acetylcholine receptors at the motor end plate. Proposed immune mechanisms include complement-mediated receptor destruction, antibody-induced accelerated receptor turnover, and simple receptor blockade. In spite of these proposed immune mechanisms, the severity of myasthenia symptoms and improvement following therapy do not correlate with antibody titers. Although the source of these autoantibodies is not proven, it is generally felt that a nonspecific thymitis may trigger the autoantibody response, the thymic myoid cells serving as the source of the antigen.

Textbook: Pages 1935–1937 ANSWER: E.

62. Which of the following statements about the relationship of the thymus and myasthenia gravis is/are true?

A. Thymic abnormalities are present in up to 80% of patients with myasthenia gravis.
B. Thymoma is present in up to 20% of patients with myasthenia gravis.
C. Myasthenia gravis will occur in up to 60% of patients with thymomas.
D. Myasthenia patients with thymoma respond more favorably to thymectomy.
E. Thymoma is the most common abnormality of the thymus in patients with myasthenia gravis.

DISCUSSION: The central role of the thymus gland in the pathogenesis of myasthenia gravis is based on the observation that more than 80% of patients have histologic abnormalities of the thymus and on the beneficial effect of thymectomy on patients' symptoms. Of the patients with documented abnormalities of the thymus the majority have B-cell lymphoid hyperplasia; only 20% have a thymoma. Conversely, up to 60% of patients with known thymoma will have or ultimately develop myasthenia gravis. In these patients, with thymoma and myasthenia gravis, the response to thymectomy is less favorable than in those without thymoma.

Textbook: Page 1937 ANSWER: A, B, C.

63. Which of the following statements about the results of thymectomy for myasthenia gravis are true?

A. Patients with ocular symptoms experience clinical improvement in 90% of cases.
B. Clinical remission can be expected in 90% of cases.
C. The response rate to thymectomy for patients with generalized symptoms is 90%.
D. Patients with thymoma experience improvement in 75%.
E. Continued medical therapy is required in 75%.

DISCUSSION: Overall, improvement can be expected in 90% of patients who undergo thymectomy for generalized myasthenia gravis. In general, the results are more favorable in patients with mild generalized myasthenia. In patients with only ocular symptoms, the benefit following thymectomy is less clear; improvement is documented in 80%. The response rate is even less (30%) in patients with thymoma. Complete remission occurs in 40% to 50% of patients following thymectomy, and the remainder require some continued medical therapy.

Textbook: Pages 1938–1939 ANSWER: C.

64. All of the following are true of the treatment of myasthenia gravis except:

A. The transcervical approach to surgical thymectomy is less likely to benefit the patient with myasthenia gravis.
B. Corticosteroids result in improvement in 80% of patients.
C. Plasma exchange is associated with improvement in up to 90% of patients.
D. Medical therapy with Mestinon (pyridostigmine) is associated with remission in approximately 10% of patients.
E. Surgical thymectomy, regardless of the approach, is associated with improved remission and response rates as compared with medical therapy

DISCUSSION: Although Mestinon therapy results in clinical improvement in most patients, complete remission can be expected in only 10%. In addition, intolerable side effects may limit their usefulness. In patients who fail to respond to Mestinon therapy, and in those who experience significant side effects, corticosteroids can be utilized, with improvement expected in 80% of patients. Plasma exchange results in improvement in 90% of patients, but the cost of therapy and its transient duration of benefit limit the use of pheresis therapy to special circumstances such as preoperative preparation or in myasthenic crisis. Overall, response rates to surgical thymectomy range from 80% to 95%, and complete remission occurs in 30% to 50%. This benefit following thymectomy has not been shown to depend on the particular technique utilized. Remission and response rates are similar for transcervical, standard transsternal, and the "maximal thymectomy" techniques.

Textbook: Pages 1939–1940 ANSWER: A.

65. Which of the following is/are acceptable alternatives in the management of malignant pericardial effusion?

A. Pericardiocentesis.
B. Subxiphoid pericardiotomy ("pericardial window").
C. Thoracotomy with pericardiectomy.
D. Instillation of tetracycline or bleomycin into the pericardial space.
E. Treatment of the underlying malignancy.

DISCUSSION: In patients with symptomatic malignant pericardial effusions, management options may be designed to establish a diagnosis, relieve symptoms, or prevent recurrence. Pericardiocentesis is very successful in removing fluid for diagnosis and alleviating symptoms; however recurrence rates are greater than 50%. This rate can be reduced to around 20% with instillation of sclerosing agents such as tetracycline or bleomycin. Surgical techniques, including subxiphoid pericardiotomy and thoracotomy with pericardiectomy, offer the highest success rates (approximately 90%) but are more invasive and usually require general anesthesia. Systemic antitumor therapy with chemotherapy or radiation therapy can be effective in controlling malignant effusions in cases of sensitive tumors such as lymphomas, leukemias, and breast cancer.

Textbook: Pages 1948–1950 ANSWER: A, B, C, D, E.

66. Which of the following statements about cardiac tamponade is/are correct?

A. At least 500 ml. of fluid must be present in the pericardium of an adult to cause symptoms of tamponade.
B. A drop in systemic blood pressure of greater than 20 mm. Hg during inspiration (pulsus paradoxus) is a finding specific to cardiac tamponade.
C. The vast majority of patients with cardiac tamponade demonstrate a low QRS voltage, nonspecific ST T-wave abnormalities, and electrical alternans (alternation of QRS amplitude) on the electrocardiogram.
D. In trauma victims with cardiac tamponade, the three components of "Beck's triad" (hypotension, elevated jugular venous pressure (JVP), and muffled heart sounds) are almost always present.
E. When the diagnosis is made, treatment must be instituted rapidly and may include pericardiocentesis, creation of a pericardial window, and identification and treatment of the underlying cause.

DISCUSSION: Development of tamponade symptoms depends on the rate of accumulation of fluid. As little as 100 to 200 ml. accumulating rapidly may cause symptoms, whereas a slowly developing pericardial effusion of over 1 liter may remain asymptomatic. Pulsus paradoxus is not specific for tamponade; it may occur in patients with severe congestive heart failure, chronic obstructive pulmonary disease, hypovolemia, acute pulmonary embolism, or shock. Electrocardiographic findings of low QRS voltage and nonspecific ST T-wave changes are common in this condition, but electrical alternans, often considered pathognomonic of cardiac tamponade, is present in only a small number of patients. Trauma victims with tamponade frequently lack one or more of the elements of Beck's triad; for example, associated hypovolemia may lead to low or normal jugular venous distention. Since cardiac tamponade is life threatening, therapy designed to drain the pericardial fluid must be provided quickly and the underlying cause must be established and controlled.

Textbook: Page 1948 ANSWER: E.

67. Which of the following statements about constrictive pericarditis is/are correct?

A. Most patients who develop constrictive pericarditis after cardiac operation present with symptoms within 6 months of the procedure.

B. Results of pericardiectomy for constrictive pericarditis are worse in patients who develop constriction after mediastinal irradiation.

C. Drainage of asymptomatic pericardial effusions arising from acute pericarditis is advised to prevent development of constrictive pericarditis.

D. If surgical treatment is planned for constrictive pericarditis it should involve total or complete pericardiectomy.

E. Echocardiography can usually make the diagnosis by imaging a thickened pericardium.

DISCUSSION: The time course in the development of constrictive pericarditis after cardiac surgery ranges from 1 month to nearly 9 years, but the mean interval from surgery to presentation is about 23 months. Most series have reported poorer outcomes from pericardiectomy for postirradiation constrictive pericarditis, possibly owing to underlying myocardial fibrosis. In this subset, 5-year survival averages 50%, as compared with 75% for constrictive pericarditis of all causes. Constrictive pericarditis is a rare complication of acute pericarditis. As a result, drainage of asymptomatic (nonpurulent) pericardial effusions from acute pericarditis is not required. Patients with significant symptoms from constrictive pericarditis should undergo total pericardiectomy, even though this procedure carries an operative mortality rate of approximately 10%. Limited pericardiectomy has proven to be ineffective for this condition. It can be difficult to distinguish constrictive pericarditis from restrictive cardiomyopathy. Echocardiography may help by demonstrating chamber dimensions and wall motion abnormalities, but CT and MRI more accurately assess pericardial thickness.

Textbook: Page 1946 ANSWER: B, D.

NOTES

NOTES

CHAPTER 23

HEART

1. Which is *not* true of cardiopulmonary resuscitation (CPR)?

A. Closed chest massage is as effective as open chest massage.
B. The success rate for out-of-hospital resuscitation may be as high as 30% to 60%.
C. The most common cause of sudden death is ischemic heart disease.
D. Standard chest massage generally provides less than 15% of normal coronary and cerebral blood flow.

DISCUSSION: Closed chest massage is not as effective as open-chest massage in normalizing blood pressure or perfusion of vital organs, and closed chest massage does generally deliver 5% to 15% of normal coronary and cerebral blood flow. The success rate for out-of-hospital resuscitation has been as high as 30% to 60% when communities are prepared to institute CPR early after a cardiac arrest. Ischemic heart disease is the most common cause of sudden death.

Textbook: Page 1952 ANSWER: A.

2. Which maneuver generally is not performed early before chest compression in basic life support outside the hospital?

A. Call for help.
B. Obtain airway.
C. Electrical cardioversion.
D. Ventilation.

DISCUSSION: Basic life support does involve calling for help, obtaining an airway, and beginning ventilation before starting chest compression. Electrical cardioversion requires special equipment and trained personnel and thus is part of advanced cardiac life support.

Textbook: Pages 1953–1954 ANSWER: C.

3. Which treatment would be least effective for asystole?

A. External pacemaker.
B. Intravenous epinephrine, 10 ml. of 1:10,000.
C. Intravenous calcium gluconate, 10 ml. of 10% solution.
D. Intravenous atropine, 0.5 mg.

DISCUSSION: Recommended treatment for asystole is administration of atropine. If atropine is unsuccessful epinephrine is given. Ultimately cardiac pacing is necessary if atropine and epinephrine do not establish an adequate heart rate. Calcium has no clear role in treating asystole.

Textbook: Page 1954 ANSWER: C.

4. The most important factor that influences the outcome of penetrating cardiac injuries is:

A. Comminuted tear of a single chamber.
B. Multiple-chamber injuries.
C. Coronary artery injury.
D. Tangential injuries.

DISCUSSION: Multiple studies in the literature confirm that injuries to the coronary arteries are the most important factor in determining outcome after a penetrating cardiac injury. Tangential injuries are the least serious. Injury to a single chamber—even if comminuted—or to multiple chambers is less likely to be fatal than are injuries that involve a major coronary artery.

Textbook: Page 1957 ANSWER: C.

5. The most useful incision in the operating room for patients with penetrating cardiac injury is:

A. Left anterior thoracotomy.
B. Right anterior thoracotomy.
C. Bilateral anterior thoracotomy.
D. Median sternotomy.
E. Subxyphoid.

DISCUSSION: The subxyphoid incision is useful for determining if there is blood in the pericardium and if there is an intracardiac injury; however, exposure is extremely limited, and definitive repair can rarely be performed through the incision. Left (or right) anterior thoracotomy is easily performed, especially in the emergency room, and gives adequate exposure to certain areas of the heart. However, each has significant limitations in exposure. Either may be extended across the thoracotomy into the other side of the chest, thus producing a bilateral anterior thoracotomy. Exposure is excellent through this incision, and most injuries can be satisfactorily repaired through this approach. Most cardiac operations today are performed through median sternotomy incisions. If the patient is in the operating room, this incision is easily performed and always provides excellent exposure for all areas of the heart.

Textbook: Pages 1958–1960 ANSWER: D.

6. In patients who present with a penetrating chest injury, injury to the heart is most likely when the following physical sign(s) is/are present:

A. Hypotension.
B. Distended neck veins.
C. Decreased heart sound.
D. All of the above.

DISCUSSION: Hypotension, increased venous pressure (distended neck veins), and decreased heart sounds make up the classic Beck's triad associated with cardiac tamponade. If these three findings are present in a person who has a penetrating chest wound, intracardiac injury is almost certain and operative intervention is mandatory.
Textbook: Pages 1957–1958 ANSWER: D.

7. Which of the following would be an acceptable method of repair for a neonate with symptomatic isolated coarctation of the aorta?

A. Resection with end-to-end anastomosis.
B. Prosthetic patch aortoplasty.
C. Subclavian flap aortoplasty.
D. Prosthetic tube graft repair.

DISCUSSION: The most commonly used methods for coarctation repair are resection with anastomosis and subclavian flap aortoplasty. Both have been shown to provide adequate relief of the obstruction with acceptable rates of restenosis. The choice of repair depends on the patient's anatomy and the surgeon's experience. Patch aortoplasty was used frequently in the past; however, because of concern over restenosis and aneurysm formation it is no longer commonly performed. Prosthetic tube graft repair is avoided except in some complex cases and some cases of recoarctation.
Textbook: Pages 1965–1967 ANSWER: A, C.

8. Which of the following constitutes a true vascular ring?

A. Pulmonary artery sling.
B. Double aortic arch.
C. Anomalous origin of right subclavian artery from the descending aorta.
D. Cervical aortic arch.

DISCUSSION: Only the double aortic arch secondary to persistence of the right and left fourth aortic arches forms a true vascular ring. Pulmonary artery sling may cause symptoms that are due to compression of the trachea, and an anomalous right subclavian may cause dysphagia, but these anomalies do not constitute complete rings. Cervical aortic arch, which is thought to be secondary to persistence of the third aortic arch, is not a complete ring and usually is asymptomatic.
Textbook: Pages 1970–1972 ANSWER: B.

9. Which of the following may be physical examination findings in a young adult with coarctation of the aorta?

A. Posterior systolic murmur between the scapulas.
B. Diminished femoral pulses.
C. Elevated blood pressure in left arm as compared with right arm.
D. Peripheral cyanosis.

DISCUSSION: A systolic murmur that radiates posteriorly is characteristic of coarctation of the aorta. Coarctation produces obstruction to aortic flow, and thus the femoral pulse has a diminished volume with delayed upstroke. Hypertension in coarctation is multifactorial, but the most important factors are diminished renal flow (single clip, single kidney-Goldblatt model) and mechanical factors. If the right subclavian artery is anomalous and arises distal to the coarctation, blood pressure may be greater in the left arm than in the right. Isolated coarctation does not produce cyanosis.
Textbook: Pages 1964–1965 ANSWER: A, B, C.

10. In a premature infant with hyaline membrane disease and inability to be weaned from mechanical ventilation, which of the following would suggest hemodynamically significant patent ductus arteriosus (PDA)?

A. Continuous murmur.
B. Hyperactive precordium with bounding peripheral pulses.
C. Jaundice.
D. Diminished femoral pulses.

DISCUSSION: PDA causes a left-to-right shunt that produces left ventricular volume overload. Physical findings include evidence of hyperdynamic circulation with a prominent apical impulse and bounding peripheral pulses. The classic murmur of PDA is a continuous or mechanical murmur heard over the precordium and radiating to the medial third of the clavicle. Diminished femoral pulses are not seen with isolated PDA and would suggest other anomalies. PDA may result in hepatomegaly but does not cause jaundice.
Textbook: Pages 1961–1962 ANSWER: A, B.

11. In an infant with suspected PDA, which of the following would be the optimal method of confirming the diagnosis?

A. Chest film.
B. Cardiac catheterization.
C. Retrograde aortography via an umbilical artery catheter.
D. Two-dimensional echocardiography with continuous-wave and color-flow Doppler echocardiography.

DISCUSSION: Echocardiography is the best method for confirming the diagnosis of a PDA. Two-dimensional echocardiography can demonstrate PDA and exclude associated anomalies. Doppler echocardiography can demonstrate the shunt, determine direction of shunting, and provide an estimate of shunt magnitude. The chest film is not particularly helpful and may be normal or show cardiomegaly with pulmonary congestion. In general, cardiac catheterization should be reserved for older patients and those with suspected associated anomalies or pulmonary hypertension.

Textbook: Pages 1961–1962 ANSWER: D.

12. Which of the following are potential complications of untreated coarctation of the aorta?

A. Endocarditis.
B. Pulmonary vascular disease.
C. Cerebrovascular accident.
D. Congestive heart failure.

DISCUSSION: Coarctation of the aorta produces an obstruction to blood flow and hypertension, turbulent flow, and increased left ventricular afterload. There is an increased incidence of coronary artery disease. Prior to the introduction of effective techniques for relief of coarctation, the most common causes of death were endocarditis, aortic rupture, congestive heart failure, and cerebrovascular accident. Pulmonary vascular disease does not occur with isolated coarctation.

Textbook: Pages 1964–1965 ANSWER: A, C, D.

13. The atrial septal defect (ASD) most commonly associated with partial anomalous pulmonary venous return (PAPVR) is:

A. Secundum defect.
B. Sinus venosus defect.
C. Ostium primum defect.
D. Complete atrioventricular (AV) canal defect.
E. Coronary sinus defect.

DISCUSSION: Although partial anomalous return of the pulmonary veins can occur with any of the ASDs listed, it is particularly common with sinus venosus defects and is considered by many to be part of this lesion. The most common anomaly is drainage of the right superior pulmonary vein to the lateral aspect of the superior vena cava.

Textbook: Pages 1976–1978 ANSWER: B.

14. The direction of an intracardiac shunt at the atrial level is controlled by:

A. The size of the defect
B. The compliance of the right and left ventricles.
C. The systemic oxygen saturation.
D. Right atrial pressure.
E. The presence or absence of an associated ventricular septal defect (VSD).

DISCUSSION: The direction of an intracardiac shunt is governed by the compliance of the downstream chambers. For an atrial level shunt, the compliance of the right and left ventricles and their ability to distend with increased volume during diastolic filling dictates the direction of the shunt flow. Since the right ventricle is usually a more compliant—and therefore more distensible—chamber than the left ventricle, flow across an ASD occurs from left to right across the open tricuspid valve during diastole. The size of an ASD does not correspond to the degree of shunt as long as the defect is large enough to be unrestrictive to flow. A large shunt can occur through a relatively small defect if the ventricular compliance is favorable.

Textbook: Pages 1979–1981 ANSWER: B.

15. The ASD most commonly associated with mitral insufficiency is:

A. Secundum defect
B. Sinus venosus defect
C. Ostium primum defect.
D. Coronary sinus defect.

DISCUSSION: Ostium primum defects, or "partial" AV canal defects, are commonly associated with a "cleft" of the anterior leaflet of the mitral valve. Depending on the deformity of the mitral valve, these defects can be accompanied by variable degrees of mitral insufficiency. This cleft of the mitral valve needs to be repaired at the same time that the defect is closed. Although other types of ASDs can be associated with mitral insufficiency, this is not as common. When mitral stenosis exists with a secundum ASD the condition is often referred to as Lutembacher's syndrome.

Textbook: Pages 1978–1979 ANSWER: C.

16. An electrocardiogram (ECG) in a patient with a systolic ejection murmur that shows an incomplete bundle branch block in the precordial lead is most consistent with:

A. A secundum ASD.
B. A sinus venosus ASD with PAPVR.
C. An ostium primum ASD.
D. A complete AV canal defect.

DISCUSSION: Many patients with secundum ASDs have an incomplete bundle branch block on their ECG. This is in contradistinction to patients with ostium primum defects, who often have a left axis deviation. Although the ECG is not pathognomonic of the defect, the findings are sometimes helpful along with other clinical and diagnostic information toward elucidating the nature of the defect.

Textbook: Pages 1982–1984 ANSWER: A.

17. ASDs can all be closed with a pericardial or prosthetic patch. Which of the following ASDs can also be safely closed primarily without the use of a patch?

A. Secundum ASD.
B. Sinus venosus ASD with PAPVR.
C. An ostium primum ASD.
D. A complete AV canal defect.

DISCUSSION: Secundum ASDs can frequently be closed primarily, although the use of a prosthetic or pericardial patch is indicated for large defects. The other types of ASDs are more safely closed with a patch.

Textbook: Pages 1984–1985 ANSWER: A.

18. Obstruction to pulmonary venous return is associated with which of the following anomalies?

A. Partial anomalous pulmonary venous connection (PAPVC) to the superior vena cava.
B. Infracardiac (Type III) total anomalous pulmonary venous connection (TAPVC).
C. Pulmonary vein stenosis.
D. Cor triatriatum.
E. Supracardiac (Type I) TAPVC.

DISCUSSION: Obstruction to pulmonary venous return is the most important factor affecting circulatory function when pulmonary venous anomalies exist. This obstruction is most prevalent and severe in patients with infracardiac TAPVC, but it also occurs in as many as 50% of patients with supracardiac TAPVC and 20% of patients with intracardiac TAPVC to the coronary sinus. Obstruction to pulmonary venous return is also the primary pathophysiologic effect of both pulmonary vein stenosis and cor triatriatum. Obstruction, however, is rare with partial anomalous pulmonary venous connection, especially with the common form of PAPVC to the superior vena cava.

Textbook: Pages 1997–1999 ANSWER: B, C, D, E.

19. Postoperative complications associated with repair of TAPVC include:

A. Complete heart block.
B. Acute pulmonary hypertensive crisis.
C. Pleural effusions.
D. Pulmonary venous obstruction.

DISCUSSION: In the early postoperative period after repair of obstructed forms of TAPVC, acute episodes of pulmonary hypertension may develop as a response to stress. To minimize this potentially fatal complication, infants are kept anesthetized with fentanyl and pancuronium for at least 48 hours. Residual or recurrent pulmonary venous obstruction occurs in only 5% to 10% of patients after TAPVC repair, but if identified it requires early reoperation. Reoperation is usually successful if the obstruction is at the level of the anastomosis. Unfortunately, in some cases, the obstruction is in the pulmonary veins and surgical relief is less successful. Although complete heart block and pleural effusions can occur after any cardiac operation, they rarely occur after TAPVC repair.

Textbook: Pages 2001–2002 ANSWER: B, D.

20. Which of the following statements about VSDs is/are correct?

A. Perimembranous lesions are located in the region of the membranous portion of the interventricular septum near the anteroseptal commissure of the tricuspid valve.
B. Muscular VSDs are holes in the interventricular septum that are bordered by muscle on three sides and by the pulmonary and the aortic valve annulus superiorly.
C. VSD, in its isolated form, is the most commonly recognized congenital heart defect.
D. The conduction bundle runs along the posteroinferior rim of a perimembranous VSD.

DISCUSSION: Perimembranous VSDs occupy the area of the membranous portion of the interventricular septum adjacent to the anteroseptal commissure of the tricuspid valve. Often a remnant of the membranous portion of the interventricular septum (the membranous flap) is left hanging on the posteroinferior rim of the defect. The annulus of the tricuspid and aortic valves often form a part of the rim of the defect, but in some patients they are separated from the VSD by a thin rim of muscle tissue that protects the conduction bundle. Muscular VSDs have exclusively muscular rims on all four sides. VSDs in the outlet septum that extend to the annuluses of the aortic and pulmonary valves are called doubly committed or juxta-arterial defects. Isolated VSDs occur at an approximate rate of 2 per 1000 live births and represent 30% to 40% of all congenital heart malformations at birth. The conduction bundle in patients with perimembranous VSDs does run along the posteroinferior rim of the defect on the left ventricular side. Sutures used for repair of a perimembranous VSD should be placed well away from this area to avoid the creation of surgically induced complete heart block.

Textbook: Pages 2005–2008 ANSWER: A, C, D.

21. Which of the following statements about VSDs is/are true?

A. When coarctation of the aorta is associated with VSD, it most commonly occurs in infants with large lesions who have to undergo repair before age 3 months.
B. In some patients with VSD, aortic valve incompetence develops over time and progresses.
C. In the United States doubly committed or juxta-arterial VSDs are most commonly associated with aortic insufficiency.
D. PDA is present in approximately one fourth of infants with a VSD and concomitant congestive heart failure.

DISCUSSION: VSD in combination with severe coarctation of the aorta occurs in approximately 17% of patients. This combination is more common among infants with large VSDs undergoing operation before age 3 months. Aortic valve incompetence does develop over time in some patients with VSD, presumably as a result of progressive prolapse of the right aortic cusp through the defect. In the United States two thirds of patients with VSD and aortic insufficiency have perimembranous lesions and one third have a doubly committed or juxta-arterial lesion. In Japan, however, the reverse is true: two thirds have doubly committed or juxta-arterial lesions and one third have perimembranous lesions. A moderate- or large-sized PDA is associated with VSD in approximately 6% of patients of all ages; however, in infants with VSD and concomitant congestive heart failure, PDA is present in approximately 25%.

Textbook: Page 2008 ANSWER: A, B, D.

22. Which of the following statements about VSD is/are correct?

A. A large VSD is approximately the size of the pulmonary valve orifice or larger.
B. Large VSDs associated with high pulmonary blood flow result in an enlarged left atrium on chest x-ray.
C. Patients with small (restrictive) VSDs tend to have normal right ventricular and pulmonary arterial pressures with normal pulmonary vascular resistance and no evidence of pulmonary vascular disease.
D. A pulmonary vascular resistance greater than 10 to 12 units per sq. m. is considered a contraindication to operation.

DISCUSSION: A large VSD is approximately the size of the aortic valve orifice or larger and causes systemic right ventricular systolic pressures. In the absence of right ventricular outflow tract obstruction, the pulmonary artery systolic pressure will also be systemic in the presence of a large VSD. Large VSDs associated with a high pulmonary blood flow do result in an enlarged left atrium because of increased pulmonary venous return. When marked enlargement of the left atrium is present in a patient suspected of having a VSD, the presence of coexisting mitral valve regurgitation should also be considered. Patients with small VSDs do have normal right ventricular and pulmonary arterial pressures. There is only a slight elevation of pulmonary blood flow relative to the systemic flow, and the pulmonary vascular resistance is normal without evidence of pulmonary vascular disease. At any age, the presence of pulmonary vascular disease so severe that the pulmonary vascular resistance is fixed and greater than 10 to 12 units per sq. m. is considered a contraindication to operation.

Textbook: Pages 2008–2009 ANSWER: B, C, D.

23. Which of the following statements about VSDs is/are correct?

A. Spontaneous closure of VSDs occurs in 25% to 50% of patients during childhood.
B. Tachypnea and failure to thrive are symptoms frequently associated with large VSDs.
C. Patients with normal pulmonary vascular resistance and left-to-right shunting across the VSD have Eisenmenger's complex.
D. Patients with a large VSD and low pulmonary vascular resistance can present with a middiastolic murmur at the apex.

DISCUSSION: Spontaneous and complete closure of VSDs, even large ones, has been estimated to occur in 25% to 50% of patients during childhood. The probability of eventual spontaneous closure is inversely related to the age at which the patient is observed. Tachypnea, poor feeding, growth failure, recurrent respiratory infections, exercise intolerance, and severe cardiac failure may develop in patients with large VSDs. Patients with Eisenmenger's complex are cyanotic, polycythemic, and severely limited in their exercise tolerance, owing to markedly elevated pulmonary vascular resistance associated with a predominantly right-to-left shunt across the VSD. A middiastolic murmur can be present at the apex in patients with a large VSD associated with low pulmonary vascular resistance. This indicates high pulmonary blood flow with a large flow across the mitral valve into the left ventricle.

Textbook: Pages 2009–2010 ANSWER: A, B, D.

24. Which of the following is/are true of the surgical treatment of VSDs?

A. A right ventricular approach is employed for the repair of most perimembranous VSDs.
B. Intracardiac repair is advisable for patients with intractable symptoms and for asymptomatic infants with evidence of increasing pulmonary vascular resistance.
C. Complete heart block is a common complication.
D. Hospital mortality after repair of VSD in infants approaches 20%.

DISCUSSION: The right atrial approach is preferred for the repair of most perimembranous VSDs. Prompt intracardiac repair is indicated for infants with large defects, large shunts, and pulmonary hypertension who present with intractable left ventricular failure, recurrent pulmonary infections, severe growth failure, or evidence of increasing pulmonary vascular resistance. In the modern era, complete heart block requiring a permanent pacemaker is a very uncommon complication of surgical closure of a ventricular septal defect. Hospital mortality after closure of a VSD currently approaches zero. While in earlier years younger age was an incremental risk factor for hospital death in some surgical experiences, this risk has been neutralized during the past decade.

Textbook: Pages 2012–2017 ANSWER: B.

25. Tetralogy of Fallot consists of all of the following features except:

A. ASD.
B. VSD.
C. Dextroposition of the aorta.
D. Pulmonary stenosis.
E. Right ventricular hypertrophy.

DISCUSSION: Although ASD is a frequent component of tetralogy of Fallot, it was not included by Fallot as part of his classic tetralogy. Occasionally, the inclusion of an ASD prompts use of the term *pentalogy* of Fallot. The other four anomalies listed were all mentioned by Fallot in his original description of this defect.

Textbook: Pages 2018–2019 ANSWER: A.

26. Which of the following has the greatest impact on the physiology of tetralogy of Fallot?

A. The size of the ASD.
B. The size of the VSD.
C. The degree of pulmonary stenosis.
D. The amount of aortic overriding.

DISCUSSION: The VSD in tetralogy of Fallot is nonrestrictive, and therefore its size does not affect the degree of shunting that can occur. Likewise, an ASD, which may or may not be a component of tetralogy of Fallot, can provide right-to-left shunting at the atrial level but is not the main contributor to the cyanosis of this disease. The degree of right-to-left shunt across the VSD is dictated by the variable compliance of the downstream chambers, and the increased resistance imposed by severe pulmonary stenosis creates greater amounts of right-to-left shunting and, therefore, more intense cyanosis. The position of the aorta in relation to the VSD is not important as long as no subaortic obstruction exists.
Textbook: Page 2020 ANSWER: C.

27. Which of the following anomalies is not associated with tetralogy of Fallot?

A. Absence of the left pulmonary artery.
B. A right aortic arch.
C. A retroesophageal subclavian artery.
D. Anomalous origin of the left anterior descending coronary artery from the right coronary artery.
E. Primary pulmonary hypertension.

DISCUSSION: The first four defects listed occasionally are associated with tetralogy of Fallot. A right aortic arch is seen in 25% of patients with that lesion. Anomalous coronary arteries or a retroesophageal subclavian artery are found in as many as 5% to 10% of patients. Absence of a pulmonary artery is unusual but can present in as many as 3% of patients. Pulmonary hypertension is distinctly unusual with tetralogy of Fallot unless the patient has had excessive pulmonary blood flow from collaterals or systemic-to-pulmonary artery shunts for a long time. It is because these patients usually do not have pulmonary hypertension that infant correction with transannular patches can be performed with such great success.
Textbook: Pages 2019–2020 ANSWER: E.

28. Surgical treatment of a patient with tetralogy of Fallot can include any of the following except:

A. Maintenance of ductal patency with prostaglandins (PGE_1) to provide pulmonary blood flow while the baby is transferred to an institution equipped to provide more definitive therapy.
B. Banding of the pulmonary artery in an acyanotic patient with tetralogy of Fallot to control pulmonary blood flow and prevent the development of pulmonary hypertension.
C. Placement of a subclavian-to-pulmonary artery shunt on the side opposite the aortic arch in a 3-day-old infant with severe cyanosis.
D. Closure of the VSD and transannular patching of the right ventricle onto the main pulmonary artery in a 2-day-old infant.

DISCUSSION: Patients with tetralogy of Fallot who do not appear cyanotic still have mild arterial hypoxemia by arterial blood gas determination. Patients with tetralogy of Fallot rarely have excessive pulmonary blood flow, and the development of pulmonary hypertension is not a concern in this population. Banding of the pulmonary artery is never a consideration in patients with tetralogy of Fallot, since the predominant physiologic effect of the defect results from too little pulmonary blood flow to begin with. Acyanotic patients with tetralogy of Fallot ("pink tets") can usually be followed for several months and their defects repaired electively as a first-stage procedure (usually by age 6 months). All of the other therapies are appropriate treatment for babies with tetralogy of Fallot. Prostaglandins maintain patency of the ductus arteriosus, providing an anatomic systemic-to-pulmonary artery shunt that sustains pulmonary blood flow until a more permanent surgical solution can be provided. The advent of prostaglandin therapy has enabled numerous critically ill infants to become stabilized enough to reach a tertiary care institution and receive proper surgical therapy who might not otherwise have survived had it not been for the ability of pulmonary blood flow to be maintained through the reversal of duct closing. The choice of palliative shunting or total anatomic correction rests largely with the experience and skill of the surgical team and is dictated in part by the anatomy of the pulmonary arteries. Either of these options is acceptable.
Textbook: Pages 2022–2029 ANSWER: B.

29. The predominant determinant of outcome for patients with pulmonary atresia and an intact ventricular septum revolves around:

A. The size of the ASD.
B. The baby's age at presentation.
C. The size of the right ventricular cavity and tricuspid valve.
D. The presence of a tricuspid—as opposed to a bicuspid—pulmonary valve.
E. The level of hypoxemia at presentation.

DISCUSSION: The long-term outcome for babies with pulmonary atresia and intact ventricular septum depends on the ability to convert the cardiac circulation into a two-ventricle versus one-ventricle physiology. Patients with a good-sized right ventricle and tricuspid valve can often be treated with pulmonary valvotomy or right ventricular outflow patching alone and can have a fairly acceptable outcome. Patients with a small right ventricle that cannot provide adequate pumping to the pulmonary bed and is often associated with a small tricuspid valve annulus may need to be staged toward a Fontan procedure—and, consequently, a less acceptable outcome. The size of an ASD is not relevant except that in patients with this syndrome, the right side of the heart will decompress across the ASD until antegrade flow can be established. Therefore, an ASD in some part is an essential feature of this lesion. The degree of arterial hypoxemia, the nature of the pulmonary valve, and the patient's age at presentation may all be factors that relate to clinical management, but they do not imply specific consequences with respect to long-term outcome.
Textbook: Pages 2029–2030 ANSWER: C.

30. Which of the following statements about double-outlet right ventricle are true?

A. A VSD is usually present.
B. In the Taussig-Bing type of double-outlet right ventricle, the VSD is usually noncommitted.
C. Patients with double-outlet right ventricle and a subaortic VSD usually have pulmonary stenosis.
D. Patients with double-outlet right ventricle with a subpulmonary VSD (Taussig-Bing malformation) tend to mimic patients with transposition of the great arteries and VSD in their presentation and natural history.

DISCUSSION: A VSD is usually present in patients with double-outlet right ventricle and is the only outlet from the left ventricle. Both great arteries may arise totally from the right ventricle, or one or both may overlie the ventricular septum immediately above the VSD. To categorize the heart as having a double-outlet right ventricle, more than 50% of each great artery must arise from the right ventricle. In the Taussig-Bing type of double-outlet right ventricle, the VSD is related to the pulmonary valve annulus and is termed a *subpulmonary defect*. Additional morphologic characteristics peculiar to this entity have been described. Most patients with double-outlet right ventricle and a subaortic VSD have concomitant pulmonary stenosis that protects the lungs from pulmonary vascular disease and also results in a clinical course similar to that of patients with tetralogy of Fallot. In the absence of pulmonary stenosis the presentation, clinical course, and natural history of the Taussig-Bing malformation are similar to those of transposition of the great arteries with VSD. Cyanosis is present, usually from birth, since streaming directs the desaturated systemic venous return toward the aorta and the oxygenated left ventricular blood toward the pulmonary artery. These patients tend to develop early congestive heart failure and can develop severe pulmonary vascular disease early in life. They usually experience symptoms within the first few months of life.

Textbook: Pages 2034–2036 ANSWER: A, C, D.

31. Which of the following statements about the surgical repair of double-outlet right ventricle are true?

A. In double-outlet right ventricle with a subaortic or doubly committed VSD, a tunnel-type repair connecting a committed VSD with its respective great artery is usually employed.
B. Repair of the Taussig-Bing malformation can be accomplished using an intraventricular tunnel technique or by performing a straight patch closure of the VSD combined with an arterial switch procedure.
C. The hospital mortality rate is highest when a subaortic VSD is present.
D. Some hearts with double-outlet right ventricle and a noncommitted VSD must be repaired using a modification of the Fontan procedure.

DISCUSSION: When the VSD is subaortic or doubly committed, the tunnel-type repair connects the left ventricle via the VSD and tunnel to the aorta. The Taussig-Bing malformation can be repaired using an intraventricular tunnel technique described by Kawashima. This repair can best be accomplished when the great arteries are in a more or less side-by-side relationship with the aorta to the right of the pulmonary artery. The infundibular septum is generously resected and the VSD is connected to the aorta by an intraventricular tunnel that runs posterior to the pulmonary artery. The most common approach for the repair of the Taussig-Bing malformation involves patch closure of the VSD to the pulmonary artery. This creates transposition of the great arteries with an intact interventricular septum. An arterial switch procedure then establishes ventriculoarterial concordance. Of all the types of double-outlet right ventricle the hospital mortality is lowest when a subaortic or doubly committed VSD is present. Double-outlet right ventricle is associated with a noncommitted VSD in approximately 10% of patients in surgical series. The repair of this subset of patients is associated with a relatively high mortality, as compared with the results obtained after repair of other forms of double-outlet right ventricle. At times, because of the remote location of the VSD and because of other compelling anatomic features, complete repair cannot be performed. In this case, a modification of the Fontan procedure must be employed.

Textbook: Pages 2035–2037 ANSWER: A, B, D.

32. Management of a patient with tricuspid atresia within the first month of life may include:

A. Creation of a systemic artery–to–pulmonary artery shunt.
B. Observation.
C. Creation of a bidirectional superior cavopulmonary anastomosis.
D. Pulmonary artery banding.
E. Fontan procedure.

DISCUSSION: Initial management of newborn infants with tricuspid atresia is determined by the anatomic and physiologic factors that affect the balance of pulmonary and systemic blood flow. Infants with severely limited pulmonary blood flow and arterial oxygen saturations of less than 70% should be stabilized with PGE_1 to maintain patency of the ductus arteriosus until a systemic-to-pulmonary artery shunt can be performed. Patients with unobstructed pulmonary blood flow may exhibit only mild cyanosis but suffer from significant congestive heart failure. Many of these patients are best managed by pulmonary artery banding to decrease the volume overload on the left ventricle and to prevent the early development of irreversible pulmonary vascular disease. Some patients with moderate restriction of pulmonary blood flow may have balanced delivery of blood to the systemic and the pulmonary circulation. These patients can be carefully followed until such time as an imbalance develops or they become candidates for a bidirectional superior cavopulmonary (Glenn) anastomosis or a Fontan procedure. The normally high pulmonary vascular resistance present in the first month of life precludes the performance of either the Glenn or the Fontan procedure in the newborn.

Textbook: Pages 2041–2042 ANSWER: A, B, D.

33. Which of the following should contraindicate performance of the Fontan procedure?

A. Patient age of 25 years.
B. Severe mitral insufficiency.
C. Left ventricular end-diastolic pressure of 18 mm. Hg.
D. Right pulmonary artery stenosis.
E. Pulmonary vascular resistance of 6 Woods units.

DISCUSSION: Good ventricular function and low pulmonary vascular resistance are essential requirements for a successful Fontan procedure. The Fontan operation should not be performed when ventricular ejection fraction is less than 30% or ventricular end-diastolic pressure is greater than 15 mm. Hg. Pulmonary vascular resistance in excess of 4 Woods units should also be considered an absolute contraindication for Fontan correction. Age at the time of Fontan procedure does not appear to be a major risk factor, except before age 2 years. Although patients who have survived into the third or fourth decade are likely to have ventricular dysfunction, a Fontan procedure can be performed successfully in these older patients if ventricular function and pulmonary vascular resistance meet the above criteria. In patients with tricuspid atresia a competent mitral valve is important for satisfactory cardiac output after the Fontan procedure. The presence of severe mitral insufficiency, however, should not necessarily contraindicate the procedure. In these cases it is recommended that the mitral valve be repaired or replaced in combination with the creation of a bidirectional superior cavopulmonary anastomosis. A completion Fontan operation is performed later. Distorted or stenosed pulmonary arteries are common sequelae of systemic-to-pulmonary artery shunts and may result in unsatisfactorily high pulmonary vascular resistance. In most cases, these stenoses can be repaired at the time of Fontan correction or with a bidirectional superior cavopulmonary anastomosis.

Textbook: Pages 2041–2042 ANSWER: C, E.

34. Initial management of a newborn infant with hypoplastic left heart syndrome should include:

A. Intravenous administration of PGE_1.
B. Supplemental oxygen.
C. Routine intubation and mechanical ventilation to achieve a P_{CO_2} between 30 and 35 mm. Hg.
D. Cardiac catheterization and balloon atrial septostomy.

DISCUSSION: Postnatal stabilization of infants with hypoplastic left heart syndrome requires patency of the ductus arteriosus and balance of the systemic and the pulmonary circulation. Because the ductus is the only pathway from the right ventricle to the systemic circulation, duct patency must be maintained with intravenous PGE_1. To minimize the workload on the single ventricle and ensure adequate delivery of oxygen to the tissues, an equal delivery of blood to both the lungs and the body is sought. The normal postnatal decrease in pulmonary vascular resistance often results in overperfusion of the pulmonary circulation and underperfusion of the systemic circulation. Maneuvers that further decrease pulmonary vascular resistance, such as the addition of supplemental oxygen, lowering the P_{CO_2} to less than 35 mm. Hg, or eliminating any resistance at the atrial septum by balloon septostomy only worsens the imbalance.

Textbook: Pages 2046–2048 ANSWER: A.

35. The performance of a bidirectional superior cavopulmonary (Glenn) anastomosis as the second stage in the reconstructive approach to hypoplastic left heart syndrome:

A. Provides early relief of volume load on the single right ventricle.
B. Increases peripheral oxygen saturations to greater than 90%.
C. Permits concomitant repair of pulmonary artery or aortic arch stenoses.
D. Improves mortality and morbidity of subsequent Fontan procedure.

DISCUSSION: After the first-stage reconstructive (Norwood) procedure, the circulation is inherently inefficient because of the obligatory recirculation of a portion of both saturated and desaturated blood. Closure of the arterial shunt and creation of a bidirectional Glenn anastomosis eliminates this inefficient recirculation and significantly diminishes the volume load on the single right ventricle. Distorted and stenosed central pulmonary arteries or aortic arch obstructions should be repaired at the same time the bidirectional Glenn procedure is performed. In almost all series the mortality of the Fontan procedure has decreased since the adoption of the three-stage approach for hypoplastic left heart syndrome. Because systemic and pulmonary venous blood continue to mix in the right atrium after a bidirectional Glenn procedure, cyanosis persists with peripheral oxygen saturations between 75% and 85%.

Textbook: Pages 2048–2049 ANSWER: A, C, D.

36. Which of the following statements about truncus arteriosus are true?

A. Most infants survive without operations until late childhood.
B. Most infants present with cyanosis.
C. Most infants present with congestive heart failure.
D. Repair requires a conduit from right ventricle to pulmonary arteries.

DISCUSSION: While an occasional child survives to age 3 or 4 years, without either palliative or totally corrective surgical treatment few live past early infancy. The lesion is one of excessive pulmonary blood flow because of the origin of the pulmonary arteries from the truncus arteriosus; physiologically, the pulmonary arteries arise directly from the aorta. Although the aortic saturation can never be 100% because of some element of bidirectional shunting at the VSD, the physiologic manifestations are congestive heart failure and excessive pulmonary blood flow rather than cyanosis. The congestive heart failure becomes severe as pulmonary vascular resistance drops. If congestive heart failure later improves spontaneously, it is because of the development of pulmonary vascular disease. Complete repair always requires closure of the VSD, detachment of the pulmonary arteries from the common trunk, and re-establishment of an outflow tract from the right ventricle to the pulmonary artery. This conduit usually contains a valve and can be either a homograft or a synthetic conduit containing a porcine valve.

Textbook: Page 2054 ANSWER: B, C, D.

37. Truncus arteriosus is a diagnosis with anatomic components including:

A. VSD.
B. Abnormal origin of pulmonary arteries.
C. Subaortic stenosis.
D. Single ventricular outflow valve.

DISCUSSION: By definition, a VSD is always present immediately beneath the truncal valve. The pulmonary arteries arise abnormally from the single trunk, which is due to failed partitioning of the embryonic conus during the first few weeks of fetal development. In the classification of Collett and Edwards, Type I truncus arteriosus has a single arterial trunk giving rise to an aorta and a main pulmonary artery; in Type II the right pulmonary arteries arise immediately adjacent to one another from the dorsal wall of the truncus; in Type III the right and left pulmonary arteries originate from either side of the truncus; and in Type IV the proximal pulmonary arteries are absent and pulmonary blood flow is by way of major aortopulmonary atresia and is no longer considered truncus arteriosus. Subaortic stenosis cannot occur in this anomaly. The single ventricular outflow valve is the truncal valve. It may contain from two to six cusps, but most often there are three and, next most often, four.

Textbook: Pages 2053–2054 ANSWER: A, B, D.

38. Optimal treatment for the neonate who presents with transposition of the great arteries {S,D,D}* and intact ventricular septum includes:

A. PGE_1 infusion to maintain duct patency.
B. Administration of intravenous fluid to increase intravascular volume.
C. Hyperventilation to decrease pulmonary resistance.
D. Oxygen administration to increase arterial oxygen tension.
E. Atrial balloon septostomy to improve atrial mixing.

DISCUSSION: Because with transposition of the great vessels the systemic and the pulmonary circulations exist in parallel rather than in series, survival depends on mixing between pulmonary and systemic circulations. Initially infants with transposition and intact atrial septum survive because of aortopulmonary flow through PDA, which may be maintained with prostaglandin infusions. Although increased pulmonary flow may cause enlargement of the left atrium and stretching of the foramen ovale resulting in atrial-level mixing of oxygenated and nonoxygenated blood, inadequate mixing at the atrial level will result in marginal tissue oxygenation, which does not improve with oxygen administration. Atrial balloon septotomy results in improved admixture and oxygen delivery in these patients and should be performed promptly if peripheral acidemia and severe cyanosis are present. Relative dehydration may decrease the degree of interatrial shunting and volume infusion often improves hemodynamics in infants. Decreased pulmonary vascular resistance may increase pulmonary blood flow at the expense of systemic blood flow and alter the loading conditions of the left ventricle, which may complicate early arterial repair.

Textbook: Pages 2061–2064 ANSWER: A, B, E.

39. Factors that preclude the use of a single-stage arterial switch reconstruction of dextrotransposition of the great vessels include:

A. Age older than 6 weeks with a left ventricular pressure of less than 50% of systemic pressure.
B. Dynamic left ventricular outflow tract obstruction.
C. Intramural coronary artery anatomy.
D. Valvar pulmonic stenosis.
E. Subpulmonary VSD.

DISCUSSION: Single-stage arterial switch procedure for reconstruction of transposition of the great vessels, with or without associated VSD has become the standard of treatment in the majority of cardiac centers. Contraindications to arterial switch repair include fixed types of left ventricular outflow tract obstruction, including valvar pulmonic stenosis, which would render the systemic semilunar valve stenotic or incompetent. Anatomic abnormalities without stenosis, such as a bicuspid valve, however, are suitable for surgical correction. The location of VSD does not affect surgical outcome, and most VSDs can be approached adequately through the right atrium or the anterior great vessel. Most dynamic forms of left ventricular outflow tract obstruction are often relieved partially or completely by realignment of the ventricular septum with the hemodynamic changes following successful arterial switch repair. When, however, the left ventricle has not been prepared to sustain the pressure load of the systemic circulation by the decrease in pulmonary vascular resistance that occurs in the first few weeks of life and when the ventricular

*The nomenclature S,D,D is based on Van Praagh's classification scheme denoting normal situs solitus (S); right-handed looping of the ventricles with the right ventricle to the right and anterior to the left ventricle (D); and dextroposition of the great arteries with the aorta anterior and to the right of the pulmonary artery (D).

pressure is less than 50% of the systemic ventricular pressure, one-stage repair is contraindicated, and staged repair with pulmonary banding and shunt followed by arterial switch must be contemplated.
Textbook: Pages 2061–2062 ANSWER: A, D.

40. Complications commonly associated with the atrial (Senning and Mustard) repairs of transposition of the great arteries include:

A. Atrial arrhythmias.
B. Systemic or pulmonary venous obstruction.
C. Right ventricular outflow tract obstruction.
D. Systemic ventricular failure.
E. Progressive elevation of pulmonary vascular resistance.

DISCUSSION: The atrial repair of transposition of the great arteries—rerouting systemic and pulmonary venous blood at the atrial level—results in the right ventricle's becoming the systemic ventricle. This results in an anatomic right ventricle with abnormal geometry sustaining the afterload of a more ideally suited left ventricle. Long-term complications of ventricular dilatation, AV valve regurgitation, and right ventricular failure have been reported in as many as 10% of patients many years following the atrial operation. The multiple suture lines in the atrium have been associated with a high incidence of late atrial arrhythmias and a low incidence of sinus rhythm following the Mustard and Senning operations. These complications do not appear to be as frequent with the arterial switch repair. In addition, the complicated interatrial baffles have been associated with pulmonary or systemic venous baffle obstruction. Because the right ventricular outflow tract is not addressed during an atrial switch operation, right ventricular outflow tract obstruction is not a recognized complication following the repair. Right ventricular outflow tract and supravalvar pulmonic stenosis, however, have been reported in patients after the arterial switch repair, owing to the reconstruction of the right ventricular outflow tract in that operation. Although progression of pulmonary arterial obstruction has rarely been reported following early repair with the atrial or the arterial switch procedure, it is an unusual complication if operation is undertaken in infancy. Delayed repair beyond age 6 months to 1 year, however, has been associated with a higher incidence of progressive development of pulmonary vascular obstructive disease. The rapidity of the development of pulmonary vascular disease is increased by the coexistence of a VSD.
Textbook: Pages 2063–2066 ANSWER: A, B, D.

41. Critical aortic stenosis in the neonate is characterized by which of the following?

A. It is most often due to commissural fusion of a trileaflet valve.
B. It may be associated with coarctation of the aorta, PDA, and mitral stenosis.
C. It can be managed medically until the child is large enough to undergo aortic valve replacement.
D. Success of valvotomy is determined by the adequacy of the left ventricle.

DISCUSSION: Critical aortic stenosis in the neonate most often presents in the first week of life with severe and progressive congestive heart failure and may be associated with coarctation of the aorta, PDA, and mitral stenosis. The prognosis is poor unless valvotomy can be performed expeditiously. Medical management cannot stabilize these infants for valve replacement at a later age. Infants whose left ventricle is too small to sustain the systemic circulation are unlikely to survive aortic valvotomy and, thus, should be managed as patients with hypoplastic left heart syndrome. The aortic valve in neonatal aortic stenosis is most commonly unicuspid or bicuspid.
Textbook: Pages 2071–2073 ANSWER: B, D.

42. Surgical management of aortic valve disease in an older child may include:

A. Enlargement of the aortic annulus.
B. Incision of fused commissures.
C. Insertion of a porcine valve prosthesis.
D. Transfer of the pulmonary valve to the aortic position.

DISCUSSION: The majority of older children with aortic stenosis and significant transvalvular gradients can be treated successfully by aortic valvotomy. This can be done percutaneously with balloon dilatation or surgically with direct visualization of the aortic valve and incision of the fused commissures. Aortic valve replacement is rarely necessary as a primary procedure but may be required in children who develop progressive aortic insufficiency after a previous intervention. When valve replacement is performed it is desirable to insert the largest prosthesis possible, to allow for growth. Enlargement of the aortic annulus is commonly performed for this purpose. If a true valve prosthesis is employed, a mechanical valve is preferred. Durability of xenograft valves in children is limited owing to early calcification and leaflet degeneration. The pulmonary autograft technique may be the best method of aortic valve replacement in children. With this operation the patient's own pulmonary valve is transferred to the aortic position and a pulmonary allograft is inserted to replace the pulmonary valve. Although the pulmonary autograft may not achieve the long-term durability of a mechanical valve, the patient does not face the long-term complications of thromboembolism and bleeding imposed by a mechanical valve and lifelong anticoagulation.
Textbook: Pages 2073–2075 ANSWER: A, B, D.

43. Which of the following statements about subvalvular aortic stenosis are true?

A. Most patients present in early infancy with severe congestive heart failure.
B. An ejection click is a specific physical sign of subaortic stenosis.
C. The subaortic membrane is approached surgically via the aorta and aortic valve.

D. A concomitant septal myectomy decreases the incidence of recurrent subaortic stenosis.

DISCUSSION: Subaortic stenosis is rarely encountered in neonates. Most often it is discovered in an asymptomatic child during a routine physical examination. A loud crescendo–decrescendo systolic murmur without an ejection click is usually noted. The presence of an ejection click is more consistent with isolated valvular aortic stenosis. Discrete subaortic stenosis is approached surgically with cardiopulmonary bypass, aortic cross-clamping, and cardioplegic arrest. The aorta is opened and the aortic valve leaflets are retracted, exposing the fibrous membrane. The fibrous ring is carefully excised, taking care to avoid injury to the anterior leaflet of the mitral valve and the penetrating conduction bundle. Once the subaortic membrane is excised a septal myectomy further opens the left ventricular outflow tract and diminishes the likelihood of recurrent subaortic stenosis.

Textbook: Pages 2075–2077 ANSWER: C, D.

44. Management of hypertrophic obstructive cardiomyopathy may include:

A. Propranolol and verapamil.
B. Aortic valve replacement.
C. Dual-chamber sequential pacing.
D. Combined septal myectomy and mitral valve plication.

DISCUSSION: The majority of patients with hypertrophic obstructive cardiomyopathy are treated medically with beta-blockers such as propranolol and calcium channel blockers such as verapamil. Patients whose symptoms do not respond to medical therapy are treated surgically with a transaortic septal myectomy. Recent reports indicate that simple plication of the anterior leaflet of the mitral valve performed in addition to the septal myectomy further opens the left ventricular outflow tract by eliminating systolic anterior motion of the mitral valve. Aortic valve replacement is not an appropriate treatment for hypertrophic obstructive cardiomyopathy. Some patients who are poor surgical candidates may experience relief of symptoms and left ventricular outflow gradients with dual-chamber permanent pacing. Appropriate pre-excitation of the ventricular septum can prompt the septum to move away from the left ventricular wall during systole and open the outflow tract.

Textbook: Pages 2077–2078 ANSWER: A, C, D.

45. Which of the following statements about supravalvular aortic stenosis are true?

A. Surgical repair is indicated only when the systolic gradient exceeds 75 mm. Hg.
B. Simple excision of the supravalvular membrane results in satisfactory relief of the stenosis in most patients.
C. The diffuse form of supravalvular aortic stenosis may cause obstruction to branches of the aortic arch.
D. Reoperation after repair of discrete supravalvular aortic stenosis is rare unless abnormalities of the valve itself also exist.

DISCUSSION: Supravalvular aortic stenosis is a progressive disease and should be repaired surgically if symptoms are present or the systolic gradient exceeds 50 mm. Hg. In addition to excision of the supravalvular membrane, a patch of dacron or pericardium must be placed across the area of narrowing and down into at least one of the sinuses of Valsalva. Reoperation is rare after this procedure unless associated aortic valve disease is also present. In the diffuse form of the disease the thickening of the aortic wall commonly results in significant luminal narrowing of the ascending aorta and its major branches.

Textbook: Pages 2078–2080 ANSWER: C, D.

46. Each year the approximate number of Americans who die from complications of coronary artery disease is:

A. 100,000.
B. 250,000.
C. 500,000.
D. 1,000,000.
E. Over 2,000,000.

DISCUSSION: It is estimated that approximately 7,000,000 Americans currently have symptomatic coronary artery disease. Of these some 1,500,000 experience myocardial infarction annually and approximately 500,000 die each year from complications.

Textbook: Page 2082 ANSWER: C.

47. Which of the following arteries is most likely to be involved with serious atherosclerosis?

A. The right coronary artery.
B. The left coronary artery.
C. The anterior descending coronary artery.
D. The circumflex coronary artery.

DISCUSSION: In order of frequency, the anterior descending coronary artery is the most commonly involved with atherosclerosis, followed by the right coronary, the circumflex, and the left main coronary artery.

Textbook: Page 2084 ANSWER: C.

48. Which of the following statements about collaterals in the normal coronary circulation is true?

A. There is a rich and quite effective collateral circulation in the coronary arterial bed.
B. The coronary arterial bed has minimal effective collaterals.
C. The coronary arterial bed is an absolute example of anatomic end-arteries.

DISCUSSION: The collateral circulation to the heart is relatively poor. In the human heart there are few natural collaterals of sufficient diameter for delivery of a significant quantity of blood. Most of the collaterals are approximately 200 μm. or smaller, and channels of this size cannot conduct significant quantities

of blood for cardiac requirements. There is no absolute example of anatomic end-arteries in humans. While the magnitude of arterial collateral circulation varies considerably, all organs have some collaterals.
Textbook: Pages 2085–2086 ANSWER: B.

49. If blood entering the normal arterial circulation of the heart is 100% saturated with oxygen, oxygen saturation of blood in the coronary sinus can be expected to be approximately:

A. 75%.
B. 60%.
C. 50%.
D. 35%.
E. Less than 20%.

DISCUSSION: The heart has an unusually high rate of oxygen utilization and consumes approximately two thirds of the oxygen in the arterial blood. The oxygen saturation of the blood in the coronary sinus is usually about 30% to 35% and varies with the magnitude of cardiac disease. The body as a whole extracts approximately 25% of the oxygen it receives, thus emphasizing the great need of the heart for oxygen at rest as well as at exercise.
Textbook: Page 2083 ANSWER: D.

50. Coronary bypass procedures have been demonstrated to:

A. Reduce the incidence of myocardial infarction.
B. Significantly relieves angina symptoms.
C. Statistically improve the life span.
D. Improve the ejection fraction of the left ventricle in many patients in whom it is significantly depressed preoperatively.

DISCUSSION: In a variety of studies, coronary bypass procedures have been demonstrated to reduce the incidence of subsequent myocardial infarction as well as to relieve significantly anginal symptoms. They also improve the life span of most patients as well as the ejection fraction of the left ventricle in those in whom it was depressed preoperatively.
Textbook: Pages 2086–2087 ANSWER: A, B, C, D.

51. The following patients are best treated with coronary artery bypass grafting (CABG):

A. A 60-year-old man with class II angina, 75% proximal right coronary artery lesion, and normal ventricular function.
B. A 60-year-old man with unstable angina, three-vessel disease, and an ejection fraction of 35%.
C. A 60-year-old nondiabetic man with class III angina symptoms and focal discrete lesions in the mid-right coronary artery and mid-left circumflex artery.
D. A 60-year-old man with diabetes, class IV angina, 75% proximal left anterior descending and 75% proximal right coronary artery obstruction, and left ventricular ejection fraction of 60%.

DISCUSSION: CABG has been shown to prolong patient survival compared with medical therapy in those patients with left main occlusive disease and those with three-vessel or two-vessel disease with proximal left anterior descending involvement in association with class III or greater anginal symptoms, impaired ejection fraction, or easily inducible ischemia with exercise. Although percutaneous transluminal coronary angioplasty (PTCA) appears to be comparable to CABG in nondiabetic patients, patients with diabetes appear to have a significant survival advantage when CABG is used. Similarly, patients with more extensive coronary artery disease are better treated with CABG than with PTCA.
Textbook: Pages 2086–2087 ANSWER: B, D.

52. Sternal wound infections that spread to the mediastinum are associated with a mortality rate of:

A. 60%.
B. 30%.
C. 25%.
D. Less than 15%.

DISCUSSION: Although the mortality rate following sternal infections with mediastinitis formerly was high, it is now greatly reduced. In most series, mediastinitis is cured in more than 90% of patients who are treated aggressively with débridement and placement of muscle flaps or omentum into the mediastinum to speed wound healing.
Textbook: Page 2092 ANSWER: D.

53. Perioperative myocardial infarction occurs following coronary bypass procedures in approximately:

A. 15%.
B. 10%.
C. 7%.
D. Less than 5%.

DISCUSSION: Following improvements in myocardial protection and coronary grafting techniques, perioperative myocardial infarction now occurs in less that 2% to 4% of patients in most series.
Textbook: Page 2093 ANSWER: D.

54. Following acute myocardial infarction, ventricular septal defects occur in:

A. 20%.
B. 10%.
C. 15%
D. 2% or less.

DISCUSSION: Postmortem studies indicate that 8% to 10% of fatal cases of myocardial infarction are due to rupture of the heart. In addition, infarction of the interventricular septum with subsequent formation of a ventricular septal defect occurs in 1% to 2% of patients with acute myocardial infarction. The usual interval between the acute infarction and septal rupture—4 to 12 days—correlates with the histologic finding of maximal cardiac muscle degeneration.
Textbook: Pages 2087–2088 ANSWER: D.

55. Which of the following clinical characteristics is/are associated with a higher mortality after emergency CABG for failed PTCA?

A. Multivessel disease.
B. Rescue atherectomy.
C. Cardiogenic shock prior to CABG.
D. Previous bypass surgery.
E. All of the above.

Textbook: Pages 2095–2096 ANSWER: A, C, D.

56. Which statement(s) about operative mortality and perioperative incidence of myocardial infarction for elective CABG (X) versus emergency CABG following failed PTCA (Y) is/are accurate?

A. The operative mortality is higher for Y but the incidence of perioperative myocardial infarction is unchanged between X and Y.
B. The operative mortality is unchanged between X and Y but the perioperative incidence of myocardial infarction is higher in Y.
C. The operative mortality and perioperative incidence is higher in X than in Y.
D. The operative mortality and perioperative incidence of myocardial infarction are no different for X and for Y.

Textbook: Pages 2097–2099 ANSWER: C.

57. Which of the following statements about patients treated by placement of an internal mammary artery (IMA) bypass graft at primary CABG is/are correct?

A. The risk for morbidity and mortality from reoperative coronary bypass grafting is increased.
B. Left ventricular function is better preserved at the time of reoperation.
C. The risk of sternal wound complications is greatly increased if the contralateral IMA is harvested at the time of reoperation.
D. A light clamp should be applied to the IMA pedicle to limit cardiac warming during cardioplegic arrest at the time of reoperation.
E. A functional study demonstrating a large portion of myocardium at risk should be obtained before reoperation.

DISCUSSION: Patients who have an intact IMA graft should have severe anginal symptoms and a significant portion of myocardium at risk before reoperative coronary bypass grafting is considered. A functional study may better define the proportion of myocardium at risk for ischemia and infarction. Patients with an intact IMA graft are less likely to require reoperation, but if stenosis distal to the IMA and disease in other vein grafts have progressed or if a large portion of myocardium is at risk, reoperation is recommended. The presence of an intact IMA is not a contraindication to reoperation; in fact, this population of patients have better-preserved ventricular function and are, perhaps, better candidates for reoperation. Placement of an IMA graft at the time of the first operation was critically important, neutralizing the adverse effects of elevated serum cholesterol, hypertension, and smoking on reoperation-free survival. The risk of damaging an intact IMA graft is 3% to 5%. A lateral projection of the IMA at cardiac catheterization will define its course, particularly in relation to the sternum, to allow more careful sternal reentry. The IMA should be minimally dissected and a light clamp applied during cardioplegic arrest to limit cardiac warming and improve myocardial protection. The IMA may be detached and recycled if needed. The use during reoperation of the contralateral IMA does not increase the risk of sternal wound complications.

Textbook: Pages 2102–2105 ANSWER: B, D, E.

58. Considering the results of coronary reoperation in comparison to primary CABG, choose the *incorrect* statement:

A. Operative morbidity and mortality are increased over those for primary CABG.
B. Mortality most often stems from cardiac causes after reoperation.
C. Survival of patients after hospital discharge following coronary reoperation is nearly equivalent to survival after primary CABG.
D. Compared to primary CABG, return of anginal symptoms is delayed after reoperative CABG.
E. Myocardial protection and the risk of myocardial infarction in reoperation are complicated by increased noncoronary collaterals, patent atherosclerotic saphenous vein grafts, and more diffuse coronary atherosclerosis.

DISCUSSION: The mortality and morbidity after reoperative CABG are approximately two to three times that of primary CABG. In contrast to primary CABG, where the majority of deaths are a result of failure of other organ systems, 75% to 85% of deaths after reoperative CABG are due to cardiac causes. The increased risk of reoperation results from more advanced native vessel disease, a longer cross-clamp time, a longer cross-clamp time per graft, a longer time to initiate cardiopulmonary bypass, and increased blood loss. The increased frequency of pulmonary complications, myocardial infarction, neurologic injury, and death, stems from the technical factors of reoperation and the characteristics of the patient population. Technical factors include difficulty in finding targets secondary to pericardial reaction and more diffusely diseased vessels, the risks of injuring the heart or great vessels on sternal re-entry, increased blood loss and risk of requiring transfusion, less available conduit for bypass, and greater difficulty in providing optimal myocardial protection. Characteristics of this patient population that increase risks include advanced age and diminished ventricular function. While survival after reoperation is nearly equivalent to that after primary CABG, angina symptoms return at twice the frequency in the first year after operation

(47% versus 20%) then return at a similar annual rate (2% to 3%).

Textbook: Pages 2104–2105 ANSWER: D.

59. Which statements are correct comparisons of gated equilibrium and initial-transit radionuclide measurements of left ventricular function?

A. Gated equilibrium techniques provide more accurate measurements of ejection fraction than initial-transit methods.
B. Left ventricular imaging time for a gated equilibrium study is at least 10 times that of an initial-transit study.
C. Both techniques require the same radiopharmaceuticals.
D. Both techniques require a bolus injection.

DISCUSSION: Both techniques are equally accurate for measuring left ventricular ejection fraction. The left ventricular imaging time for gated equilibrium studies is at least 10 times that of initial-transit radionuclide angiocardiography. Initial-transit techniques use data from fewer than 10 heartbeats, whereas equilibrium studies require more than 100 heartbeats to acquire data with similar information density. The initial-transit study can be performed with any radioactive substance, but the gated equilibrium technique requires a radiopharmaceutical that remains within the blood pool for imaging. The initial-transit radionuclide study requires a bolus injection, but an equilibrium study can be acquired up to several hours after injection and must be acquired while the tracer is at equilibrium.

Textbook: Pages 2106–2108 ANSWER: B.

60. The radionuclide variable that contains the greatest amount of prognostic information in patients with coronary artery disease is:

A. Exercise ejection fraction.
B. Change in regional wall motion from rest to exercise.
C. Maximal cardiac output during exercise.
D. Change in heart rate during exercise.

DISCUSSION: The exercise ejection fraction is the single most important radionuclide variable relating to subsequent cardiac death or myocardial infarction, and this single variable contains 80% of the prognostic information in the test.

Textbook: Pages 2109–2110 ANSWER: A.

61. Which of the following statements about left ventricular aneurysm is/are correct?

A. Ventricular aneurysms are commonly associated with systemic arterial embolization.
B. Absent collateral circulation in an area of myocardium supplied by an acutely occluded artery favors aneurysm formation.
C. Posterobasal aneurysms are more common than those located in the anteroapical region.
D. Aneurysm repair can improve associated cardiac valve dysfunction.
E. Persistent ST segment elevation after acute myocardial infarction suggests aneurysm formation.

DISCUSSION: The mural thrombus frequently present on the endocardial surface of an aneurysm is usually adherent and rarely embolizes. Collateral circulation, when present, often prevents transmural necrosis following arterial occlusion. Since the left anterior descending coronary artery is the vessel most commonly occluded in patients with ventricular aneurysms, most of the aneurysms are anteroapical. Improvements in ventricular contour and reduction in ventricular volume accompany aneurysm repair. Although persistent elevation of ST segments following myocardial infarction is very suggestive of aneurysm formation, the diagnosis should be confirmed by more definitive tests.

Textbook: Pages 2111–2112 ANSWER: B, D, E.

62. Which of the following factors does/do not increase early mortality associated with repair of left ventricular aneurysm?

A. Class IV cardiac status.
B. Size of aneurysm.
C. Presence of left main coronary disease.
D. Emergent operation.
E. Location of aneurysm.

DISCUSSION: Class IV cardiac status and emergent operation both imply extensive myocardial damage and in most reported series are associated with increased operative mortality. Similarly, the presence of significant stenosis of the left main coronary artery increases the operative mortality of virtually all cardiac procedures. On the other hand, neither the size of the aneurysm nor its location affect early operative mortality, despite the fact that posterior aneurysms are technically more difficult to repair and are much less common.

Textbook: Pages 2112–2113 ANSWER: B, E.

63. The most effective medical therapy in ameliorating the symptoms of Kawasaki's disease and preventing the development of giant coronary artery aneurysms is administration of:

A. Antibiotics.
B. Antiviral agents.
C. Aspirin.
D. Gamma globulin.
E. Glucocorticoids.

DISCUSSION: Kawasaki's disease is a multisystemic disorder of unknown cause and is the leading cause of acquired heart disease in children in both Japan and the United States. Although many clinical aspects of Kawasaki's disease suggest an infectious agent, the search for a single agent has been unsuccessful; neither antibacterials nor antivirals have a role in the therapy of Kawasaki's disease. The goal of initial therapy of Kawasaki's disease is the reduction of inflammation, including coronary and myocardial inflammation. After the diagnosis of Kawasaki's disease is secured, patients are treated with intravenous gamma globulin and large doses of aspirin. Gamma globulin, 2 gm. per kg., is administered as a single infusion over 12 hours. Treatment with intravenous immune globulin has been shown to decrease the duration of fever, to decrease the prevalence of cardiovascular complications, and to prevent the progression to giant coronary aneurysms. High-dose aspirin therapy contributes to the resolution of the acute manifestations of Kawasaki's disease. When Kawasaki's disease is diagnosed, children are given a regimen of aspirin, 100 mg. per kg. per day, which is continued until defervescence. Thereafter, they are maintained on small doses of aspirin, 3 to 5 mg. per kg. per day, for 8 weeks. The goal of aspirin therapy is amelioration of symptoms and prevention of the thrombotic and embolic complications of Kawasaki's disease. Aspirin does not decrease the risk of the development of coronary aneurysms. There is no role for glucocorticoids in the treatment of Kawasaki's disease.

Textbook: Pages 2115–2117 ANSWER: D.

64. Indications for surgical intervention in Kawasaki's disease include which of the following?

A. The presence of multiple coronary artery aneurysms.
B. Myocardial infarction and severe left ventricular dysfunction.
C. The presence of a 5 mm. aneurysm in the right coronary artery.
D. Progressive stenosis in the left anterior descending coronary artery.
E. None of the above.

DISCUSSION: The indications for surgical treatment of Kawasaki's disease include: (1) progressively stenotic coronary lesions demonstrated on coronary arteriography, with no distal coronary aneurysms with stenosis; (2) localized aneurysm with significant stenosis in the left main coronary artery; (3) significant stenosis in two coronary arteries; (4) presence of collateral vessels arising from a coronary artery with a proximal aneurysm; (5) progressive stenosis in the left anterior descending coronary artery; and (6) presence of a left ventricular aneurysm. Advanced thrombosis of coronary aneurysms causing critical stenoses in multiple coronary arteries is the most common indication for surgical intervention.

Textbook: Pages 2116–2117 ANSWER: D.

65. Which of the following statements about the pathophysiology of Ebstein's anomaly is/are true?

A. The tricuspid valve is usually insufficient.
B. Typically there is a left-to-right shunt across the ASD.
C. The redundant anterior leaflet of the tricuspid valve may cause obstruction of the right ventricular outflow tract.
D. Pulmonary hypertension is a common late complication.
E. High pulmonary vascular resistance in neonates exacerbates tricuspid regurgitation and cyanosis.

DISCUSSION: Ebstein's anomaly is characterized by downward displacement of the tricuspid valve into the right ventricular cavity. The anterior leaflet is large and "sail-like," while the other two leaflets are rudimentary. Although the tricuspid valve occasionally may be stenotic, it is usually regurgitant. The tricuspid regurgitation and functional right ventricular outflow tract obstruction caused by the large anterior leaflet lead to right-to-left shunting across the ASD. Systemic venous hypertension is often present, but pulmonary hypertension almost never occurs with this malformation. Finally, neonates that present with Ebstein's anomaly are markedly cyanotic, owing to their high pulmonary vascular resistance. This causes a functional pulmonary atresia, which increases right-to-left shunting across the ASD.

Textbook: Page 2119 ANSWER: A, C, E.

66. In the surgical treatment of Ebstein's anomaly, which of the following is/are true?

A. In neonates, the tricuspid valve orifice may be oversewn and a systemic-pulmonary shunt created to provide pulmonary blood flow.
B. Techniques in repair of the tricuspid valve do not utilize plication of the atrialized right ventricle.
C. Closure of the ASD alone is adequate repair of the malformation.
D. If tricuspid valve replacement is performed, the valve should be sutured above the coronary sinus to avoid injury to the conduction system.
E. Currently, mechanical prostheses are recommended for tricuspid valve replacement because the durability of bioprosthetic valves in the tricuspid position is so poor.

DISCUSSION: In a recent report on the surgical treatment of Ebstein's anomaly in neonates, Starnes described a technique consisting of oversewing the tricuspid valve, atrial septectomy, and placement of a systemic-pulmonary shunt. These patients are then later staged to a modified Fontan procedure when they outgrow their shunts. Repair of the ASD alone was performed early in the treatment of Ebstein's anomaly and was associated with high mortality rates. It is not considered an adequate repair. Most techniques in tricuspid valve repair for Ebstein's malformation utilize plication of the atrialized right ventricle in addition to excision of redundant atrial tissue. If tricuspid valve replacement is necessary, current approaches utilize bioprosthetic valves because of their excellent durability in the tricuspid position. Placement of the valve ring above the coronary sinus has been associated with a lower rate of postoperative heart block.

Textbook: Pages 2120–2123 ANSWER: A, D.

67. Which of the following congenital lesions of the coronary circulation causes a cardiac murmur that is similar to the murmur produced by a PDA?

A. Origin of the left coronary artery from the pulmonary artery.
B. Origin of the right coronary artery from the pulmonary artery.
C. Coronary artery fistula.
D. Membranous obstruction of the ostium of the left main coronary artery.

DISCUSSION: The major clinical finding with a coronary artery fistula is a continuous murmur over the site of the abnormal communication. This murmur may closely resemble that of PDA.

Textbook: Page 2125 ANSWER: C.

68. The congenital coronary lesion most likely to cause death in infancy is:

A. Coronary artery fistula.
B. Origin of the left coronary artery from the pulmonary artery.
C. Origin of the right coronary artery from the pulmonary artery.
D. Congenital coronary aneurysm.

DISCUSSION: The prognosis for most patients with origin of the left coronary artery from the pulmonary artery is poor. It has been estimated that 95% of patients with this anomaly die within the first year of life unless surgical therapy is undertaken. Patients whose right coronary artery originates from the pulmonary artery are usually asymptomatic. Patients with coronary fistulas occasionally suffer congestive heart failure early. Congenital aneurysms of the coronary arteries are most often asymptomatic until complications occur, usually later in life.

Textbook: Pages 2126–2127 ANSWER: B.

69. The congenital coronary lesion associated with minimal or absent clinical manifestations and nearly normal life expectancy is:

A. Congenital origin of both coronary arteries from the pulmonary artery.
B. Congenital coronary artery fistula.
C. Membranous obstruction of the ostium of the left main coronary artery.
D. Congenital origin of the right coronary artery from the pulmonary artery.

DISCUSSION: Clinical manifestations of congenital origin of the right coronary artery from the pulmonary artery are usually minimal or absent. This malformation is thought to have been associated with death. The oldest reported patient with this malformation died at age 90 years from unrelated problems.

Textbook: Pages 2126–2127 ANSWER: D.

70. Which of the following is/are indications for aortic valve replacement for aortic stenosis?

A. Syncope.
B. Congestive heart failure.
C. Angina.
D. Transvalvar gradient of 35 mm. Hg without symptoms.

DISCUSSION: With progressive narrowing of the aortic valve area from the normal 3 to 4 sq. cm. to 1 sq. cm., patients become symptomatic. The classic symptoms produced by aortic stenosis are syncope, congestive heart failure, and angina. Once symptoms occur, life expectancy is limited to 2 to 5 years. Therefore, symptomatic aortic stenosis is an indication for aortic valve replacement. The risk of death with asymptomatic aortic stenosis is quite low, and aortic valve replacement is not indicated for asymptomatic patients with a transvalvar gradient less than 50 mm. Hg.

Textbook: Pages 2136–2138 ANSWER: A, B, C.

71. Under which of the following circumstances is medical management logical?

A. Moderate aortic insufficiency seen on echocardiography with normal left ventricular end-systolic dimensions.
B. Moderate to severe aortic insufficiency seen on echocardiography with cardiomegaly on chest roentgenography.
C. Moderate aortic insufficiency seen on echocardiography with symptoms of congestive heart failure.
D. Moderate aortic insufficiency with an end-systolic left ventricular dimension of 70 mm. as seen on echocardiography.

DISCUSSION: The left ventricle is usually able to compensate for a long time for the increased volume load imposed by aortic insufficiency. The natural history of asymptomatic aortic stenosis is excellent; 10-year survival for moderate aortic insufficiency managed medically is as high as 85% to 95%. Medical management typically consists of diuretics and afterload reduction; however, once the compensatory mechanisms begin to fail, survival is limited. Half of patients with signs or symptoms of congestive heart failure die within 2 years. Therefore, evidence of left ventricular dilation by echocardiography (left ventricular end-systolic dimension greater than 55 mm., cardiomegaly on chest roentgenography) or symptoms of congestive heart failure are indications for aortic valve replacement.

Textbook: Pages 2138–2140 ANSWER: A.

72. Which of the following may be indications for operation for mitral stenosis?

A. Systemic embolization.
B. Infective endocarditis.
C. Onset of atrial fibrillation.
D. Worsening pulmonary hypertension.

DISCUSSION: Although each is only a relative indication for operation for mitral stenosis, systemic embolization, infective endocarditis, onset of atrial fibrillation, and worsening pulmonary hypertension may each be an indication for operation for mitral stenosis. Systemic embolization, infective endocarditis, and onset of atrial fibrillation are each complications of mitral stenosis that portend a risk of further complication with continued medical therapy. Patients older than

40 years with mild class II congestive heart failure stand to gain symptomatically from operation for significant mitral stenosis and do not run excessive risk of multiple reoperative procedures.

Textbook: Pages 2144–2146 ANSWER: A, B, C, D.

73. Which of the following is/are *not* true?

A. Operation improves survival in patients with severe, symptomatic mitral valve disease.
B. Left ventricular dilatation with class I or class II heart failure is an indication for operation with mitral regurgitation.
C. Tricuspid regurgitation is most commonly caused by abnormalities of the leaflets themselves.
D. Mitral valve replacement requires resection of the mitral valve leaflets and chordae.

DISCUSSION: Relative to medical therapy alone, surgical therapy has been shown to improve survival in patients with severe, symptomatic mitral valve disease. In mitral regurgitation, left ventricular dilatation *is* an indication for surgical intervention regardless of failure symptoms. The most common cause of tricuspid regurgitation is tricuspid annular dilatation *without* abnormalities of the leaflets themselves. Mitral valve replacement with preservation of both leaflets or at least the posterior leaflet is well described and is probably advisable for most patients to preserve left ventricular function and reduce the probability of ventricular-annular separation.

Textbook: Pages 2146–2148 ANSWER: C, D.

74. Which of the following generally are *not* symptoms of tricuspid valve disease?

A. Pulmonary edema.
B. Hepatic failure.
C. Anasarca.
D. Hoarseness.

DISCUSSION: Hepatic failure and anasarca are indeed common symptoms of severe, long-standing tricuspid valve disease with increased venous pressure. Pulmonary edema is a consequence of left-sided heart disease and does not result from a tricuspid lesion. Similarly, hoarseness is most common after mitral valve disease with left atrial enlargement and is rarely due to tricuspid valve disease alone.

Textbook: Pages 2148–2150 ANSWER: A, D.

75. Which of the following are relative indications for mitral valve replacement, as opposed to mitral valve repair?

A. Extensive leaflet calcification.
B. Mitral regurgitation.
C. Chordal rupture of the anterior mitral leaflet.
D. Significant annular dilatation.

DISCUSSION: Extensive mitral valve calcification is a relative indication for mitral valve replacement. Mitral regurgitation or significant annular dilatation may, however, be amenable to mitral valve repair. Chordal rupture of the anterior leaflet is generally reparable using chordal transposition or polytetrafluoroethylene (PTFE) chordae.

Textbook: Pages 2152–2154 ANSWER: A.

76. Which of the following are *not* true?

A. Tricuspid regurgitation due to annular dilatation alone generally does not require valve replacement.
B. Mitral valve replacement with either a bioprosthesis or a mechanical valve requires warfarin anticoagulation.
C. Tricuspid valve replacement is generally an indication for using a tissue valve.
D. Chronic renal failure is a relative indication for tissue valves.

DISCUSSION: Tricuspid regurgitation due to annular dilatation alone generally can be treated with tricuspid annuloplasty or with correction of associated mitral valve disease. Mitral valve replacement with a mechanical valve does require warfarin anticoagulation; however, mitral valve replacement with a bioprosthesis may be managed with aspirin alone. Tricuspid valve replacement is an indication for using a tissue valve because of the significant incidence of valve thrombosis when a mechanical valve is in the tricuspid position. Chronic renal failure is a relative indication for tissue valves because valve calcification is rare and because anticoagulation of patients on dialysis carries high risks of morbidity and mortality.

Textbook: Pages 2150–2155 ANSWER: B.

77. Which of the following are relative indications for mechanical, as opposed to tissue, valve replacement?

A. Patient younger than 30 years.
B. Young female patient who desires children.
C. An elderly patient.
D. Tricuspid valve replacement.

DISCUSSION: Age younger than 30 years is a relative indication for mechanical valves because of an increased incidence of calcification of tissue valves in younger persons. A young female who desires children would be a relative contraindication to mechanical replacement because of the risk of teratogenesis and hemorrhage during pregnancy secondary to warfarin therapy. Advanced age is a relative indication for biologic valves to avoid complications of anticoagulation and because the probability of reoperation is low. Tricuspid valve replacement is a relative contraindication to mechanical valve replacement, owing to the increased incidence of tricuspid valve thrombosis with a mechanical prosthesis.

Textbook: Pages 2154–2155 ANSWER: A.

78. Which of the following statements are *not* true?

A. Bioprosthetic valves have a relatively high incidence of hemolysis.

B. Bioprosthetic valves have a lower incidence of postoperative prosthetic valve endocarditis.
C. Mechanical valves develop structural failure after an average of 7 to 10 years.
D. Mortality attributable to warfarin therapy approaches 5% per patient-year.

DISCUSSION: Bioprosthetic valves have a relatively low incidence of hemolysis. Bioprosthetic and mechanical valves do not differ significantly in the associated incidences of postoperative prosthetic valve endocarditis. Bioprosthetic valves develop structural failure after an average of 7 to 10 years, whereas mechanical valves have a life span of well beyond 10 years. The mortality attributable to warfarin therapy approaches 1% per patient-year.

Textbook: Pages 2154–2155 ANSWER: A, B, C, D.

79. Which of the following are *not* generally associated with mitral stenosis without regurgitation?

A. Pulmonary hypertension.
B. Pulmonary edema.
C. Left ventricular dilatation.
D. An opening snap after the second heart sound.

DISCUSSION: Pure mitral stenosis without regurgitation may be associated with pulmonary hypertension, pulmonary edema, and an opening snap after the second heart sound. Left ventricular dilatation would be rare in pure mitral stenosis and generally occurs with volume or pressure overload of the left ventricle, as with mitral regurgitation.

Textbook: Page 2144 ANSWER: A, B, D.

80. The most common location of accessory pathways in patients with the Wolff-Parkinson-White syndrome is the:

A. Left free wall.
B. Right free wall.
C. Posterior septum.
D. Anterior septum.

DISCUSSION: All major published series of the Wolff-Parkinson-White syndrome indicate that the majority of all accessory pathways appear in the left free wall space. In one series, approximately 60% of all accessory pathways occur in the left free wall space. In Ebstein's anomaly, pathways are usually located in the posterior septum and/or right free wall spaces. If these patients are excluded, approximately 70% of pathways occur in the left free wall space.

Textbook: Pages 2158–2159 ANSWER: A.

81. The anatomic electrophysiologic basis of AV node re-entry tachycardia is dual AV node conduction pathways. AV node re-entry tachycardia is most likely to occur with which of the following electrophysiologic aberrations?

A. Proximal antegrade block in the slow conduction pathway.
B. Proximal retrograde block in the slow conduction pathway.
C. Proximal antegrade block in the fast conduction pathway.
D. Proximal retrograde block in the fast conduction pathway.

DISCUSSION: A retrograde conduction block in either the slow or fast pathway would be likely to prevent a re-entrant circuit from developing. A proximal antegrade block in the slow conduction pathway is extremely unusual because of the short refractory period of the slow conduction pathway. The most common conduction block that occurs in patients with dual AV node physiology is a proximal antegrade conduction block in the fast pathway because of its longer refractory period. This antegrade block in the fast conduction pathway allows AV conduction to occur via the slow pathway and to return in retrograde fashion up the fast pathway to establish the re-entrant circuit responsible for AV node re-entry tachycardia.

Textbook: Pages 2161–2162 ANSWER: C.

82. Match the four surgical procedures that have been developed for the treatment of atrial fibrillation with the major detrimental sequela(e) of atrial fibrillation that each corrects.

A. His bundle ablation.
B. Left atrial isolation procedure.
C. Corridor procedure.
D. Maze procedure.

1. Patient's sensation of irregular heart rhythm.
2. Hemodynamic compromise because of loss of AV synchrony.
3. Increased vulnerability to thromboembolism.

DISCUSSION: The surgical procedure most commonly employed for the treatment of atrial fibrillation is catheter ablation of the His bundle. The International Catheter Ablation Registry reveals that more than 60% of patients who undergo elective catheter ablation of the bundle of His do so for the treatment of atrial fibrillation. His bundle ablation is an isolation procedure, in that it confines the atrial fibrillation to the atria and protects the ventricles from the unpleasant sensation of an irregular heartbeat. Because the atria continue to fibrillate there is no restoration of AV synchrony, and therefore there is no improvement in cardiac hemodynamics. Moreover, the continuing fibrillation of the left atrium means that postoperatively the patient is still at the same risk for thromboembolism. Thus, His bundle ablation corrects only one of the three detrimental sequelae of atrial fibrillation, namely the arrhythmia problem.

The left atrial isolation procedure confines atrial fibrillation to the left atrium, allowing the sinus node to drive the remainder of the heart in a normal sinus rhythm. Thus, it alleviates the unpleasant sensation of an irregular heartbeat. In addition, because AV synchrony is re-established between the right atrium and right ventricle, right-sided cardiac output is restored to normal. This means that normal cardiac output is delivered through the lungs to the left side of the heart. In the presence of a normal left ventricle the left-sided cardiac output is also normal, despite the fact that left-sided AV synchrony is not present; however, because the left atrium is allowed to fibrillate, the vulnerability to thromboembolism remains unchanged postoperatively.

The corridor procedure allows the sinus node to drive the heart in normal sinus rhythm, but because of the total isolation of the sinoatrial and AV nodes from the remainder of the atria, the atria may continue to fibrillate. Even if they do not, in effect they are isolated from their respective ventricles so that AV synchrony is lost on both sides of the heart. As a result, the corridor procedure alleviates the sensation of arrhythmia but does not restore normal hemodynamics, nor does it decrease vulnerability to thromboembolism. The maze procedure ablates the re-entrant circuits responsible for atrial fibrillation and restores the normal sinus rhythm. Thus, it alleviates the sensation of arrhythmia, restores normal hemodynamics, and alleviates the vulnerability to thromboembolism.

Textbook: Pages 2157–2158 ANSWER: A-1; B-1,2; C-1; D-1,2,3.

83. All of the following statements about nonischemic ventricular tachyarrhythmias are true *except:*

A. They usually occur in the right ventricle.
B. They are usually associated with a left bundle branch block pattern during the tachycardia.
C. They are usually more refractory to medical therapy than ischemic ventricular tachyarrhythmias.
D. They usually occur as a result of automaticity rather than re-entry.

DISCUSSION: Nonischemic ventricular tachyarrhythmias usually occur in the right ventricle, and as a result the ECG shows a left bundle branch block–type pattern during ventricular tachycardia. These arrhythmias are notoriously refractory to medical therapy and they occur almost exclusively on a re-entrant basis.

Textbook: Page 2164 ANSWER: D.

84. Which of the following statements about left atrial myxoma are true?

A. This lesion, by site and histology, is the most common primary cardiac tumor.
B. It is best diagnosed by cardiac catheterization and angiography.
C. The symptom complex can mimic collagen vascular disease.
D. It has an intracavitary growth pattern.
E. It has a multicentric origin in the chamber wall.

DISCUSSION: Eighty per cent of primary cardiac tumors are benign, and half of these benign tumors are myxomas. Seventy-five per cent of myxomas arise in the left atrium in the region of the fossa ovalis. Echocardiography is the technique of choice in the evaluation of intracardiac tumors, and findings suggestive of myxoma occur in 95% of patients examined. Invasive procedures, with the attendant risk of tumor embolization, are not warranted. Owing to an autoimmune phenomenon, left atrial myxomas can present with systemic constitutional symptoms of fever, malaise, weight loss, polymyositis, and blood dyscrasias that mimic collagen vascular disease. Of surgical significance is the fact that most myxomas rarely extend deeper than the endocardium but grow as polypoid, intracavitary masses. Attachment by a vascular stalk thus allows tumor mobility, predisposing to embolization and interference with mitral valve competence and causing characteristic echocardiographic findings.

Textbook: Pages 2171–2173 ANSWER: A, C, D.

85. Which of the following statements about malignant cardiac tumors are true?

A. Sarcomas are the most frequent primary malignancy.
B. Metastatic tumors are usually asymptomatic.
C. Adjuvant chemotherapy and irradiation are efficacious in prolonging survival.
D. Intra-atrial extension of renal neoplasms is a contraindication for surgical resection.
E. Constrictive physiology is an indication for operation.

DISCUSSION: Twenty per cent of primary cardiac tumors are some variant of sarcoma. Precise histologic classification is not imperative, as all have a similar clinical picture with rapid systemic dissemination and aggressive local invasion. In contrast, metastatic tumors cause symptoms in only 10% of patients. Unfortunately, most primary and secondary cardiac malignancies infrequently respond to systemic chemotherapy or mediastinal irradiation. Surgical treatment is most successful with renal tumors extending into the right atrium. Significant 5-year survival can be achieved with concomitant nephrectomy and intra-atrial resection of the tumor thrombus. Relief of tamponade is worthwhile; however, extensive decortication provides little help.

Textbook: Pages 2173–2174 ANSWER: A, B.

86. Disadvantages of temporary pacing through skin electrodes applied to the anterior chest wall include all of the following except:

A. Skin burns.
B. Painful chest wall muscle contractions.
C. Ventricular fibrillation.
D. Inability to pace.

DISCUSSION: In 1952 Zoll first described successful pacing through external metal electrodes applied to the anterior chest wall. Clinical experience with this technique has shown that it is both feasible and lifesaving for temporary pacing; however, disadvantages of the external pacing technique include skin burns when too little electrode jelly is applied, painful chest wall muscle contractions, and inability to pace in thick-chested or emphysematous patients. Ventricular fibrillation induced by external temporary cardiac pacing is exceedingly rare.

Textbook: Page 2176 ANSWER: C.

87. In adults the most common cause of acquired complete heart block is:

A. Ischemic heart disease.
B. Sclerodegenerative disease.
C. Traumatic injury.
D. Cardiomegaly.

DISCUSSION: Before permanent pacemakers were available, 50% of patients with complete heart block died within 1 year. The most common cause of acquired complete heart block in adults is sclerodegenerative disease of the cardiac skeleton and AV conduction system. Other less common causes of complete heart block include ischemic heart disease, cardiomyopathic processes, Chagas' disease, and traumatic injury.

Textbook: Page 2176 ANSWER: B.

88. The most common indication for permanent pacing is:

A. Complete heart block.
B. Second-degree AV block.
C. Chronic bifascicular block.
D. Sick sinus syndrome.

DISCUSSION: Patients with sinus node dysfunction may develop a number of arrhythmias, such as inappropriate sinus bradycardia, chronotropic incompetence, sinoatrial exit block, and sinus arrest. This group of rhythm disorders typically occurs in older patients with or without underlying heart disease and is collectively known as the "sick sinus syndrome." In addition, many patients with sick sinus syndrome have associated atrial tachyarrhythmias, particularly atrial fibrillation. This association of atrial tachyarrhythmias in patients with the sick sinus syndrome is called the tachycardia-bradycardia (or tachy-brady) syndrome. The most common indication for permanent pacing occurs in patients with the sick sinus syndrome.

Textbook: Pages 2176–2178 ANSWER: D.

89. Decreasing pacemaker electrode tip size results in:

A. Lower pacing thresholds.
B. Improved electrogram sensing.
C. Decreased battery life.
D. Less patient discomfort.

DISCUSSION: Decreasing pacemaker electrode tip size results in lower pacing thresholds, both at the time of implant and subsequently, because of higher current density. However, better sensing function is directly related to electrode area and is adversely affected by small electrode size. Therefore, a compromise between pacing and sensing efficiency is required. Typical electrode surface areas for pacing are between 8 and 10 sq. mm.

Textbook: Pages 2181–2182 ANSWER: A.

90. At the time of ventricular pacemaker implantation, lead resistance is determined at a voltage near that of the pacemaker's output. The calculated resistance at 5 volts should range from:

A. 10 to 100 ohms.
B. 125 to 250 ohms.
C. 300 to 800 ohms.
D. 1000 to 1500 ohms.

DISCUSSION: At the time of pacemaker implantation, in addition to measuring pulse amplitude (voltage and current) and pulse width, resistance is also determined. As described by Ohm's law, resistance is calculated by dividing voltage by current. Resistance calculations are made at a voltage near that of the pacemaker's output. The calculated resistance at 5 volts should range from 300 to 800 ohms. An unsatisfactorily low resistance is unsatisfactory because current is wasted and battery life is shortened. Conversely, excessively high resistance (more than 800 ohms) increases battery life but decreases the current delivered to the heart for pacing.

Textbook: Page 2185 ANSWER: C.

91. A ventricular inhibited-demand pacemaker using the Intersociety Commission for Heart Disease Resources (ICHD) code is designated as:

A. DVI.
B. VVI.
C. VOO.
D. VDD.

DISCUSSION: A ventricular inhibited-demand pacemaker using the ICHD code is designated as VVI. As the ICHD code states, the pacemaker senses intrinsic ventricular activity and is inhibited when this activity exceeds the standby or escape rate of the pacemaker. When the intrinsic ventricular rate falls below the escape rate of the pulse generator, the pacemaker begins to function at its programmed rate.

Textbook: Pages 2185–2186 ANSWER: B.

92. In rate-modulated pacing, the pacing rate is determined by a physiologic parameter other than atrial rate and is measured by a special sensor in the pacemaker or pacing lead. The most commonly used physiologic parameter in rate-modulated pacemakers is:

A. QT interval.
B. Venous blood temperature.
C. Mixed venous oxygen saturation.
D. Body motion.

DISCUSSION: During exertion, the required increase in cardiac output is obtained mostly by the increase in paced heart rate, although increased venous filling and maintenance of AV synchrony are also important contributors. The most commonly used physiologic parameters in rate-modulated pacemakers at the present time are body motion and minute ventilation.

Other parameters that are less commonly used or under evaluation include QT interval, venous blood temperature, mixed venous oxygen saturation, contractility, stroke volume, venous pH, and the paced depolarization gradient.

Textbook: Pages 2187–2188 ANSWER: D.

93. The most common pacing mode used in patients with symptomatic bradycardia and an underlying sinus rhythm is:

A. AAI.
B. DVI.
C. DDD.
D. VVI.

DISCUSSION: "Universal," or DDD, pacing has been shown to have many benefits over other pacing modalities, including the ability to track the intrinsic sinus rate, pace the atrium and ventricle, maintain atrioventricular synchrony, and avoid the pacemaker syndrome. Recognition of these benefits has steadily increased the use of DDD pacemakers in the last decade, and at the present time DDD is the most common pacing mode.

Textbook: Pages 2188–2189 ANSWER: C.

94. A transvenous pacemaker generator pocket should be placed on the patient's nondominant side over the:

A. Anteromedial chest wall.
B. Anterolateral chest wall.
C. Inferomedial chest wall.
D. Inferolateral chest wall.

DISCUSSION: Bipolar impulse generators can be placed either in the subcutaneous tissue or beneath the muscle. Migration of the impulse generator most commonly occurs in infraclavicular pacemakers pockets. Migration tends to follow the curvature of the chest wall, and the impulse generator tends to migrate laterally. This can be prevented by creating an anteromedial pocket large enough to contain the impulse generator and lead. In susceptible persons the impulse generator can be further secured to the chest wall to prevent migration.

Textbook: Pages 2182–2183 ANSWER: A.

95. Pacemaker-mediated tachycardia is caused by:

A. Pacemaker induction of atrial fibrillation.
B. Sensing of retrograde atrial activation.
C. Inappropriate ventricular sensing.
D. Lead fracture.

DISCUSSION: Pacemaker-mediated tachycardia occurs in the setting of intact ventriculoatrial conduction. Typically, premature ventricular contractions may be conducted retrogradely through the AV conduction system and cause retrograde activation of the atrium. If this retrograde atrial activation occurs after completion of the programmed pacemaker ventriculoatrial refractory period, the atrial event is sensed by the DDD pacemaker and evokes a paced ventricular event that may cause further VA conduction. If each ventricularly paced event results in atrial activation sensed by the pacemaker, pacemaker-mediated tachycardia will be generated.

Textbook: Pages 2195–2196 ANSWER: B.

96. Which cardiovascular pharmacologic agents are safe to use during routine abdominal surgery in a 75-year-old woman with documented hypertension and mild coronary artery disease?

A. Nifedipine.
B. Atenolol.
C. Hydralazine.
D. Captopril.
E. Reserpine.

DISCUSSION: Nifedipine is tolerated fairly well by elderly patients and is safe to use in the perioperative period with close hemodynamic monitoring. Atenolol is a safe beta-blocker to use during the perioperative period and provides protection from cardiac rhythm disturbances and rebound hypertension. Hydralazine, if given without a beta-blocker, often elicits reflex tachycardia, which limits its usefulness. Captopril is a safe agent that does not appear to interfere with the normal cardiovascular response to anesthesia, and abrupt withdrawal of this agent may result in severe hypertension and should be avoided. Reserpine is an adrenergic inhibitor that may depress cardiac output and result in hypotension, so its use in the perioperative setting is limited.

Textbook: Pages 2199–2201 ANSWER: A, B, D.

97. Which inotropic drugs are safe for use in elderly patients with mild congestive heart failure in the postoperative period?

A. Digitalis compounds.
B. Dopamine.
C. Amrinone.
D. Melrinone.
E. Dobutamine.

DISCUSSION: Dopamine and dobutamine stimulate cardiac beta-receptors and are very useful in providing inotropic support for patients in the postoperative period. Melrinone and amrinone are phosphodiesterase inhibitors that have strong inotropic effects while causing arterial and venous dilation. Melrinone and amrinone are useful in patients with low cardiac output, especially in the setting of congestive heart failure. Digitalis compounds can be troublesome in the postoperative period owing to the toxic effects of these agents. Furthermore, perioperative hypoxia and hypokalemia increase myocardial susceptibility to digitalis-induced ventricular arrhythmias.

Textbook: Pages 2201–2202, 2203, 2205 ANSWER: B, C, D, E.

98. Which anticoagulation treatment plan(s) is/are appropriate for a 72-year-old man with a mechanical heart valve in place who takes Coumadin (warfarin) and now requires elective left colon resection?

A. Discontinuation of Coumadin therapy on the day of the operation.
B. Discontinuation of Coumadin therapy on the day of the operation with replacement of clotting factors with fresh frozen plasma (FFP) before the start of the surgical procedure.
C. Discontinuation of Coumadin therapy 5 days before operation with no further anticoagulation therapy before surgery.
D. Discontinuation of Coumadin therapy 5 days before operation with the institution of intravenous heparin as the prothrombin time normalizes.
E. Discontinuation of Coumadin therapy 2 days before operation followed by large doses of aspirin.

DISCUSSION: Many patients who require anticoagulation with Coumadin for underlying cardiac disease need to undergo routine general surgical procedures. The current recommendations for patients who have been on long-term Coumadin therapy is to discontinue Coumadin 5 days before an operative procedure. As the patient's prothrombin time normalizes intravenous heparin should be started. The patient should be maintained on a therapeutic dose of heparin with an activated partial thromboplastin time (aPTT) of at least 60 seconds. Heparin should then be withheld approximately 4 to 6 hours before the surgical procedure. The operation is then performed in a "heparin window," where the level of anticoagulation can easily be titrated or totally reversed with protamine if necessary.

Textbook: Page 2206 ANSWER: D.

99. Which of the following treatment plans is appropriate for a 68-year-old patient with moderate to severe congestive heart failure following a major abdominal surgical procedure?

A. Aggressive use of inotropic support with epinephrine.
B. Aggressive diuresis with furosemide and inotropic support with dopamine.
C. Afterload reduction with nitroprusside and inotropic support with dopamine.
D. Close perioperative monitoring and inotropic support with melrinone.
E. Intravenous digitalis with diuresis using furosemide as needed.

DISCUSSION: Treatment of congestive heart failure using epinephrine alone is contraindicated owing to the profound vasoconstrictive properties of epinephrine, which only exacerbate the heart failure. Diuresis with furosemide and inotropic support with dopamine is acceptable for patients with mild congestive heart failure; however, in the postoperative period pharmacologic diuresis can lead to profound hypovolemia requiring continuous invasive hemodynamic monitoring. The ideal choice for the postoperative management of patients with severe congestive heart failure is afterload reduction using nitroprusside and inotropic support with dopamine. This helps to stimulate the failing heart while decreasing the afterload pressure against which the heart must pump. Melrinone is a useful phosphodiesterase inhibitor, which has been shown to be useful in the treatment of mild to moderate congestive heart failure. Digitalis along with a diuretic in the postoperative period can be troublesome owing to the potential toxicity of digitalis while the patient has ongoing fluid and electrolyte shifts.

Textbook: Pages 2201–2202, 2203–2205 ANSWER: C, D.

100. Which of the following steps is/are appropriate for a 65-year-old woman who develops atrial fibrillation with associated mild hypotension and rapid ventricular response following partial gastric resection?

A. Correction of electrolytes and blood chemistries.
B. Evaluation for possible myocardial infarction.
C. Treatment with intravenous lidocaine.
D. Attempt to limit the ventricular response with digitalis.
E. Immediate cardioversion.

DISCUSSION: When a patient develops postoperative atrial fibrillation following an extracardiac procedure, correction of the patient's blood chemistries and electrolytes is essential. The patient must also undergo evaluation for a possible myocardial infarction as the cause of the atrial dysrhythmia. The first rule in treatment is to slow the ventricular response and attempt to limit hemodynamic instability. Digitalis is effective in slowing down the ventricular response and thus improving the hemodynamic status of the patient. Lidocaine has little use in controlling atrial dysrhythmias but is very effective in decreasing ventricular ectopy. Immediate cardioversion is rarely indicated for new-onset atrial fibrillation. Only after correction of all underlying metabolic and electrolyte defects as well as an attempt at medical conversion and ventricular rate control is cardioversion recommended.

Textbook: Pages 2204–2206 ANSWER: A, B, D.

101. The damaging effects of cardiopulmonary bypass are, to a large degree, due to activation of the humoral amplification system. The humoral amplification system includes which of the following?

A. The coagulation cascade.
B. The fibrinolytic cascade.
C. Complement activation.
D. A and C.
E. A, B, and C.

DISCUSSION: Cardiopulmonary bypass stimulates a whole-body inflammatory response, and the concentrations of several inflammatory mediators (e.g., complement fraction C5a) have been associated with subsystem dysfunction following cardiopulmonary bypass. This inflammatory response is complex and has several arms, including the coagulation, fibrinolytic, and complement systems. Simply blocking one pathway is unlikely to completely prevent bypass-induced injury.

Textbook: Pages 2211–2214 ANSWER: E.

102. Adequate flow during cardiopulmonary bypass is best indicated by:

A. Systemic blood pressure of 90/50 mm. Hg.
B. Arterial P_{O_2} of 230 mm. Hg.
C. Mixed venous hemoglobin saturation of 78%.
D. Central venous pressure of 1 mm. Hg.
E. Plasma lactate value of 6 mg. per dl.

DISCUSSION: The purpose of cardiopulmonary bypass is to provide adequate circulation of blood to sustain aerobic metabolism. Oxygen consumption during bypass depends on bypass flow until a critical flow is attained. With higher flows there is no further increase in oxygen consumption (i.e., oxygen consumption becomes flow independent), and the mixed venous hemoglobin saturation increases. A mixed venous hemoglobin saturation of 78% indicates that bypass flow is above the critical level and that flow is adequate. The other variables do not ensure adequate bypass flow.

Textbook: Pages 2210–2211 ANSWER: C.

103. Which of the following does not typically occur during the first few minutes of cardiopulmonary bypass?

A. Interstitial fluid increases.
B. Blood flow becomes nonpulsatile.
C. Platelet count decreases.
D. Complement is activated.
E. Systemic vascular resistance falls.

DISCUSSION: Several events occur during the first few minutes of bypass. The tubing and oxygenator surfaces are coated by serum proteins that in turn activate platelets. This reduces the platelet count. The roller pump produces nonpulsatile flow, which is different from the usual pulsatile cardiac flow. Serum complement is activated by exposure of blood to the nonphysiologic surfaces of the pump-oxygenator, and systemic vascular resistance falls. Interstitial fluid accumulates during bypass; however, this occurs later during bypass.

Textbook: Pages 2211–2214 ANSWER: A.

104. Which of the following are physiologic benefits of intra-aortic balloon counterpulsation to the ischemic ventricle?

A. Preload reduction.
B. Afterload reduction.
C. Coronary blood flow enhancement.
D. Decreased ventricular end-diastolic pressure.

DISCUSSION: In general, preload relates to the volume of blood or fluid presented to the left ventricle. Although wall tension does increase with increased volume, Starling properties are called forth for added efficiency. Preload is controlled by volume status as well as capacity of the venous system. The effects of balloon counterpulsation on cardiac preload are minimal and secondary to other changes. As the balloon collapses in the aorta, the absence of the balloon volume, or "abyss," creates a decrease in ventricular afterload. In effect this decreases ventricular wall tension, reducing myocardial oxygen consumption significantly. During counterpulsation, the intra-aortic balloon inflates in diastole, elevating coronary perfusion pressure significantly. Maximal coronary artery perfusion occurs in this part of the cardiac cycle. Thus, ischemic ventricles benefit especially from balloon pumping. The balloon pump does not directly decrease the left ventricular end-diastolic pressure. However, in ventricles failing from ischemia the combination of afterload reduction and improved coronary blood flow usually augments cardiac function, producing decreased cardiac filling pressure or left ventricular end-diastolic pressure.

Textbook: Pages 2218–2219 ANSWER: B, C, D.

105. Which of the following are the major indications for instituting intra-aortic balloon pumping?

A. Medically refractory angina.
B. Acute papillary muscle rupture.
C. Left main coronary artery lesion.
D. Ventricular failure after cardiac surgery.
E. PTCA failure.

DISCUSSION: Medically refractory angina is one of the major indications for implementing the intra-aortic balloon pump. When intravenous nitroglycerin becomes ineffective at relieving chest pain or results in early hypotension, the balloon pump should be used in preparation for surgical revascularization or percutaneous angioplasty. By reducing left ventricular afterload, the pump reduces regurgitation into the left atrium. Thus, balloon counterpulsation is very helpful for treating patients with acute mitral insufficiency secondary to papillary muscle rupture. Patients should undergo valve surgical procedures emergently, as balloon pump support is only temporizing. The mere presence of a left main coronary lesion is not an indication for use of the balloon pump. In former years such pumps were inserted prophylactically before induction of anesthesia for coronary bypass surgery. Newer anesthetic techniques have largely obviated this; however, in the presence of a left main lesion and medically refractory angina the balloon pump should be used. The balloon pump is quite effective in helping to wean patients who have postcardiotomy left ventricular failure from cardiopulmonary bypass. This is one of the major uses of this device. The Emory University group was the first to expound on the efficacy of the balloon pump in stabilizing patients following percutaneous angioplasty failure. With the pump inserted, most patients can be transported to the operating room safely, many being stable enough to harvest an internal mammary graft instead of having to defer to the more accessible but less preferable saphenous vein.

Textbook: Pages 2219–2222 ANSWER: A, B, D, E.

106. Which of the following are the most frequent complications of intra-aortic balloon counterpulsation?

A. Stroke.
B. Limb ischemia.
C. Arrhythmias.
D. Aortic thrombosis.

DISCUSSION: Stroke rarely occurs secondary to intra-aortic balloon pump use. The balloon must be positioned well below the aortic arch vessels and never proximal to the left subclavian artery origin. Strokes have been reported from emboli being thrown retrograde from the balloon; however, this is very rare. Limb ischemia is one of the most frequent complications of balloon pumping. The combination of iliofemoral atherosclerosis and catheter luminal obstruction may impede distal flow. This may require catheter removal to re-establish flow. In 2% to 10% of patients, arterial reconstruction is necessary to repair balloon-related complications. Smaller catheters have helped prevent limb ischemia. Arrhythmias in general are not complications of balloon pumping. In fact, arrhythmias related to ischemia may be controlled by the balloon pump. Aortic thrombosis can occur very rarely with pump use. A more frequent occurrence is distal embolization with limb ischemia. Patients should be heparinized while the balloon catheter is in place. Following cardiac surgery heparinization is usually delayed for 12 to 24 hours.

Textbook: Pages 2225–2226 ANSWER: B.

107. Permanent artificial hearts are being developed that are electrically powered. Wireless techniques are used to transmit the electrical energy across the body wall using the principle of:

A. Infrared sensor.
B. Inductive coupling.
C. Thermionic coupling.
D. High-pressure liquid chromatography (HPLC).
E. Infrared spectroscopy.

DISCUSSION: Electrical energy can be transmitted across the body wall by tunnelling an electric wire; however, experience has shown that infection, starting at the skin line and burrowing deeper into the body, will occur over time. This infection can be delayed, but not stopped, by the use of a velour covering on the wire. Wireless electrical energy transmission was first used in clinical surgery by W.W.L. Glenn in the 1950s for powering pacemakers. The remarkable advances in electronics have facilitated this technique; however, the placement of the two coils parallel to one another (with the skin between), as opposed to interlocking as in an industrial transformer, reduces the efficiency of transmission from approximately 99% to 70%.

Textbook: Pages 2230–2232 ANSWER: B.

108. The following statements about the pneumatic artificial heart is/are correct:

A. It can support the circulation for over 1 year.
B. It may be complicated by infection or thromboembolism.
C. When further developed, it will be an ideal permanent heart substitute.
D. It is an ideal "bridge" for transplantation.
E. It can be implanted using techniques similar to those used for heart transplantation.

DISCUSSION: The pneumatic artificial heart was developed as a permanent cardiac substitute, but the need for two tubes to pass through the chest wall and the bulky power unit have relegated the pneumatic heart to short-term use as a bridge to transplantation. The heart is implanted using similar techniques as a heart transplantation. The presence of foreign surfaces and crevices make the device prone to thromboembolism and infection. Most surgeons feel that left ventricular support or biventricular assist pumps represent a better option for those patients with end-stage congestive heart failure who require use of a bridge device.

Textbook: Pages 2229–2230 ANSWER: A, B, E.

NOTES

NOTES